N

Medical Dictionary

THOMAS NELSON PUBLISHERS
Nashville • Camden • New York

REVISED EDITION

Illustrations taken from the Medical Aid Encyclopedia For The Home, copyright 1965, 1972 by Stravon Publishers, Inc., and used by permission.

Library of Congress Cataloging in Publication Data
Main entry under title:

Nelson's new compact medical dictionary.

1. Medicine—Dictionaries. I. Urdang, Laurence.
II. Title: Medical dictionary. [DNLM: 1. Dictionaries, Medical. W 13 N432]

R121.N37 1985 610'.3'21 85-7239

ISBN 0-8407-5980-0

8 9 10 11 12 13 14 15 16 17 / 00 99 98 97 96 95 94 93 92

FOREWORD

The purpose of this dictionary is to provide a handy, quick-reference guide to the names of parts of the body and of common treatments, drugs, conditions, and ailments. One of its unique features is the brevity of its definitions. Almost at a glance, Nelson's New Compact Medical Dictionary gives the user accurate information about thousands of the terms most commonly heard in doctors' offices and in hospitals, as well as those words referred to in newspaper and magazine articles.

In addition to its being useful around the house, this pocket dictionary will serve beginning students in nursing, medicine, surgery, and pharmacology by giving concise meaning of words they are most likely to encounter in the field of medicine.

This revised edition contains much that is new, including definitions for terms of recent note, such as *anorexia, ibuprofen,* and *occupational therapy*.

These additions and many other revisions make this edition even more accurate and up-to-date, while still retaining the concise format of the original.

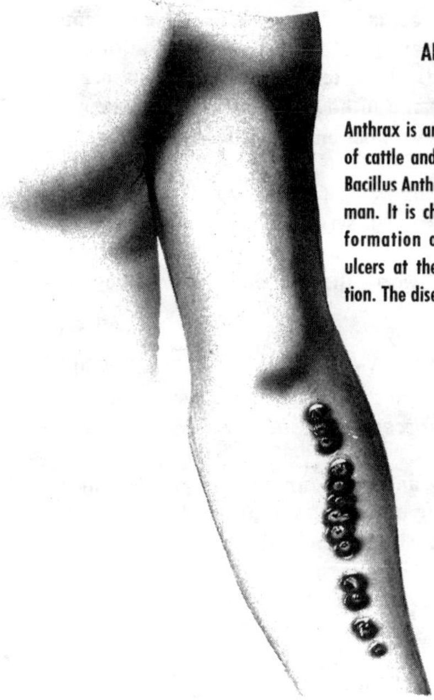

ANTHRAX

Anthrax is an infectious disease of cattle and sheep, due to the Bacillus Anthracis. It can occur in man. It is characterized by the formation of hard edema or ulcers at the point of inoculation. The disease can be fatal.

A

a *abbr.* accommodation; anterior; asymmetric; area; total acidity.

A one of the four blood types. See **ABO blood groups.**

a- *or* **an-** *prefix* without; lacking; wanting: asexual, anesthesia.

Å *abbr.* Ångstrom; Ångstrom unit.

āā *abbr.* (in prescriptions) of each.

ab- *prefix* from; deviating from: *abnormal.*

AB a blood type in which both A and B antigens are present. See **ABO blood groups.**

abactio induced abortion.

abactus venter induced abortion.

abalienated mentally incapable.

abalienation the state of being mentally deranged or incapable.

abapical opposite the extremity or apex.

abaptiston a conical-shaped trephine, designed to minimize damage to the brain tissues while removing a section of the skull.

abarognosis inability to estimate the weight of something.

abarthrosis a movable joint; synovial joint.

abarticular not directly involving a joint; at some distance from a joint.

abarticulation 1. diarthrosis. 2. a dislocated joint.

abasia difficulty in walking owing to faulty motor control.

abaxial 1. not within the axis of any body or part. 2. located at the opposite extremity of some axis.

abdient tending to move away from the point of a stimulus.

abdomen the section of the front part of the body lying between the pelvis and the thorax and containing many major organs; belly. —**abdominal** *adj.*

abdominalgia pain in the abdomen; bellyache.

abdomino- *combining form* relating to or associated with the abdomen.

abdominoscopy examination of the abdominal contents.

abduce abduct.

abduct to draw away from a median or center line.

abduction the manipulation of a limb away from the middle line of the body.

abductor a muscle, as the deltoid, that draws a limb away from the middle line of the body.

aberration deviation from or variation of the normal condition or course.

abiogenesis spontaneous generation of a living organism.

abionarce lack of energy and drive due to chronic illness.

abiotic not compatible with life; nonliving.

abirritant an agent that soothes or relieves irritation.

ablastin an antibody that inhibits the multiplication or growth of certain microorganisms.

ablation the detachment or removal of a bodily part, esp. by cutting.

ablatio retinae detachment of the retina of the eye.

ablepsia blindness.

abluent any agent capable of cleansing.

ABO blood groups the main classification system for types of blood, depending on the presence of antigen A or B, or of both (AB), or of neither (O) on the surface of the erythrocyte. See also **Rh factor.**

abortifacient an agent, as a drug, for inducing abortion. —**abortifacient** *adj.*

abortion spontaneous or induced expulsion of a fetus from the uterus, esp. during the first 12 weeks of pregnancy. —**abortive** *adj.*

abortus an aborted fetus.

abrasion a superficial cut or scrape on the skin or mucous membrane.

abreaction the release of tension and anxiety by the reliving of repressed painful experiences and the understanding of their meaning through the psychoanalytic process.

abruptio a tearing away or premature detachment, especially of the placenta (abruptio placentae).

abscess a localized accumulation of pus in a tissue or organ that is surrounded by inflamed tissue.

absinthism a nerve disorder caused by the excessive consumption of absinthe.

absorbefacient 1. causing absorption. 2. an agent that causes absorption.

absorbent taking in or up by capillary action. —**absorbency** *n.*

acalculia the inability or loss of ability to solve even a simple mathematicial problem.

acampsia abnormal stiffness or rigidity of a joint; ankylosis.

acantha the spine or a spinous process of a vertebra.

acanthosis abnormal thickening of the outermost layer of the epidermis.

acapnia a diminished amount of carbon dioxide in the blood.

acardia absence of the heart from birth.

acariasis any disease caused by infestation with mites (acarids).

acaricide an agent that kills mites.

Acarus a genus of mites including those causing scabies.

acatalepsy absence of comprehension or understanding. —**acataleptic** *adj.*

acataphasia a speech disorder characterized by an inability to express thoughts in clear, logical sequence.

acataposis inability to swallow liquids or great difficulty in doing so.

acathexis a mental disorder characterized by the absence of normal emotional reactions towards objects or ideas, esp. those that are subconsiously significant to the patient.

accepted daily intake the largest quantity of a substance, as a drug, that can be taken by a person without toxic effect. Also, **ADI.**

accessorius relating to any of various muscles, glands, nerves, etc., that have an accessory or auxiliary function; assisting.

accommodation the ability of the eye to focus on near and far objects by contraction of the ciliary muscles to control the curvature of the lens.

accouchement childbirth; labor and delivery.

acephaly absence of the head from birth.

acescent slightly acid.

acetabuloplasty an operation on the acetabulum to correct a deformity or treat osteoarthritis.

acetabulum the cuplike socket of the hipbone.

acetaminophen a substitute for aspirin that acts to reduce pain and fever.

acetic acid the acid contained in vinegar, used esp. in urine testing.

acetone a colorless, volatile solvent liquid produced synthetically and found in minute quantities naturally in the body and in larger amounts in the condition diabetes mellitus.

acetonemia abnormal presence of large amounts of acetone in the blood.

acetonuria abnormal presence of large amounts of acetone in the urine.

acetylcholine a chemical compound released at autonomic nerve endings to aid in the transmission of nerve impulses.

acetylsalicylic acid chemical name for aspirin.

achalasia failure of various visceral openings or sphincters, as the pylorus, to relax normally.

Achilles tendon the large strong tendon joining the muscles of the calf of the leg with the bone of the heel.

achillorrhaphy surgical repair of a ruptured Achilles tendon.

achillotomy surgical division of the Achilles tendon.

achiria 1. absence of the hands from birth. 2. loss of sensation in one or both hands.

achlorhydria lack of hydrochloric acid in the stomach.

achluophobia fear of being in the dark.

acholia a lack of bile secretions.

achondroplasia abnormal development of cartilage leading to dwarfism.

achromasia the absence of normal skin pigmentation.

achylia absence of chyle in the intestinal tract.

acid any of various water-soluble, sour compounds that combine with alkalis to form salts and turn blue litmus paper red.

acidemia an abnormally high acid level of the blood.

acid-fast not decolorized easily by acids.

acidity the quality or degree of being acid.

acidosis a condition of decreased alkalinity of the blood and body tissues below normal levels.

aciduria the condition of an acid urine.

acinus *pl.* **acini** one of the small, secreting, saclike structures lining a compound gland.

acmesthesia sensitivity to a sharp point on the skin, as a pinprick.

acne a disorder of the skin esp. of the face, shoulders, and back that occurs chiefly during adolescence, is marked by pustules and blackheads, and is caused by hyperactivity of the sebaceous glands.

acnemia 1. wasting of the calf muscles. 2. absence of the legs from birth.

acomia baldness.

acoprosis absence or virtual absence of waste matter in the large intestine.

acorea absence of the pupil of the eye at birth.

acoustic of or relating to sound or hearing.

acquired assumed or contracted after birth; not congenital or hereditary.

acquired immune deficiency syndrome. See **AIDS.**

acriflavine a yellow dye used as an antiseptic esp. on wounds.

acrocentric having the centromere closer to one arm of the chromosome than to the other.

acrocephaly a malformation of the skull in which the crown is pointed.

acrocyanosis a severe form of chilblains, resulting from an inadequate blood supply to the hands and feet.

acrodynia painful inflammation of the nerves of the fingers or toes.

acrogeria premature wrinkling and aging of the skin of the hands and feet.

acromegaly abnormal enlargement of the facial features,

hands, and feet owing to hypersecretion of growth hormone by the pituitary gland after puberty. Compare *gigantism.*

acromicria abnormal smallness of the bones of the skull and extremities, thought to be caused by a deficiency of growth hormone secreted by the pituitary gland.

acromion the outward projection of the spine of the scapula forming the high point of the shoulder.

acronyx an ingrown fingernail or toenail.

acroparesthesia an abnormal numbness or tingling sensation in the hands or feet.

acrophobia an abnormally severe dread of being at a great height.

acrosome part of the head of a sperm cell.

ACTH adrenocorticotrophic hormone.

actinism the property of radiant energy that produces chemical changes.

actinodermatitis dermatitis resulting from exposure to radiant energy, esp. sunlight.

Actinomyces a genus of rod-shaped bacteria including disease-producing parasites.

actinomycin an antibacterial agent esp. active against Gram-positive bacteria, obtained from a species of *Actinomyces.*

actinomycosis disease produced by bacteria of the genus *Actinomyces* and characterized chiefly by discharging abscesses.

actinomyoca a swelling caused by infection with bacteria of the genus *Actinomyces.*

actinoneuritis inflammation of nerves caused by chronic exposure to radium or X-rays.

actinophage a virus capable of destroying bacteria of the genus *Actinomyces.*

actinotherapy treatment with infra-red or ultra-violet radiation.

activated charcoal a form of charcoal used as an antidote in conditions where it is necessary to adsorb quantities of a gas or other substance, as in flatulence.

activator a substance serving to effect a physical or chemical change in another substance while remaining itself inactive.

actomyosin a complex of actin and myosin that with ATP is responsible for muscular contraction and relaxation.

acupressure. pressure acupuncture.

acupuncture a technique of Chinese origin of puncturing the body with needles to relieve pain or cure disease.

acute (of a disease) having a sudden onset, swift rise, and brief course.

acute alcoholism inebriation from drinking too many alcoholic beverages. See also **alcoholism, chronic alcoholism.**

acute childhood leukemia a malignant cancer of the blood affecting children between two and five years of age, of whom about 20 to 30 percent survive.

acute lymphocytic leukemia a malignant disease of the blood and bone marrow affecting mostly children between two and five years of age, of whom 83 to 92 percent survive.

acute myelocytic leukemia a malignant cancer of the blood-forming tissues affecting mostly adolescents and young adults, of whom few survive because of other infections.

acystia absence of the bladder from birth.

adactylia absence of fingers or toes from birth. —**adactylous** *adj.*

adamantinoma a highly destructive tumour of the jaw.

Adam's apple a prominence at the front of the neck (esp. in men), formed by the largest laryngeal cartilage.

adaptation an adjustment to environmental conditions or to variations or intensity of stimulation.

addiction compulsive physical or psychological dependency on a habit-forming drug.

Addison's disease a disease resulting from deficient secretions of the adrenal cortical hormone and being typically characterized by weight loss, nausea, low blood pressure, malaise, and brownish pigmentation of the skin and mucous membranes, esp. of the mouth.

adduct to draw (a limb) toward or past the median axis of the body. —**adduction** *n.*

adductor a muscle serving to draw a bodily part toward the median line of the body or toward the axis of a bodily extremity.

adenalgia pain originating in a gland.

adenectomy the surgical removal of a gland.

adenectopia the presence of a gland in an abnormal site.

adenine a purine chemical base coding hereditary data in the genetic code in DNA and RNA.

adenitis inflammation of a gland or a lymph node.

adenocarcinoma a malignant tumor in or composed of glandular cells.

adenocyte one of the cells forming a gland.

adenofibroma a benign tumor of connective tissue composed largely of glandular tissue.

adenoidectomy surgical removal of the adenoids.

adenoids an enlarged mass of glandular tissue in the nasopharynx that can potentially inhibit breathing. —**adenoidal** *adj.*

adenoma a benign tumor of glandular tissue.

adenosarcoma a malignant tumor of glandular tissue.

adenosine a nucleoside yielding adenine and ribose.

adenosine diphosphate ADP.

adenosine monophosphate AMP.

adenosine triphosphate ATP.

adenovirus any of various DNA-containing viruses that cause infections of the upper respiratory tract.

ADH antidiuretic hormone.

adhesion tissues joined abnormally by fibrous tissue chiefly as the result of inflammation.

ADI accepted daily intake.

adiaphoresis inadequate ability to perspire.

adipoma a lipoma.

adipometer a device for measuring skin thickness.

adiponecrosis necrosis of fatty tissues.

adiposalgia painful areas of fatty tissue beneath the skin.

adipose relating to animal fat; fatty.

adiposis an excessive accumulation of body fat; liposis.

adiposity fatness; obesity.

aditus an anatomical passage or opening for entry.

adjuvant an ingredient that adds to the effectiveness of a remedy.

ad lib. as much as required (of a drug, remedy, etc.).

admedial near the median plane.

adnexa associated anatomical parts; appendages.

adolescence the period of life between puberty and maturity.

ADP adenosine diphosphate; an ester of adenosine converted to ATP for storing energy in the form of a high-energy phosphate bond.

adrenal 1. adjacent to the kidneys. 2. relating to or derived from the adrenal glands.

adrenalectomy surgical removal of one or both adrenal glands.

adrenal glands a pair of endocrine glands adjacent to the anterior medial border of the kidney, consisting of a cortex and a medulla.

adrenaline epinephrine.

adrenalopathy any disease or disorder of the adrenal glands.

adrenergic activated or transmitted by epinephrine (adrenaline).

adrenocorticotrophic hormone a hormone that is secreted by the anterior lobe of the pituitary gland and stimulates the secretion of hormones by the adrenal cortex.

adrenolytic a substance that inhibits the action of epinephrine (adrenaline) or the function of the adrenal glands.

adrenomegaly abnormal enlargement of the adrenal glands.

adrenopause a supposed period of reduced activity of the adrenal glands.

adrenosterone an androgen secreted by the adrenal cortex.

adrenotoxin any substance that is poisonous to the adrenal glands.

adsorbent relating to or characterized by adsorption.

adsorption the adhesion of a thin molecular layer of a substance, as a gas or liquid, to the solid or liquid surface with which it is in contact.

adult polycystic disease (APD, APKD). See **polycystic kidney disease.**

adventitia the outermost covering or coat of a vein, artery or other structure, not forming an integral part of it.

aerogen a bacillus that produces intestinal gas.

afebrile lacking fever; having a normal body temperature.

affect the consciously apprehended aspect of an emotion regarded as distinct from bodily reactions.

afferent carrying toward; said of nerves carrying impulses to a nerve center and of blood and lymph vessels supplying a particular organ or part.

affinity a force of attraction between particles or substances that brings them into a chemical combination.

African trypanosomiasis an often fatal form of sleeping sickness caused by the bite of the tsetse fly.

afterbirth the placenta, umbilical cord, and fetal membranes expelled from the uterus after the birth of the infant.

afterbrain the metencephalon.

aftercare treatment and supervision of a patient discharged from a hospital.

afterdischarge the extension or prolongation of a reflex response after removal of the original stimulus.

afterimage a visual impression that remains after the stimulation causing it has ceased.

afterpain pain arising from uterine contractions following expulsion of the placenta.

aftosa foot and mouth disease.

agalactia the absence of milk secretion following the birth of a child.

agalorrhea the sudden stopping of the flow of milk from the breast.

agammaglobulinemia a rare condition in which gamma globulin is absent, resulting in reduced ability to produce antibodies.

agamous relating to reproduction by budding, fission or other nonsexual means.

agar *or* **agaragar** a gelatinous, colloidal extractive of a red alga, used esp. in bacteriology as a culture medium.

agenesis failure or lack of development, esp. of a bodily part.

agenosomia the absence or severe malformation of the genital organs in a fetus.

agerasia youthful appearance of an elderly person.

ageusia loss of the sense of taste.

agglutination the clumping together of particles, as blood cells or bacteria, suspended in a liquid.

agglutinin a substance, as an antibody, causing agglutination.

agglutinogen an antigen stimulating the production of an agglutinin.

aggression hostile or destructive behavior or attitude arising chiefly from frustration or feelings of inadequacy.

agitophasia abnormally rapid but impaired speech.

aglutition an inability to swallow.

agnea the inability to recognize objects.

agnosia a disturbance in the ability to comprehend the nature of a sensory impression.

agonist relating to or describing a muscle in a state of contraction, compared with its opposing (antagonist) muscle.

agoraphobia a fear of open spaces or of crossing an open area.

agraffe a device for holding the edges of a wound together without the use of sutures.

agrammatism loss of the ability to use words in a normal or meaningful pattern as the result of brain damage or disease.

agranulocytosis a destructive condition characterized by severe reduction in the number of granulocytes in the blood.

agraphia the psychological loss of the ability to express oneself in writing.

ague a malaria-like condition marked by fever, chills, and sweating recurring in paroxysms at regular intervals.

agyria a congenital defect of the brain in which the normal cerebral folds are undeveloped or absent.

AHG antihemophilic globulin; a blood-coagulating protein factor in which hemophiliacs are deficient.

AID. artificial insemination with donor semen.

AIDS acquired immune deficiency syndrome; a disease formerly usually fatal, first identified among homosexuals but more recently diagnosed among all segments of the population, in which the patient loses immunity to disease, often dying as a result of an acquired infection.

AIH. artificial insemination with the husband's semen.

air embolism embolism resulting from air entering the circulatory system.

akathisia a psychological condition marked by restlessness, hyperactivity, and anxiety.

akinesis loss or impairment of movement.

Al *symbol* aluminum.

ala a wing or winglike part or anatomical process.

alalia the inability to talk due to impairment, as by disease, of the organs of speech.

alba the white matter of the brain, composed mainly of the myelinated axons of nerve cells.

albinism congenital deficiency in skin pigment resulting typically in milky skin, white hair, and eyes with red pupils and pink or blue irises.

albino one affected with albinism.

albocinereous relating to both the white and the gray matter of which the brain and spinal cord are composed.

albumin any of various water-soluble proteins found in blood plasma or serum, muscle, and the whites of eggs and other animal substances.

albuminuria the abnormal presence of albumin (or other proteins) in the urine, usually a sign of some kidney disorder.

alcohol a colorless, flammable, volatile liquid constituting the intoxicating agent in distilled and fermented liquors; ethyl alcohol.

alcoholism an abnormal physiologic or psychological dependence on alcoholic drinks, commonly characterized by excessive solitary or secret drinking and various withdrawal symptoms should drinking cease abruptly; poisoning of the body with alcohol.

alcoholophilia an unnatural craving for alcohol.

alcoholuria the presence of alcohol in the urine.

aldehyde an oxidation product of alcohol, being intermediate in composition between an acid and an alcohol.

aldosterone a hormone of the adrenal cortex regulating the body's salt and water balance.

aldosteronism a condition characterized by weakness, tetany, high blood pressure, irregular heartbeat, and excessive secretion of urine, associated with the production by the adrenal cortex of abnormally large amounts of aldosterone.

aleukocytosis a condition of greatly diminished numbers of white blood cells in the circulation or, rarely, their absence.

alexia an inability to read.

alga *pl.* **algae** any of a group of aquatic plants, as seaweeds, containing chlorophyll often with a brown or red pigment.

algesia sensitivity to pain.

algogenic producing or causing pain.

alimentary of or relating to nutrition or nourishment.

alimentary canal a tubular passage from the mouth to the anus serving to digest and absorb food and eliminate bodily waste.

alimentation the process of giving nourishment; the state of being nourished.

alinasal relating to the flaring part of the nostrils (alae nasi).

alinjection the preservation of tissue specimens by hardening with an injection of alcohol.

aliphatic oily or fatty.

aliquot a measured portion of something.

alkalemia excessive alkalinity of the blood.

alkalescence mild alkalinity or the process of becoming alkaline.

alkali a substance that combines with acids to form salts and turns red litmus paper blue.

alkalimeter an instrument for measuring the alkalinity of a mixture or the strength of alkalis alone.

alkaline relating to or having the properties of an alkali.

alkalinity the amount of alkali in a given substance.

alkaloid any of various complex, bitter, nitrogen-containing organic bases, as morphine or quinine, that are derived from plants and have potent pharmacological activities.

alkalosis a condition in which the body fluids become abnormally alkaline due to the withdrawal of acid or chlorides from the blood or an excess of alkalis in the blood or other body fluids.

allele allelomorph.

allelomorph any of a group of genes occurring alternatively at a given locus.

allergen a substance that induces allergy.

allergic relating to, inducing, or showing allergy.

allergist a physician specializing in allergy.

allergy hypersensitive reaction to a substance (allergen), as by the swelling of mucous membranes or sneezing or itching.

allochromasia a change in the color of the skin or hair.

allocortex the part of the cerebral cortex that is phylogenetically oldest.

allopath one who practices allopathy.

allopathy a system of medicine characterized by treating diseases by the induction of a dissimilar morbid reaction in some part of the body.

alloplasty the surgical repair of the human body using nonhuman tissue.

alloy a mixture of two or more metals.

alopecia loss of hair; baldness.

altitude sickness the effects, as nausea or nosebleed, of reduced oxygen in the blood resulting from exposure to rarefied air at high altitudes.

alveolotomy the surgical incision into the socket of a tooth to drain an abscess or gain access for other treatment.

alveolus 1. the socket of a tooth. 2. an air sac in the lungs.

alvine relating to the abdomen or intestines.

alvus the abdomen and its contents.

alymphia lack or deficiency of lymph.

Alzheimer's disease acute senility in a person of late middle age, usually considered too young to be senile.

amalgam an alloy of mercury and another metal used esp. for filling dental cavities.

amarillic relating to yellow fever.

amaroidal having a slightly bitter taste.

amastia congenital absence of one or both breasts.

amathophobia fear of dirt, dust or filth.

amaurosis progressive degeneration of sight, esp. in the absence of any pathological change to the eye.

ambidextrous using both hands with equal skill and ease.

ambivalence simultaneous attraction toward and repulsion from a person, object, or goal.

amblyopia dimness of vision not of apparent organic origin and attributed esp. to dietary deficiency or toxic effects. —**amblyopic** *adj.*

ambulant ambulatory.

ambulatory (of a patient) able to walk about.

ameba amoeba.

amebiasis amoebiasis.

amebicide amoebicide.

ameburia the presence of amoebas in voided urine.

ameiosis cell division in which gametes are formed without a reduction in their chromosome number.

amelanotic relating to certain types of growths on the skin that do not contain the pigment melanin.

amelia absence of one or more limbs from birth.

amelification formation of tooth enamel.

amelioration improvement in the condition of a patient or symptom.

amenorrhea abnormal cessation or absence of menstruation.

amentia mental deficiency.

ametria congenital absence of the uterus.

ametropia a defective refractive condition of the eye in which the image received fails to focus on the retina.

amino acid an amphoteric organic acid; esp., any of such acids that are the chief components of proteins and are obtained as essential components of the diet or are synthesized by living cells.

amitosis cell division by simple cleavage of the nucleus and division of the cytoplasm.

ammonia a volatile alkali with an extremely pungent odor.

ammoniemia the abnormal presence in the blood of

ammonia or its breakdown products, resulting in various symptoms including weak pulse and coma.

ammoniuria the presence of an excessive amount of ammonia in voided urine.

amnesia loss of memory esp. from shock, brain injury, psychological repression, illness, or fatigue.

amnesiac one who suffers from loss of memory.

amnestic an agent that induces amnesia.

amniocentesis the drawing off of amniotic fluid for diagnostic purposes.

amnioclepsis the unrecognized escape of small amounts of amniotic fluid.

amnion the thin, membranous sac enclosing an embryo.

amniotic fluid the serous fluid surrounding and cushioning the embryo inside the amnion.

amniotic sac the thin sac containing the fetus and the amniotic fluid. It consists of the amnion and the chorion.

amniotomy deliberate rupture of the amnion to induce or facilitate labor.

amobarbital a barbiturate drug used to depress the central nervous system, induce sleep, etc., given by injection or as capsules.

amoeba *also* **ameba** a unicellular microscopic protozoan that moves by extending its membranous walls. —**amoebic, amebic** *adj.*

amoebiasis *also* **amebiasis** disease caused by infection with amoebas.

amoebicide *also* **amebicide** a substance lethal to amoebas.

amor lesbicus lesbianism.

amorphous having no definite shape; formless.

amotio retinae detachment of the retina.

AMP adenosine monophosphate; adenosine containing only one phosphoric acid group.

amphetamine a synthetic drug that is a stimulant to the central nervous system and is potentially addictive, once widely used to suppress appetite.

amphiarthrosis a joint with surfaces connected by disks of fibrocartilage.

amphiblestritis inflammation of the retina; retinitis.

amphicrania neuralgia affecting both sides of the head.

amphigenetic produced by both male and female.

amphodiplopia double vision affecting both eyes simultaneously.

amphoteric capable of acting either as an acid or as a base.

ampule *also* **ampul, ampoule** a small, hermetically sealed glass vial for holding a solution, esp. for hypodermic injection.

ampulla a flask-shaped swelling or pouch esp. of a duct.

amputate to perform an amputation.

amputation the cutting off of a limb or other bodily appendage.

amusia loss of the ability to recognize musical tones.

amyelencephalia congenital absence of both the brain and spinal cord.

amyelia congenital absence of the spinal cord.

amyelination loss of the protective myelin sheath that covers the axon of a nerve.

amyelineuria paralysis of the spinal cord.

amygdala a mass of gray matter in the front part of the brain's temporal lobe.

amygdaloid resembling a tonsil or an almond in shape.

amylase any of the enzymes that aid in the hydrolysis of starch and glycogen.

amyloid 1. a waxy, translucent glycoprotein deposited in some organs under unnatural conditions. 2. resembling starch.

amyloidosis the deposition of amyloid in bodily tissues or organs.

amyotrophic lateral sclerosis a degenerative, fatal disease in which the arms and legs atrophy. Also called **Lou Gehrig's disease.**

ana (in prescriptions) of each in equal amount.

anabolism constructive metabolism in which an organism synthesizes complex molecules from simpler ones.

anaerobe an organism living, thriving, or occurring in the absence of free oxygen. —**anaerobic** *adj.*

anal relating to or situated near the anus.

analeptic 1. a medication that is restorative or stimulating to the central nervous system. 2. relating to such a medicine or remedy; invigorating.

analgesia insensitivity to pain without loss of consciousness.

analgesic 1. a drug that relieves pain, such as aspirin. 2. relating to analgesia.

analgia freedom from pain.

anallergic 1. not causing the production of hypersensitivity or anaphylaxis. 2. a serum, etc., that is not anaphylactic.

analogous similar or comparable in many respects.

analysand one who is undergoing psychoanalysis.

analysis 1. separation of a whole into its component parts; identification or separation of the ingredients of a substance. 2. psychoanalysis.

analyst 1. one who is skilled in making analyses. 2. psychoanalyst.

ananaphylaxis a condition in which anaphylaxis is neutralized.

anaphase a stage in cell division in which the chromosomes move toward the poles of the cell.

anaphoresis reduction in activity of the sweat glands.

anaphylaxis extreme and sometimes fatal allergic response to the injection of a drug or foreign protein resulting from previous sensitization to the substance; anaphylactic shock.

anaplasia reversion of cells to a more primitive or less differentiated form.

anastate any product or substance formed as the result of anabolism.

anastole the separation, shrinking back or retraction of the edges of a wound.

anastomosis the uniting of blood vessels or tubular internal organs so as to create communication between them.

anatherapeusis treatment characterized by the gradual increase in the dose of a drug.

anatomical snuff-box the natural depression or hollow formed between the index finger and the base of the thumb when the latter is abducted.

anatomy a branch of medical science dealing with the form and structure of organisms, esp. the human body.

ancipital having two edges or heads.

anconad in the direction of the elbow.

ancylostomiasis an infection caused by the hookworm.

androgen a hormone producing male sex characteristics. **—androgenic** *adj.*

androsterone an androgenic hormone occurring in male urine.

anemia *also* **anaemia** a condition in which the blood has a deficiency in red blood cells, in hemoglobin, or in volume. **—anemic, anaemic** *adj.*

anencephaly impaired development of the brain with absence of neural tissue in the cranium.

anergic marked by an abnormal degree of inactivity; unenergetic.

anesthesia *also* **anaesthesia** loss of sensitivity to pain with or without loss of consciousness, achieved through any of various means.

anesthesiologist *also* **anaesthesiologist** a physician specializing in anesthesiology.

anesthesiology *also* **anaesthesiology** a branch of medicine concerned with anesthesia and anesthetics.

anesthetic *also* **anaesthetic** 1. a substance producing anesthesia. 2. relating to or capable of producing anesthesia.

anesthetist *also* **anaesthetist** one who administers anesthetics.

anetic relaxing or soothing.

anetus intermittent fever.

aneuria lack of energy and drive.

aneurine vitamin B_1; thiamine.

aneurysm a permanent, blood-filled, abnormal dilation of the wall of a blood vessel.

aneurysmectomy surgical removal of the sac formed by an aneurysm.

aneurysmotomy surgical incision into the sac of an aneurysm.

anfractuosity a fissure or sulcus in the cerebrum.

angel's wing a deformity in which the shoulder blades project posteriorly.

angialgia pain in a blood vessel.

angiasthenia vascular weakness or instability.

angiectasis dilation of a blood vessel.

angiectomy surgical removal of a section of a damaged or diseased blood vessel, usually followed by suturing together the remaining ends or (in larger vessels) replacement of the segment with a graft.

angiitis *also* **angitis** inflammation of a blood vessel or lymph vessel.

angina a condition marked by spasmodic attacks of suffocating pain.

angina pectoris a condition marked chiefly by brief paroxysmal attacks of chest pains resulting from an insufficient supply of blood to the heart.

angiocardiography X-ray photography of the heart and its blood vessels after injection of a radiopaque contrast medium.

angiocardiopathy any disease that involves both the heart and blood vessels.

angiocarditis inflammation of the heart and blood vessels.

angiocholecystitis inflammation of the gallbladder and bile vessels.

angioclast a surgical instrument for controlling arterial bleeding; arterial forceps.

angioedema angioneurotic edema.

angiofibrosis fibrous thickening of the walls of blood vessels.

angiography X-ray photography of the blood vessels after injection of a radiopaque contrast medium.

angiohypertonia spasm of the blood vessels; angiospasm.

angiology the branch of anatomy concerned with the study of the blood vessels and lymphatics.

angioma a tumor composed of blood vessels or lymph vessels.

angioplasty plastic repair of blood vessels or lymphatic glands.

angiotomy surgical separation of a blood vessel.

anhidrotic an agent that checks sweating.

anhydrase an enzyme that acts in the removal of water from a compound.

anhydrous free from water.

animalcule a minute or microscopic organism.

anion an ion with a negative electric charge.

anisocoria inequality in the pupils of both eyes.

anisogamous marked by the fusion of heterogamous gametes or of gametes differing chiefly in size. —**anisogamy** *n.*

anisometropia marked inequality in refractive power in the two eyes.

ankle 1. the joint between the foot and the leg. 2. the region surrounding this joint.

ankyloblepharon adhesion or fusion of the edges of the eyelids.

ankyloglossia restricted mobility of the tongue resulting from a foreshortened frenum.

ankylosis 1. abnormal stiffness or immobilization of a joint through disease or surgery. 2. fusion of separate bones to form a single bone. —**ankylose** *vb.*

annular *also* **anular** ring-shaped, as a muscle.

annulorrhaphy the closure of the circular opening around a hernia by suturing.

anode the positive pole of a primary cell or of a storage battery that is delivering current.

anodontia the absence of teeth.

anodyne 1. a drug that eases pain. 2. serving to lessen pain.

anomia loss of the ability to recognize objects or recognize names.

anoperineal relating to or situated near the anus and perineum.

Anopheles any member of a large genus of mosquitoes including all those that transmit malaria to man.

anophelicide any agent that kills *Anopheles* mosquitoes.

anophelifuge an insect repellent effective against *Anopheles* mosquitoes.

anophthalmus 1. congenital absence of the eyes. 2. one born without eyes.

anorectal relating to or situated within the anus and the rectum.

anorectic 1. relating to anorexia. 2. a drug that suppresses appetite; anorexiant.

anorexia loss of appetite.

anorexia nervosa prolonged loss of appetite esp. when of neurotic origin.

anorexiant a drug or agent that causes a loss of appetite; anorectic.

anoscope proctoscope.

anosigmoidoscopy medical examination of the anus, rectum and lower part of the large intestine.

anosmia impairment or loss of the sense of smell.

anotia absence of the ear from birth.

anotus one without ears.

anovulant a drug that suppresses ovulation.

anovular *also* **anovulatory** 1. not related to or accompanied by ovulation. 2. without ovulation.

anovulation cessation or suppression of ovulation.

anoxemia a condition of the blood marked by insufficient oxygenation.

anoxia severe lack of oxygen causing permanent damage.

ansa 1. (in bacteriology) a small wire loop used to pick up and transport bacteria, protozoa, etc., suspended in a liquid film. 2. any bodily structure or part shaped like or resembling a loop or arc.

ansate *also* **ansiform** loop-shaped.

ansotomy surgical division of a constricting loop.

Antabuse a trade name for disulfiram.

antacid 1. neutralizing an acid. 2. a substance that counteracts acidity, such as sodium bicarbonate or aluminum hydroxide.

antagonist 1. a muscle that contracts with and limits the action of another muscle with which it is paired. 2. a drug that counteracts the action of another drug.

antalgesic a drug or agent that eases pain; anodyne.

antalkaline neutralizing or counteracting alkalinity.

antasthmatic 1. preventing asthma or relieving the symptoms of an asthmatic attack. 2. an agent that prevents asthma or relieves its symptoms.

antefebrile occurring before the onset of a fever.

antemortem preceding death.

antenatal of or relating to an unborn child or to pregnancy; prenatal.

antepartum before birth.

anterior situated before or toward the front; reverse from posterior.

anterograde proceeding or pointed forward.

antero-inferior lying or situated in front and below.

antero-interior lying or situated toward the front and internally.

anterolateral lying or situated in front and to the side.

anteromedian lying or situated in front and toward a midline.

anteroposterior lying or situated from front to back.

anterosuperior lying or situated in front and above.

anthelmintic *also* **anthelminthic** an agent for expelling or destroying parasitic intestinal worms.

anthema any skin eruption.

anthocyanin any of various blue to red pigments that color plants.

anthracosilicosis a disease of the lungs resulting from prolonged inhalation of carbon dust and fine particles of silica.

anthracosis a disease of the lungs resulting from prolonged inhalation of carbon dust alone.

anthrax an acute, infectious disease chiefly of cattle and sheep that is caused by a spore-forming bacterium, is transmissible to man, and is characterized by external ulcerating nodules or by lesions in the lungs.

anthropoid 1. resembling man. 2. resembling an ape.

anthropology the study of the physical, cultural, and environmental aspects of mankind.

anthropometry the branch of anthropology concerned with comparative physical measurements of the body.

anthropophobia a fear of human companionship or an aversion to people generally.

antiagglutinin a specific antibody that counteracts, inhibits or destroys the activity of an agglutinin.

antianaphylaxis desensitization to the potentially harmful effects of a specific antigen, as by a series of very small but progressively increased doses of the antigen.

antiarrhythmic a drug used for treating cardiac arrhythmia, as lidocaine.

antiasthmatic 1. preventing asthma or relieving the symptoms of an asthmatic attack. 2. an agent that prevents asthma or relieves its symptoms.

antibacterial killing or inhibiting the growth of bacteria.

antibiotic 1. tending to or capable of preventing or destroying life. 2. a substance, as penicillin, produced by a microorganism and able to inhibit the growth of or kill another microorganism.

antibody a specific protein substance produced by the body to attack invading bacteria or other foreign matter.

anticholinergic repelling or annulling the physiologic action of acetylcholine.

anticoagulant a drug that prevents or delays the coagulation of the blood, as heparin, used in the treatment of thrombosis and embolism.

anticonvulsant a drug that prevents or reduces the severity of a convulsive seizure, as in epilepsy; an antiepileptic.

antidepressant a drug that relieves or prevents depression.

antidiuretic 1. relating to the reduction of urinary excretion. 2. an agent that acts to reduce the excretion of urine.

antidiuretic hormone (ADH) vasopressin.

antidote an agent that counteracts the effects of a poison or neutralizes the poison before it takes effect.

antiemetic a drug that prevents or relieves the intensity of nausea and vomiting.

antiepileptic relating to a drug that prevents or relieves the severity of an epileptic seizure.

antifebrile reducing fever or relieving its symptoms.

antifungal a drug that prevents the growth of fungi or kills them.

antigen a substance, as a foreign protein or microorganism, that stimulates the production of an antibody when introduced into the body. **—antigenic** *adj.* **—antigenicity** *n.*

antihistamine any drug that counteracts the effects of histamine, used in the symptomatic treatment of various allergies.

antilipidemic a drug or system of treatment for reducing the amount of lipids in the blood serum.

antineoplastic a drug that prevents the growth or increase of neoplasms.

antipruritic a drug that prevents or reduces itching.

antipyretic a drug for reducing fever.

antitoxin an antibody formed in response to the presence of a specific toxin and able to neutralize that toxin. —**antitoxic** *adj.*

antitussive a drug for reducing or eliminating the reflex to cough.

antivenim a prepared substance used in emergency aid for victims of snakebite and insect bites.

anuria the reduction or stoppage of output of urine, indicative of kidney dysfunction and often fatal.

aorta the main artery leading from the heart to supply blood to the body.

apastia failure to eat.

APD, APKD. adult polycystic disease. See **polycystic kidney disease.**

aphasia loss or impairment of the faculty of speech, due to some disease of or injury to the brain.

aphonia loss of the voice, esp. caused by laryngitis or some disease of the vocal cords or their nerve supply.

apnea breathlessness; inability to catch one's breath.

apneumia congenital absence of the lungs.

apodal without feet.

apodia congenital absence of the feet.

apoplexy stroke.

appendectomy surgical removal of the vermiform appendix.

appendicitis inflammation of the vermiform appendix.

appendix 1. any bodily appendage. 2. the wormlike (vermiform) appendage attached to the blind pouch at the beginning of the large intestine.

appestat the part of the brain (thought to be in the hypothalamus) responsible for governing the sensations of hunger and satiety.

aqueous humor the watery fluid filling the space between the cornea and lens of the eye.

arachnoid one of the three membranes (meninges) that cover the brain and spinal cord, lying between the pia mater below and the dura mater above.

arboviral infection an infection, as dengue and yellow fever, caused by virus carried by arthropods, which include the crabs, lobsters, mites, ticks, spiders, and insects.

areola the pigmented circular area surrounding the nipples.

arrhythmia any abnormal rhythm, esp. of the heartbeat.

arteriography X-ray photography of the arteries following injection of a radiopaque contrast medium.

arterioles the smallest vessels of the arterial system, linked by the capillaries to the venous system.

arteriosclerosis a disease marked by thickening and hardening of arterial walls. —**arteriosclerotic** *adj.*

artery a blood vessel that carries blood away from the heart.

arthritis inflammation of a joint.

arthrocentesis the process of withdrawing a sample of synovial fluid from a joint by means of a needle for diagnostic purposes.

artificial insemination the fertilization of an ovum by means other than coitus, such as the introduction of spermatozoa into the vagina with a syringe.

artificial respiration any of various means of forcing air into and out of the lungs of a person who has stopped or nearly stopped breathing.

asbestosis a lung disease caused by chronic inhalation of tiny particles of asbestos.

ascariasis intestinal infestation with parasitic roundworms of the species *Ascaris lumbricoides.*

ascorbic acid vitamin C.

ASD. atrial septal defect.

asepsis a germ-free condition.

Asian flu a severe epidemic of influenza that took place in 1957, caused by a virus strain that is thought to have originated in Singapore.

aspermia inability to produce or ejaculate semen.

asphyxia loss of consciousness from too little oxygen and overabundance of carbon dioxide in the blood.

aspirate to draw off fluid or gas (as from a body cavity) by means of suction.

aspirator an instrument for drawing off fluid or gas by means of suction.

aspirin a drug used to reduce pain and fever; acetylsalicylic acid.

astasia the inability to stand due to loss of motor coordination.

astatine a radioactive halogen element.

asteatosis loss of activity of the sebaceous glands or gross diminution of their secretions.

astereognosis loss of the ability to recognize shapes by the sense of touch.

asterixis involuntary jerking movements of various muscle groups caused by advanced liver disease or some disturbance of cerebral metabolism.

asternia absence of the breastbone (sternum).

asthenia loss of strength or stamina; debility. **—asthenic** *adj.*

asthenocoria retarded reaction of the pupil when stimulated by light, caused by a disorder of the adrenal glands.

asthenopia eyestrain; weak sight, caused by fatigue of the muscles that control the eyeball.

asthenospermia loss of movement or impaired motility of sperm cells.

asthma a condition that is marked by severely labored

breathing, wheezing, and sensations of chest constriction along with periods of respite and is often thought to be of allergic origin.

astigmatism a defect of vision in which light rays entering the eye are abnormally bent before reaching the retina, thus producing a blurred image.

astomia congenital absence of the mouth.

astragalus former term for the ankle bone (talus).

astraphobia fear of lightning and thunder.

astringent 1. causing contraction of soft tissues. 2. an agent that causes contraction of tissues, used to check hemorrhage, arrest secretion, etc.

astrocyte a star-shaped cell of nervous tissues.

astrocytoma a tumor of nerve tissue composed of astrocytes.

asymmetry lack of symmetry; imbalance.

asynergy poor coordination among organs or muscles that normally function harmoniously.

asystole cessation of the heartbeat; cardiac standstill.

atactilia loss of the sense of touch.

ataraxia calmness of mind; total relaxation; imperturbability.

atavism recurrence in an organism of a characteristic typical of its distant ancestors.

ataxia an inability to coordinate voluntary muscular movement.

ataxiophemia impaired coordination of the muscles concerned with speech production.

atelectasis 1. collapse or incomplete expansion of a lung. 2. defective expansion of the pulmonary alveoli at birth.

atelocardia incomplete development of the heart.

atelochilia harelip.

atelochiria incomplete or imperfect development of the hands.

athelia congenital absence of the nipples.

atherogenic of or relating to the production of degenerative changes in arterial walls.

atheroma degeneration of arterial walls resulting from the deposit of fatty esters.

atheromatosis widespread vascular disease characterized by atheroma.

atherosclerosis abnormal thickening of arterial walls resulting from fatty deposits and fibrosis. **—atherosclerotic** *adj.*

athetosis a nervous disorder chiefly of children that is usually the result of brain lesion and is characterized by continuous slow movements of the hands and feet. **—athetotic, athetosic** *adj.*

athlete's foot a fungus infection (ringworm) of the feet, typically of the areas between the toes, characterized by itching, cracking and scaling of the skin and the formation of watery blisters.

atlas the first vertebra of the neck, shaped like a ring and supporting the skull.

atom the smallest particle of an element existing either alone or in combination. **—atomic** *adj.*

atomizer an instrument for dispensing a liquid in a spray of fine droplets.

atony lack or insufficiency of muscular tone.

ATP adenosine triphosphate; an adenosine ester derivative supplying energy for many biochemical cellular processes.

atresia absence or closure of a natural bodily passage.

atrial fibrillation very rapid spasmodic contractions of the atria, a form of arrhythmia that occurs in rheumatic heart disease and other disorders.

atrial septal defect a congenital abnormality in which there is an opening between the atria of the heart.

atrium *pl.* **atria** either of the two upper chambers of the heart. Also called *auricle.* —**atrial** *adj.*

atrophy the wasting away or decrease in size of a body part or tissue; degeneration.

atropine a white, poisonous, crystalline compound derived chiefly from belladonna and used to control spasms and dilate the pupil of the eye.

audiogram a graph tracing the relationship between frequency of vibration and the minimal level at which a person can hear.

audiology the study of hearing and hearing disorders. —**audiologist,** *n.*

audiometer an instrument for measuring keenness of hearing. —**audiometric** *adj.* —**audiometry** *n.*

auditory relating to or experienced through the sense of hearing.

aura a subjective sensation sometimes experienced before the onset of a neurological attack, as of epilepsy.

aural relating to the ear or the sense of hearing.

auricle 1. pinna. 2. atrium.

auricular 1. of or relating to the sense of hearing. 2. of or relating to the auricles (atria) of the heart.

auriscope an instrument for examining the ear; otoscope.

auscultation the diagnostic technique of listening to and analyzing sounds produced by organs within the body.

autism an emotional disorder found chiefly in young children and marked by alternating periods of extreme withdrawal and irrational violence. Also called *infantile autism.* —**autistic** *adj.*

autoclave 1. an electric appliance using superheated steam under pressure to sterilize dental or surgical instruments and other operating room equipment. 2. to subject to the action of an autoclave.

autoerotism *also* **autoeroticism** sexual desire and the seeking for its gratification directed toward oneself.

autogenous 1. originating within an organism. 2. produced independently of external influences or aid. —**autogenic** *adj.* —**autogeny** *n.*

autograft an organ or tissue transplanted from one part to another part of the same body.

autohypnosis hypnosis that is self-induced.

autoimmunity a condition in which the body is abnormally sensitive to some of its own tissues as the result of forming antibodies against them.

autoinfection reinfection resulting from the presence of pathogenic microorganisms already present in the body.

autointoxication poisoning resulting from toxins already within the body.

autolysis the disintegration of cells or tissues by enzymes produced within the body.

automatism repetitive, unconscious motor activity, as that sometimes following an epileptic seizure.

automyosophobia fear of being dirty or of smelling bad.

autonomic 1. acting independently: *autonomic reflexes.* 2. resulting from internal influences or causes.

autonomic nervous system the part of the nervous system that supplies smooth and cardiac muscle and glandular tissue and regulates involuntary actions.

autonomotropic acting on the autonomic nervous system, as a drug.

autophagia 1. the self-consumption of a cell. 2. the biting of one's own flesh.

autophilia love of self; narcissism.

autopsy a post-mortem examination; necropsy.

autoradiograph a photographic image produced by the

radiation of a radioactive substance contained in a subject in close contact with the emulsion. **—autoradiography** *n.*

auxesis an enlargement resulting from the expansion of cells rather than from an increase in their number.

avascular 1. lacking blood vessels. 2. relating to an inadequate blood supply.

avirulent not virulent.

avitaminosis disease resulting from a dietary deficiency of any of various vitamins.

avulsion the tearing away or separation of a bodily structure or part either accidentally or surgically.

axanthopsia inability to see yellow hues or tints.

axenic (of a culture) free from contamination by foreign organisms.

axilla armpit.

axis *pl.* **axes** the second vertebra of the neck, serving as the pivot for turning the head.

axon a long nerve cell process that conducts impulses away from the cell body.

azoospermia inability to produce spermatozoa; absence of live sperm cells in the semen.

azotemia the abnormal accumulation of urea in the blood; uremia.

B

B one of the four blood types. See **ABO blood groups.**

Babinski reflex *or* **Babinski's reflex** a reflex movement of the foot in which when the sole is tickled the great toe turns upward, indicative of organic lesion of the brain or spinal cord.

baccate resembling a berry; berrylike.

bacciform having the shape of a berry.

bacillary 1. rod-shaped. 2. relating to or produced by bacilli.

bacille Calmette-Guérin (BCG) a vaccine commonly used against tuberculosis.

bacillemia the presence in the blood of rod-shaped bacteria.

bacilli *pl. of* bacillus.

bacillicide any agent capable of killing bacilli.

bacilliform rod-shaped; resembling a bacillus in form.

bacilliparous producing bacilli.

bacillogenic *or* **bacillogenous** 1. of bacillary origin; originating in bacilli. 2. producing bacilli; bacilliparous.

bacillophobia abnormal fear or dread of bacilli.

bacillosis a condition caused by infection with bacilli.

bacilluria the presence of bacilli in the urine.

bacillus *pl.* **bacilli** 1. any of a genus (*Bacillus*) of rod-shaped, aerobic bacteria including saprophytes and some parasites. 2. a disease-producing bacterium.

bacitracin an antibacterial drug.

bacteremia the presence of bacteria in the blood.

bacteria *pl. of* bacterium.

bacterial relating to or caused by bacteria.

bacterial plaque plaque

bactericholia the presence of bacilli in the bile.

bactericidal destructive of bacteria.

bactericide a drug or agent that destroys bacteria.

bacteriogenous 1. caused by bacteria or of bacterial origin. 2. producing bacteria.

bacteriology a science concerned with bacteria and their importance to medicine, agriculture, and industry.

bacteriolytic destroying or dissolving the cellular structure of bacteria.

bacteriopathology the study of diseases caused by bacteria or their toxic products.

bacteriophage a bacteriolytic virus.

bacteriophobia an abnormal fear of bacteria and other microorganisms.

bacteriosis widespread bacterial infection.

bacteriostasis prevention of the growth and multiplication of bacteria. —**bacteriostatic** *adj.*

bacteriostat any agent that inhibits the growth or multiplication of bacteria.

bacterium *pl.* **bacteria** any of a class of microscopic plantlike organisms lacking chlorophyll that have single-celled bodies, live in water, soil, organic matter, or in the bodies of animals and plants, and are significant as pathogens or for their chemical effects.

BAL British anti-lewisite; dimercaprol.

balanitis inflammation of the glans penis.

balanoplasty plastic surgery involving repair or reconstruction of the glans penis.

balanoposthitis inflammation of the glans penis and foreskin (prepuce).

balanorrhagia a constant discharge from the glans penis.

balanorrhea inflammation of the glans penis accompanied by the discharge or formation of pus.

balanus glans penis.

ball-and-socket joint enarthrosis.

ballistocardiogram a recording of minute movements of the body during systole, used in measuring cardiac output.

balm 1. a soothing ointment or other application. 2. balsam.

balneology the branch of medical science concerned with balneotherapy.

balneotherapy the therapeutic use of baths, esp. using natural mineral waters, in treating disease or pain.

balsam 1. a fragrant, resinous exudate obtained from various trees. 2. balm.

bandage a strip of cloth or plastic fabric for binding and dressing wounds.

Band-Aid a trademark for a small adhesive bandage with a gauze pad affixed to the center of the adhesive side.

Banting treatment *or* **Banting diet** a low-carbohydrate, high-protein diet to reduce obesity.

baragnosis inability to sense the weight of a hand-held object.

barbiturate any of various derivatives of barbituric acid used extensively as antispasmodics, sedatives, and hypnotics.

barbituric acid a synthetic crystalline acid that is derived from pyrimidine.

barbiturism chronic poisoning by derivatives of barbituric acid, characterized by fever, chills and headache.

barbula hirci the hairs that grow in the outer part of the external ear in men.

baresthesia the sense of pressure.

baresthesiometer a delicate instrument for measuring the sense of pressure.

barium a silver-white bivalent toxic metallic element.

barium enema a procedure for rendering the rectum and lower part of the large intestine visible on X-ray photographs by first introducing barium sulfate into the rectum under gentle pressure.

barium meal a procedure for rendering the esophagus and upper part of the digestive tract visible on X-ray photographs by first swallowing a quantity of barium sulfate.

barium sulfate a colorless insoluble compound used esp. as an opaque medium in X-ray photography of the alimentary canal.

baroreceptor a nerve ending, as in the arterial walls, responsive to changes in pressure.

bartholinitis inflammation of Bartholin's glands.

Bartholin's gland either of two glands, located one on each side of the vagina, that secrete a mucous lubricating fluid.

basad toward a base.

basal metabolic rate the rate at which an organism at rest releases heat.

basal metabolism the amount of energy required for the maintenance of basic body functions, as breathing, circulation, etc.

base 1. the lowest or underlying part; foundation. 2. a chemical compound capable of reacting with an acid to form a salt.

basement membrane a thin single-layered membrane of connective tissue cells underlying the epithelium of many organs.

basic reacting as an alkali.

basilar of or relating to a base or basal area.

basiphobia fear of walking.

basophil *or* **basophile** a white blood cell with basophilic granules.

basophilia 1. an increased number of basophils in the blood. 2. a tendency to stain with basic dyes.

basophilic susceptible to staining with basic dyes.

bathmotropic affecting the excitability of nerves or muscles in response to stimuli.

bathophobia fear of looking down into deep places or a fear of being in a deep place.

bathycardia a condition in which the heart is located abnormally low in the thoracic cavity.

bathyesthesia sensation in muscles and other deep structures.

bathyhyperesthesia abnormal sensitivity of muscles and other deep structures.

bathyhypesthesia impairment or partial loss of sensation in muscles and deeper structures.

battered child syndrome the complex of severe physical harm to a child resulting from the brutality of a parent or other adult guardian.

BCG bacille Calmette-Guérin.

BCG vaccine a vaccine prepared from living tubercle bacilli used to vaccinate against tuberculosis.

B complex vitamin B complex.

bdelygmia nausea.

bear down to contract the abdominal muscles and diaphragm during childbirth.

bedbug a wingless bloodsucking bug that feeds on human blood and sometimes infests houses.

bedpan a shallow receptacle used for urination or defecation by someone confined to bed.

bedsore an ulcerated lesion of tissue, esp. that overlying bony prominences, resulting from deprivation of nutrition through prolonged pressure.

behavior the conduct and response of an organism to outside stimuli.

behaviorism the psychological study of human behavior exclusive of the study of the mind and consciousness.

belch to raise gas or air from the stomach; eructate.

belladonna 1. a poisonous plant of the nightshade family that yields atropine. Also called *deadly nightshade.* 2. a medical extract, as atropine, of the belladonna plant.

Bell's palsy paralysis of the facial nerve, most often of unknown cause.

belly 1. the thick central area of a muscle. 2. the abdomen.

belonephobia fear of sharp-pointed objects, such as needles or pins.

Benadryl a trademark for diphenhydramine hydrochloride (an antihistamine).

bends caisson disease; decompression sickness.

benign not malignant or a threat to life; innocent.

Benzadrine a trademark for amphetamine.

benzocaine a local anesthetic used in many over-the-counter remedies for itching and pain.

beriberi a vitamin deficiency disease affecting the nerves, heart, and digestive system and resulting from a lack of thiamine.

berylliosis poisoning from prolonged exposure to the element beryllium, as by direct contact or inhalation.

beryllium a white metallic bivalent element.

bestiality sexual intercourse between a human being and an animal.

betacism a relatively rare speech defect in which the sound of the letter B is given to other consonants.

beta globulin a globulin of plasma or serum with electrophoretic mobilities between alpha globulin and gamma globulin.

between-brain the diencephalon.

bhang a powdered preparation of cannabis which is smoked or chewed for its intoxicating effects in some Eastern countries.

bi- *prefix* 1. two. 2. twice. 3. double.

bicarbonate an acid salt of carbonic acid.

bicarbonate of soda sodium bicarbonate.

biceps either of two two-headed muscles, situated at the front of the upper arm or at the back of the upper leg.

bicornuate having two horn-shaped processes: *a bicornuate uterus.*

bicuspid 1. ending in or having two points: *bicuspid teeth.* 2. a premolar tooth.

bifid divided into two sections or parts by a median cleft: *a bifid chin.*

biforate having two openings.

bifurcate divided into two branches or parts. —**bifurcation** *n.*

bigeminal paired or consisting of two parts.

bilabe delicate forceps for removing calculi, as those lodged in the urethra.

bilateral having or affecting two sides.

bile a greenish or yellowish alkaline viscid fluid secreted by the liver and serving chiefly as an aid to digestion.

bilharziasis *pl.* **bilharziases** schistosomiasis.

biliary relating to bile.

biliary cirrhosis a condition caused by obstruction of the flow of bile through ductules in the liver.

bilious 1. of or relating to bile. 2. suffering from or marked by disordered liver function.

bilirachia the presence of bile in the spinal fluid.

bilirubin a reddish-yellow pigment found in bile, urine, and blood.

bilirubinemia the presence of abnormally large amounts of bilirubin in the blood.

bilirubinuria the presence of bile in the urine.

biliverdin a green pigment found in bile.

bilobulate *or* **bilobular** having two lobes or lobules.

bimanual using or requiring both hands.

binary fission the division of a cell into two daughter cells.

binaural relating to or using both ears.

binocular relating to, using, or designed for use by both eyes.

binomial having two names, esp. for both genus and species.

bioassay analysis of the strength of a substance by comparing its effect on a test organism with the effect of a standard preparation.

bioastronautics the branch of science concerned with the effects of space travel on biological processes.

biochemistry chemistry that deals with life processes and compounds. —**biochemical** *adj.*

bioelectricity electrical activity in living organisms or tissues.

biofeedback a technique for making a person aware of his autonomic processes by sight or sound to enable him to control them consciously.

biogenesis the development of life from life already in existence. —**biogenetic** *adj.*

biogravics the branch of science concerned with studying the effects on living organisms of weightlessness and excessive gravitational force.

biology the scientific study of living organisms and their life processes. —**biologic, biological** *adj.*

biomechanics the study of the relationship between mechanical engineering and the body's system of locomotion.

biometry the statistical analysis of biological problems. —**biometric** *adj.*

bionics the science of using electronic devices, as pacemakers, to solve medical problems. —**bionic,** *adj.*

biophage a parasite.

biophagous (of certain parasites) feeding on living organisms.

biophysics the application of the principles and methods of physics to biological problems. —**biophysical** *adj.*

biopsy the examination of tissues, fluids, or cells removed from the living body.

biorhythm a rhythmic, or cyclical biological phenomenon, as sleeping, menstruation, etc.

biosynthesis the production by a living organism of a chemical compound. —**biosynthetic** *adj.*

biotin a member of the vitamin B complex found in all forms of life.

biotoxicology the branch of science concerned with the study of toxins produced by living organisms.

biotoxin a toxin formed and shown to be present in the tissues of a living animal.

biparous having given birth to two young.

birth the emergence of a new individual from the body of its parent; parturition.

birth control the prevention or delay of pregnancy by a device, drug, or practice.

birth defect an abnormality present at birth.

birthmark any skin blemish present at birth; nevus.

bisexual 1. having characteristics of both sexes; hermaphroditic. 2. erotically attracted to both sexes.

bisferious (of the pulse) beating twice.

bismuth a red, metallic, trivalent element.

bistoury a long knife-like instrument for draining abscesses, etc.

bite the way the teeth of the jaws meet.

bitewing an x-ray film holder that can be held between the clenched teeth.

bivalent having a valence of two.

biventer (of a muscle) having two bellies.

blackhead comedo.

blackwater fever an often fatal complication of malaria.

bladder a membranous sac functioning as a receptacle for a liquid, esp. the urinary bladder.

blain a sore or blister on the skin; blotch.

bland non-irritating; mild: *a bland diet.*

blastin a substance that stimulates the growth of cells.

blastogenesis 1. reproduction by budding. 2. embryonic development during cleavage and the formation of the germ layers.

blastoma a tumor composed mainly of undifferentiated or immature cells.

blastomere any of the cells into which the ovum divides after fertilization.

blastomycosis a skin disease caused by a yeast-like fungus.

blastula *pl.* **blastulas** *or* **blastulae** an early stage in the cleavage of a fertilized ovum.

bleeder a hemophiliac.

blennadenitis inflammation of the mucus-secreting glands.

blennemesis the vomiting of mucus.

blennogenic forming mucus.

blennoid resembling mucus; having a viscid consistency.

blennostatic relating to a reduction in mucus secretion.

blennothorax accumulation of mucus in the bronchi.

blennuria the presence of excessive amounts of mucus in the urine.

blepharal relating to the eyelids.

blepharectomy surgical removal of part of the eyelid.

blepharedema swelling of the eyelids.

blepharism twitching of the eyelid.

blepharitis inflammation of the eyelid, esp. the margin.

blepharoadenoma a glandlike tumor of the eyelid.

blepharoatheroma a sebaceous cyst of the eyelid.

blind fistula a fistula open at only one end.

blindness lack of visual perception; loss of sight.

blind spot a point in the retina of the eye that is insensitive to light.

blister a usually circular elevation of the epidermis containing a watery liquid. —**blistery** *adj.*

blood the fluid circulating in the heart, arteries, veins and capillaries and carrying oxygen and nourishment to all parts of the body and bringing away waste products.

blood bank an establishment for storing blood or plasma.

blood cell a cell present normally in blood; a white blood cell, red blood cell or platelet.

blood clot a fibrous substance that forms, usually when blood is exposed to air.

blood count the determination of the number and type of blood cells present in a specific volume of blood.

blood group any of various classes into which human beings are grouped according to the presence or absence in their blood of certain antigens. Also called *blood type.*

blood poisoning septicemia.

blood pressure the pressure exerted by the blood flowing through the blood vessels, esp. the arteries.

blood sugar glucose present in the blood.

blood vessel any tube-like part of the circulatory system.

blue baby an infant with a circulatory defect that imparts a bluish tint to the skin.

boil the common name for a furuncle.

bolus a soft, rounded mass of chewed food.

bone one of the hard structures forming the skeleton of a vertebrate. —**bony** *or* **boney** *adj.*

booster injection *or* **booster shot** an additional injection given to maintain immunization, usually smaller than the original injection.

boric acid a white powder used in solution as a mild antiseptic.

boss a rounded swelling.

bosselated characterized by or having several rounded protuberances. —**bosselation** *n.*

botulin a toxin sometimes occurring in imperfectly canned food.

botulism acute food poisoning caused by the presence of botulin.

bougie a tapering surgical instrument for introduction into a bodily passage.

bougienage the use of a bougie in the examination or treatment of a bodily passage or canal.

bouton a knoblike swelling or structure.

boutonneuse fever an infectious, rickettsial disease, similar to Rocky Mountain spotted fever.

bowel the intestine or one of its divisions.

bowleg a leg that bows outward at the knee. —**bowlegged** *adj.*

B.P. blood pressure.

brachialgia intense pain in the arm.

brachiocyllosis the condition of having a crooked arm.

brachiotomy incision into or removal of an arm.

brachium the upper part of the arm. —**brachial** *adj.*

brachycephalic having an abnormally short head or skull. —**brachicephaly** *or* **brachycephalia** *n.*

brachycnemic having abnormally short legs.

brachydactylic having abnormally short fingers.

brachydont having short teeth.

brachygnathia a receding lower jaw. —**brachygnathous** *adj.*

brachypodous having short feet.

Bradley method a method of natural childbirth

bradycardia relatively slow heartbeat.

brain the part of the central nervous system located within the skull and serving as the organ of thought and neural and muscular coordination.

brain death permanent loss of consciousness and of brain function; irreversible coma.

brain stem the part of the brain consisting of the pons, medulla oblongata and midbrain; all of the brain except the cerebrum and cerebellum.

brain tumor a neoplasm of the central nervous system that does not spread to the spinal cord.

breast either of two protuberant, glandular, milk-secreting organs on the front of the female chest; mammary gland.

breast cancer a neoplasm in the breast tissue, malignant in many women

breech birth delivery of a baby in which the feet, knees, or buttocks emerge first, sometimes dangerous.

bregma the point on the skull where the coronal and sagittal sutures meet.

Bright's disease a kidney disease marked by albumin in the urine; a form of nephritis.

Brill's disease an acute infectious disease similar to but milder than typhus.

broad-spectrum effective against many microorganisms or insects: *broad-spectrum antibiotics; broad-spectrum insecticides.*

Broca's area the speech center in the brain.

bromhidrosis a condition marked by abnormally unpleasant-smelling body odor.

bromide a salt of hydrobromic acid, esp. one used as a depressant drug.

bromine a liquid nonmetallic element obtained from sea water and natural brines, whose compounds are of medical use.

bromism *also* **brominism** poisoning caused by the chronic use of bromides.

bronchi *pl. of* bronchus.

bronchi- *or* **bronchio-** *prefix* bronchial tubes.

bronchiectasis *also* **bronchiectasia** dilation of a bronchus or of the bronchi.

bronchiogenic originating in or coming from the bronchi.

bronchiole *also* **bronchiolus** one of the smallest divisions of the bronchial tree, having no cartilaginous walls and being less than 1 mm in diameter.

bronchiostenosis the abnormal narrowing of a bronchial tube.

bronchitis inflammation of the bronchi.

bronchodilator 1. causing an increase in the internal diameter of a bronchial tube or bronchus. 2. a drug or agent that causes dilation of a bronchial tube or bronchus.

bronchoscope an instrument for insertion to view the bronchi. —**bronchoscopy** *n.*

bronchus *pl.* **bronchi** either of two primary tubes of the trachea leading to the right and left lung respectively. —**bronchial** *adj.*

brontophobia an abnormal fear of thunder.

brucellosis undulant fever.

bruise an epidermal injury with discoloration from ruptured blood vessels but without a break in the skin.

bruit any abnormal sound discovered during auscultation, such as a gurgling or splashing sound heard when both fluid and air are present in the pericardium.

bruxism involuntary grinding of the teeth.

bubo *pl.* **buboes** an inflammatory swelling of a lymph gland, esp. in the groin. —**bubonic** *adj.*

bubonic plague plague marked especially by buboes of the groin.

buccal relating to, occurring in, or situated in the cheeks or the oral cavity.

buffer a chemical substance that can be added to a drug, as aspirin, to make it more digestible.

bulbourethral glands two small glands on both sides of the prostate that lead to the urethra and secrete the fluid in semen.

bulimia *or* **boulimia** an abnormal craving for food resulting in episodes of voracious eating. —**bulemic,** *adj.*

bulla *pl.* **bullae** blister; vesicle.

bundle of His a fibrous band in the myocardium that transmits the cardiac impulse.

bunion an inflammation with swelling over the first bursa of the big toe.

burn damage to the skin from exposure to fire, heat, radiation, caustics, or electricity. —**burn** *vb.*

burnout physical or emotional exhaustion resulting from overwork.

bursa *pl.* **bursas** *or* **bursae** a small sac filled with serous fluid between movable parts, as between a bone and a tendon. —**bursal** *adj.*

bursitis inflammation of a bursa, esp. of the shoulder or the elbow.

buttock the back of the hip forming one of two fleshy protuberances on which one sits.

THE BRAIN
(CROSS SECTION)

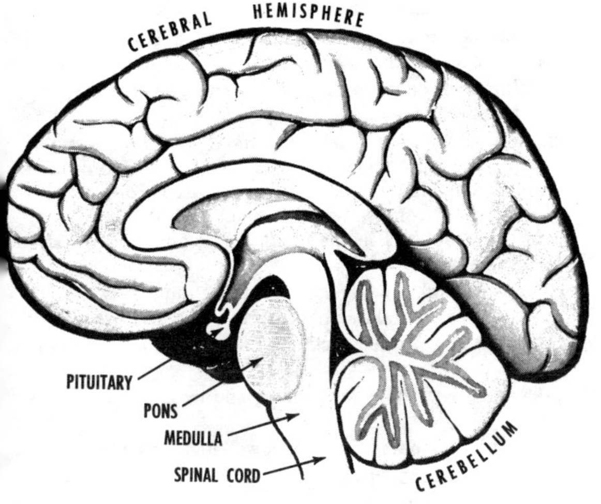

C

cachexia malnutrition and physical wasting associated with chronic disease.

cadaver a dead body; corpse, esp. one intended for dissection.

caesarean *or* **caesarian** cesarean.

caffeine a bitter compound used as a stimulant and diuretic and found in coffee, tea, and kola nuts.

caffeinism chronic poisoning by caffeine, characterized by irritability, insomnia, and palpitations.

caisson disease a condition marked typically by pain, paralysis, asphyxia, and collapse, caused by too rapid a shift from a high-pressure atmospheric environment to a normal environment, which results in the release of nitrogen bubbles in the bloodstream and tissues. Also called *bends.*

calamine a pink powder used in lotions, ointments, etc., to relieve itching and as an astringent.

calcaneal *or* **calcanean** relating to the heel bone or calcaneus.

calcaneus a tarsal bone forming the major bone of the heel.

calcanodynia pain in the heel on walking or standing.

calcar a spurlike projection.

calcareous containing calcium or calcium carbonate.

calcarine spurlike.

calcariuria the presence of calcium salts in the urine.

calcaroid resembling lime salts.

calcemia the presence of abnormally large amounts of calcium in the blood.

calcicosis a lung disease caused by the inhalation of limestone dust.

calciferol vitamin D_2.

calcification the deposit of insoluble lime salts in tissue.

calciphilia a condition in which the tissues tend to absorb an abnormally large amount of calcium salts, leading to their calcification.

calciprivia lack of dietary calcium.

calciprivic deprived of calcium.

calcitonin a thyroid hormone important in the metabolism of calcium.

calcium a metallic element occurring only in combination, forming about 85 per cent of the mineral matter of bones.

calcium carbonate a compound used in medicine as an antacid.

calcodynia pain in the heel.

calcoid a tumor of the dental pulp.

calculary relating to a calculus or to the formation of calculi.

calculosis the tendency or predisposition to form calculi.

calculus *pl.* **calculi** *or* **calculuses** a concretion of mineral salts in a hollow organ or a duct; stone.

calicectomy surgical removal of a calyx.

caligo dimness of vision.

calipers an instrument with two adjustable legs for measuring the distance, diameter, or thickness between surfaces.

callosal relating to the corpus callosum.

callosity a callus.

callous thickened and hardened esp. from friction and pressure.

callus 1. a thickening of or hard thickened area of the skin; callosity. 2. a mass of tissue forming around a break in a bone and converted to bone during healing.

calor heat, one of the signs of inflammation.

Calorie a unit of heat; the amount of heat required to raise the temperature of one kilogram of water one degree centigrade: used to express heat- or energy-producing value of food oxidized in the body. Also called *kilocalorie.* —**caloric** *adj.*

calorifacient producing or generating heat.

calorimeter a device for the measurement of the amount of heat given off by a body.

calvarium the upper, domelike part of the skull.

calvities baldness; alopecia.

calyx one of the cuplike divisions of the renal pelvis.

canaliculus *pl.* **canaliculi** a small channel or passage.

cancellous tissue spongy, porous tissue, as normal inside some bones.

cancer a malignant tumor of potentially limitless growth. —**cancerous** *adj.*

cancerocidal able to destroy cancer cells; cytotoxic.

cancerophobia an abnormal fear of getting cancer.

cancriform resembling cancer or the manifestations of a malignant growth.

cancroid 1. resembling a crab. 2. resembling a cancer.

Candida any of a genus of yeast-like fungi that are the causative agents of thrush.

candidiasis an infection caused by *Candida.*

canine any of four pointed, conical teeth situated between the lateral incisors and first premolars in the upper and lower jaws.

canker a small ulcer of the lips, mouth, or tongue.

cannabis the dried flowering spikes of the hemp plant (*Cannabis sativa*), which yield hashish; marijuana.

cannabism severe hallucinations and other symptoms associated with cannabis poisoning.

cannula a small tube for insertion into a body cavity.

cannulation insertion of a cannula.

canthal relating to a canthus.

cantharides a counterirritant drug prepared from the dried bodies of the blister beetle (*Cantharis vesicatoria*), now no longer in use because of its dangerous irritant effects on the urinary tract; Spanish fly.

canthectomy surgical incision into a canthus to increase the width of the slit between the lids.

canthus *pl.* **canthi** either of the angular junctures of the eye formed by the meeting of the upper and lower eyelids.

capiat an instrument for removing foreign objects from the uterus or other body cavities.

capillarectasia dilation of the capillaries.

capillaritis inflammation of the capillaries.

capillarity the spontaneous rise or depression of liquids placed in very narrow tubes; an effect of surface tension.

capillary *pl.* **capillaries** any of the very small blood vessels forming a network throughout the body and connecting arterioles and venules.

capillary hemangioma a birthmark that is filled with blood; common in babies, it usually disappears in childhood.

capitate 1. having a round or head-shaped extremity. 2. one of the carpal bones.

capitium a special bandage made to fit the head.

capitopedal relating to both the head and feet.

capitulum a small projection on a bone where it articulates with another bone.

capnogram a record of the amount of carbon dioxide in exhaled air.

caprizant denoting a bounding pulse beat.

capsule 1. an enveloping membrane around an organ, joint or other structure. 2. a small container made of soluble material, such as gelatin, for enclosing powdered drugs, medicated pellets, etc. 3. any bodily structure or part resembling a capsule.

capsulitis inflammation of an anatomical capsule.

capsuloma cancer of a bodily capsule, esp. that of the kidney.

caput *pl.* **capita** 1. the head. 2. any structure or part resembling a head; the rounded end of an organ or part.

carbohydrate any of various compounds of oxygen, hydrogen, and carbon, as sugars and starches, that are the principal energy-producing foods in the diet.

carbolic acid a disinfectant and poison derived from coal tar; phenol.

carbolize to mix with or add carbolic acid.

carboluria the presence of carbolic acid in the urine.

carbon dioxide a colorless, heavy gas, CO_2, that is noncombustible, is absorbed from the air by plants, and is formed in the tissues during respiration and expelled by the lungs.

carbon monoxide a colorless, odorless gas, CO, that is formed by incomplete combustion of carbon and is lethal in sustained amounts.

carbon monoxide poisoning poisoning by inhalation of carbon monoxide, marked by dizziness, headache, convulsions, paralysis, coma, and, eventually, death.

carbonuria the presence of carbon compounds, esp. carbon dioxide, in the urine.

carbophilic requiring carbon dioxide for efficient growth.

carbuncle a painful staphylococcal inflammation of the skin and subcutaneous tissue characterized by necrosis of the deeper tissues and multiple openings for the discharge of pus.

carbunculosis the presence of multiple carbuncles.

carcinectomy the surgical removal of a malignant tumor.

carcinogen an agent or substance producing or conducive to cancer. —**carcinogenesis** *n.* —**carcinogenic** *adj.* —**carcinogenicity** *n.*

carcinoma *pl.* **carcinomas** *or* **carcinomata** a malignant tumor of epithelial tissue. —**carcinomatous** *adj.*

carcinomatosis a condition marked by the spreading of carcinomas from a primary source.

carcinosarcoma a mixed malignant growth exhibiting features of both carcinoma and sarcoma.

carcinostatic 1. arresting the growth of a carcinoma. 2. an agent that arrests or inhibits the growth of a carcinoma.

cardi- *or* **cardio-** *prefix* heart; cardiac.

cardiac 1. of, near, or acting on the heart. 2. relating to the part of the stomach into which the esophagus opens.

cardiac arrest *or* **cardiac standstill** sudden stoppage of the heart functions.

cardiac arrhythmia an abnormal heartbeat.

cardiac massage massage of the heart through the chest wall or directly, during surgery, to restore circulation in cardiac arrest or fibrillation.

cardiac murmur heart murmur.

cardiac output the amount of blood pumped by the heart.

cardiac standstill cardiac arrest.

cardialgia a burning sensation in the stomach or seeming to come from the region of the heart, usually caused by indigestion; heartburn.

cardiasthenia a condition in which the action of the heart is weak.

cardiataxia severe abnormalities or irregularities in the heart action.

cardiatelia failure of the heart to develop normally.

cardiectasia dilation of the heart.

cardiectopia abnormal location of the heart within the thoracic cavity.

cardioangiology the branch of science concerned with the heart and blood vessels.

cardioaortic relating to both the heart and aorta.

cardioarterial relating to the heart and the arteries.

cardiocele protrusion of the heart through a space in the diaphragm or other opening, such as a wound.

cardiocentesis a surgical procedure involving puncture of the heart.

cardiodynamics the forces, movements and actions of the beating heart.

cardiodynia pain originating in the heart.

cardiogenesis the embryonic formation of the heart.

cardiogenic originated by the heart; of cardiac origin.

cardiogram a tracing made by a cardiograph.

cardiograph an instrument that traces graphically the electrical events and movements taking place within the heart. **—cardiographer** *n.* **—cardiography** *n.*

cardiohepatomegaly abnormal enlargement of both the heart (cardiomegaly) and the liver (hepatomegaly).

cardioinhibitory slowing down or inhibiting the normal action of the heart.

cardiokinetic influencing the heart action.

cardiology the branch of medicine concerned with the heart and its disorders. **—cardiological** *adj.* **—cardiologist** *n.*

cardiomegaly abnormal enlargement of the heart.

cardiomuscular relating to the heart muscle.

cardiomyopathy a chronic disease of heart muscle.

cardiomyotomy surgical incision into the heart muscle.

cardionecrosis necrosis of part of the heart muscle, as in severe myocardial infarction.

cardiopalmus palpitation of the heart.

cardiopathy any disease of the heart.

cardiopericarditis inflammation of both the heart muscle and its surrounding sac (pericardium).

cardiophobia abnormal fear of heart disease.

cardiophone a specially adapted stethoscope for listening to heart sounds, usually consisting of a microphone and amplifier.

cardiopulmonary of, relating to, or involving the heart and the lungs.

cardiopulmonary resuscitation (CPR) an emergency measure involving artificial respiration and external cardiac massage.

cardiospasm painful spasm of the stomach at its upper (cardiac) part or of the esophagus near the point where it joins the stomach, typically causing regurgitation.

cardiothrombus a blood clot within a heart chamber.

cardiotomy 1. surgical incision into the heart muscle. 2. surgical incision into the upper (cardiac) part of the stomach in the area of the esophageal opening.

cardiotoxic exerting a toxic or harmful effect on the action of the heart or its tissues.

cardiovalvulitis inflammation of the heart valves.

cardiovascular relating to or involving the heart and blood vessels.

cardioversion the delivery of an electrical shock to the heart to restore its normal rhythm.

carditis inflammation of the heart muscles.

caries 1. tooth decay (dental caries). 2. bone decay.

cariogenesis the process or mechanism of producing caries.

cariogenic (of certain dietary constituents, esp. sugar) producing tooth decay; causing caries.

carminative a substance, as oil of peppermint, aiding in the expulsion of gas from the alimentary canal.

carotene a yellow or red pigment occurring in some plants that is convertible to vitamin A.

carotenemia the presence in the blood of unusually large quantities of carotene, sometimes resulting in a yellowish-red pigmentation of the skin resembling jaundice; pseudo-jaundice.

carotenoid 1. any one of a group of plant pigments that includes carotene. 2. resembling carotene; yellowish.

carotid either of two great arteries passing up the neck and supplying the head with blood.

carpal of, relating to, or involving the wrist.

carpoptosia dropping of the wrist; wrist drop.

carpus the eight bones between the hand and the forearm; wrist.

carrier an agent who harbors pathogenic microorganisms transmittable to others while remaining personally immune to the disease.

cartilage translucent elastic tissue which, with bone, comprises the basic structure of the skeleton. —**cartilaginous** *adj.*

caruncle a small fleshy protuberance often of abnormal origin.

cascara sagrada a cathartic drug.

caseation necrosis in which damaged tissue is converted into a cheesy soft substance.

casein a phosphoprotein derived from milk.

cassette a special holder for photographic or X-ray film.

cast a mass of fibrous matter that takes the shape of the organ in which it is formed and is ejected from the body.

castor oil a cathartic drug.

castration removal of the testes or the ovaries. —**castrate** *vb.*

CAT See **computerized axial tomography.**

catabolism a destructive phase of metabolism resulting in the breakdown of complex materials within the organism. —**catabolize** *vb.*

catalepsy a condition marked by suspended animation and a tendency for the limbs to remain in whatever position they are placed.

catalyst an agent or substance that speeds up a chemical reaction without itself taking part of it. —**catalysis** *n.*

catamenia menses. —**catamenial** *adj.*

catamnesis the medical history or follow-up of a patient after treatment of an illness.

cataphasia a speech disorder characterized by involuntary repetition of the same word.

cataphoresis electrophoresis.

cataplasm a poultice.

cataplexy a sudden loss of muscular strength following an emotional crisis.

cataract a clouding of the lens of the eye that obstructs the transmission of light.

catarrh inflammation of the mucous membranes and especially those of the nose and respiratory passages. —**catarrhal** *adj.*

catatonia a schizophrenic condition marked chiefly by stupor and immobility with occasional attacks of hyperactivity and excitability. —**catatonic** *adj.*

catecholamine a natural or synthetic chemical that affects the sympathetic nervous system, as dopamine and epinephrine.

catgut a tough cord made from sheep intestines and used chiefly for absorbable sutures and ligatures.

catharsis 1. purgation. 2. the psychoanalytic resolution of an emotional conflict through verbal release.

cathartic 1. relating to catharsis. 2. an agent used to purge the bowels; purgative.

catheter a tubular instrument for introduction into a body cavity or passage esp. to permit withdrawal of fluids or maintain an opening.

catheterize to introduce a catheter into.

cat scratch fever *also* **cat scratch disease** a mild disease thought to be typically caused by the scratch of a cat and marked by malaise, fever, and swelling of the lymph glands.

cauda a structure or part resembling a tail or having a tapering extremity. —**caudal** *adj.*

cauda equina a bundle of nerve roots that extend downward from the spinal cord.

caudal anesthesia injection of an anesthetic into the lower end of the spinal canal; spinal anesthesia.

caudalis toward the tail; caudal.

caul the inner fetal membrane sometimes covering the head at birth.

caustic a chemical substance, as a strong acid or alkali, that has a corrosive action on other substances.

cauterization the application of a caustic agent to sear or destroy tissue and esp. to stop hemorrhage. —**cauterize** *vb.* —**cautery** *n.*

cavernous relating to or filled with hollow spaces: *cavernous tissue.*

cavitation the development of cavities in bodily tissue or organs esp. as a result of disease.

cavity a popular term for dental caries.

cavum a hole or hollow; cavity.

cecectomy surgical removal of the cecum of the large intestine.

cecitis inflammation of the cecum.

cecocolostomy the surgical formation of an artificial connection between the cecum and colon.

cecoptosis an abnormal downward displacement of the cecum.

cecotomy surgical incision into the cecum.

cecum the blind pouch forming the first part of the large intestine, to which the vermiform appendix is attached.

celiac *also* **coeliac** related to, situated in, or affecting the abdominal cavity.

celiac disease a chronic disease of young children marked by defective digestion and absorption of gluten and by persistent diarrhea.

celialgia abdominal pain; colic.

celiodynia celialgia; colic.

celiopathy the branch of pathology concerned with the study of abdominal diseases.

celiotomy laparotomy.

celitis peritonitis.

cell a microscopic mass of protoplasm containing a nucleus and other elements and constituting the basic reproducible structural unit of living organisms.

cellulitis a spreading inflammation of cellular or connective tissue, resulting from a failure of the body's immune mechanism to contain an originally localized infection.

celluloneuritis inflammation of nerve cells.

cellulose a polysaccharide that constitutes the chief structural part of the cell walls of plants.

celology the branch of surgery concerned with the study and repair of hernias.

celoscopy examination of any body cavity.

Celsius centigrade; relating to or having a thermometric scale divided into 100 degrees, with 0° representing freezing point and 100° representing boiling point. Abbreviated *C*

cementum the hard tissue covering the root of a tooth.

cenesthesia *or* **coenesthesia** awareness of one's existence and, through all stimuli reaching the brain, of one's general condition.

centesis surgical puncture of a body cavity, as for the draining off of contained fluid.

centigrade Celsius. Abbreviated *C*

central nervous system the part of the nervous system consisting of the brain and spinal cord and serving to coordinate the entire nervous system of the body.

centrifuge a machine that uses centrifugal force to separate substances, as the cellular components of blood from plasma, having different densities.

centriole either of a pair of cellular organelles near the nucleus and during mitosis forming the poles of the spindle.

centromere the clear cytoplasm containing a centriole.

centrum the center of any structure or part, as the body of a vertebra.

cephalalgia headache.

cephalic relating to or situated on or near the head.

cephalitis inflammation of the brain; encephalitis.

cephalogenesis the embryonic formation of the head.

cephalomegaly abnormal enlargement of the head.

cephalometry the science of measuring the head.

cephalomyitis inflammation of the muscles of the head and scalp.

cercus *pl.* **cerci** any stiff structure resembling a hair.

cerebellitis inflammation of the cerebellum.

cerebellospinal relating to both the cerebellum and spinal cord.

cerebellum one of the major divisions of the brain, situated underneath the rear part of the cerebrum and controlling muscular coordination and (together with the inner ear) bodily equilibrium. —**cerebellar** *adj.*

cerebral of or relating to the cerebrum.

cerebral accident sudden, severe injury within the cerebrum, esp. the rupture of a blood vessel.

cerebral cortex the topmost layer of gray matter that covers the cerebrum.

cerebral hemisphere either of the two halves into which the brain is divided front to back.

cerebral hemorrhage rupture of and loss of blood from a blood vessel in the brain.

cerebral palsy a disorder resulting from brain damage before or during birth and marked typically by muscular incoordination and speech difficulties.

cerebration mental activity, conscious or subconscious.

cerebrifugal (of efferent nerve fibers or impulses) proceeding away from the cerebrum.

cerebripetal (of afferent nerve fibers or impulses) proceeding toward the cerebrum.

cerebritis a general, nonpurulent inflammation of the cerebrum or brain.

cerebromeningitis inflammation of both the brain and its covering membranes (meninges).

cerebropontile relating to the brain and pons.

cerebrospinal of or relating to the brain and spinal cord.

cerebrospinal fluid a watery, clear fluid surrounding the spinal cord and brain and filling the lateral ventricles of the brain.

cerebrovascular relating to or affecting the cerebrum and the blood vessels that supply it.

cerebrovascular accident hemorrhage or embolism in a blood vessel in the brain.

cerebrum the largest division of the brain, overlying the cerebellum and brain stem (medulla oblongata, midbrain and pons).

cerumen a yellowish waxy substance secreted by the glands of the external ear; earwax.

cervical relating to or affecting the neck or a cervix, esp. of the uterus.

cervical cancer *or* **cervical carcinoma** a common malignant cancer of the uterine cervix which may spread to other parts of the body.

cervical vertebra a segment of the vertebral column, one of the seven at the neck.

cervicitis inflammation of the cervix of the uterus.

cervix the neck-like part of the uterus that protrudes into the vagina.

cesarean *or* **caesarean section** delivery of a baby by surgery, in which the abdomen and uterus are incised.

cestode any of a subclass of flatworms comprising the tapeworms.

Chagas' disease a form of trypanosomiasis, transmitted by bloodsucking insects.

chalk calcium carbonate.

chancre an initial lesion, esp. of the primary stage of syphilis. —**chancrous** *adj.*

chancroid a venereal disease characterized by an initial genital lesion resembling that of the primary stage of syphilis. —**chancroidal** *adj.*

change of life menopause; climacteric.

chapping a rough, red, dried condition of the skin, usually as a result of cold, dry conditions.

charas hashish.

charley horse a severely painful muscle cramp in the leg.

cheilitis inflammation of the lips.

cheilosis a condition of the lips and mouth in which the skin is scaly and fissured, owing to a deficiency of vitamin B_2 (riboflavin).

chem- *or* **chemo-** *or* **chemi-** *prefix* chemical; chemistry; chemically.

chemopallidectomy chemical destruction of part of a structure in the brain (globus pallidus), once widely used in the treatment of parkinsonism and related diseases.

chemoprophylaxis the prevention of disease by the administration of drugs.

chemoreceptor a sensory nerve-ending that receives chemical stimuli. —**chemoreception** *n.* —**chemoreceptive** *adj.*

chemosis a conjunctival edema resulting from any of a number of causes.

chemosurgery the removal of tissue by chemical means, as in the treatment of gangrene and some skin cancers.

chemotherapy the use of chemical agents in controlling or treating disease.

chest thorax.

chiasma a crossing of two tendons, nerves or other structures.

chickenpox an acute, contagious viral disease marked chiefly by low-grade fever and the formation of vesicles and occurring usually in children.

chilblain an inflammatory sore occurring esp. on the hands or feet as the result of exposure to cold.

chilitis *also* **cheilitis** inflammation of the lips.

chilophagia chronic biting of the lips.

chiropodist podiatrist. —**chiropody** *n.*

chiropractic a system of treating disease by manipulation, esp. of the spinal column.

chloasma a temporary, permanent, or recurring brownish discoloration of the skin, esp. of the face, common in pregnancy and as a result of taking oral contraceptives.

chloral hydrate a sedative, hypnotic drug, commonly known as "knock-out drops."

chloramphenicol a broad-spectrum antibiotic.

chloroform a clear, volatile, toxic liquid that has an odor like ether and is used as a solvent and (esp. formerly) as a general anesthetic.

Chloromycetin a trademark for chloramphenicol.

chlorophyll *also* **chlorophyl** the green pigment of plants, preparations of which are used for their ability to soothe and remove odors.

chloropsia a rare visual defect in which everything appears to have a green or yellowish-green hue.

chlorpheniramine maleate a common antihistamine used in many over-the-counter cold remedies.

chlorpromazine an antiemetic and tranquilizer.

chlortetracycline a broad-spectrum antibiotic.

chloruretic relating to the action or effect of increasing the excretion of chloride in the urine.

cholagogue 1. an agent that causes contraction of the gallbladder, thereby stimulating the flow of bile into the duodenum. 2. relating to an agent that stimulates the flow of bile.

cholalic relating to bile.

cholangiography X-ray examination of the bile ducts. —**cholangiographic** *adj.*

cholangiotomy surgical incision into a bile duct.

cholangitis inflammation of a bile duct.

cholecyst a rare name for the gallbladder.

cholecystectomy surgical removal of the gallbladder.

cholecystitis inflammation of the gallbladder.

cholecystostomy surgical formation of an artificial opening into the gallbladder.

cholecystotomy surgical incision into the gallbladder.

cholelithiasis the presence or production of gallstones.

cholemesia the vomiting of bile.

cholemia the abnormal presence of bile salts in the bloodstream.

choleperitonitis inflammation of the peritoneum caused by the presence of bile in the abdominal cavity.

cholera an acute, infectious bacterial disease usually caused by drinking contaminated water and marked by vomiting and severe gastrointestinal disturbance.

choleriform resembling cholera; choleroid.

cholerrhagia the excessive flow of bile into the small intestine.

cholestasia *also* **cholestasis** cessation of the flow of bile.

cholesterol a steroid alcohol found in animal cells and body fluids and implicated as a contributing factor in arteriosclerosis and atherosclerosis.

cholesterolemia the presence in the bloodstream of unusually large amounts of cholesterol.

cholic relating to the bile.

choline an organic base that is a B-complex vitamin vital to liver function.

cholinergic relating to nerve endings that release acetylcholine.

choloplania the abnormal presence of bile salts in the tissues or bloodstream.

cholopoiesis the formation of bile.

cholorrhea excessive secretion of bile into the small intestine.

chondr- *or* **chondri-** *or* **chondro-** *prefix* cartilage.

chondral relating to cartilage.

chondrectomy surgical removal of a piece of cartilage.

chondritis inflammation of cartilage.

chondrodynia pain in cartilage.

chondrogenesis the formation of cartilage.

chondromalacia the abnormal softening of cartilage.

chondromatosis a condition in which there are many tumors in the cartilage.

chondroplasty surgery of the cartilage.

chondrosarcoma a malignant tumor derived from cartilage cells, usually near the extremities of long bones.

chondrotome a strong knife used to cut cartilage.

chondrotomy surgical separation or division of a cartilage.

chondrotrophic influencing the growth and development of cartilage.

chorda a tendon or tendinous structure or part.

chordee painful erection of the penis, often with a downward curvature, usually occurring as a sympton of gonorrhea.

chorditis inflammation of a cord, esp. a vocal cord.

chorea a disease marked by spastic movements of the muscles of the limbs and face and progressive mental deterioration.

chorioangioma a benign tumor of blood vessels, esp. those of the placenta.

chorion the outer embryonic membrane, part of which contributes to the placenta. —**chorionic** *adj*.

chorionitis inflammation of the outermost of the fetal membranes (chorion).

chorioretinitis inflammation of the choroid and retina of the eye.

choroid a vascular membrane between the retina and the sclerotic coat of the eye that contains pigment cells.

choroid plexus a complex of small blood vessels in the brain.

chromatid either of the paired complex strands of a chromosome.

chromatin strands of DNA that form chromosomes.

chromatopsia color blindness.

chromaturia any abnormal discoloration of the urine.

chromesthesia 1. the stimulation of taste, smell, etc., by the perception of color. 2. color sense.

chromhidrosis the secretion of colored sweat.

chromophile *or* **chromophilic** (of certain tissues or cells) easily stained.

chromophobe *also* **chromophobic** (of certain tissues or cells) resistant to stain or incapable of receiving stains.

chromophobia an abnormal aversion to colors.

chromopsia incomplete or partial color blindness.

chromoscopy the procedure of testing for color perception.

chromosome one of the rod-shaped bodies of a cell nucleus containing the genes (each human cell has 46 chromosomes). **—chromosomal** *adj.* **—chromosomic** *adj.*

chromotrichial relating to colored hair.

chronic (of a condition or disease) persisting for a relatively long time, sometimes for a lifetime.

chronic alcoholism a complex of physical and psychological conditions resulting from the habitual, excessive drinking of alcoholic beverages.

chronic lymphocytic leukemia cancer of the white blood cells.

chronognosis time sense; the ability to appreciate the passage of time.

chronotaraxis the inability to appreciate the passage of time; impaired time sense.

chyle a milky fluid found in lymph vessels and formed in the small intestine during the digestion of fats.

chyme a virtually liquid mass of partially digested food and secretions that is formed in the stomach and passes to the small intestine during the process of digestion.

cicatricial of or relating to a cicatrix.

cicatrix a scar remaining from a healed wound.

cilium *pl.* **cilia** a minute protoplasmic thread projecting from the surface of a cell and capable of lashing movements. —**ciliary** *adj.*

cimex *pl.* **cimices** a bedbug.

cinchona the dried bark of a tree (cinchona tree) from which quinine can be obtained, formerly used in the treatment of malaria; Peruvian bark.

cinchonism poisoning by cinchona, quinidine or quinine, characterized by headache, ringing in the ears or loss of hearing, and sometimes a severe allergic reaction.

cineradiography the technique of making moving pictures of images appearing on the screen of a fluoroscope.

circadian involving or based on 24-hour periods or intervals.

circinate (of certain structures or parts) shaped like a ring; circular.

circulation the movement of blood through the vessels resulting from the pumping action of the heart.

circulus a circular or ringlike structure or part.

circumcision the surgical removal of all or part of the foreskin. —**circumcise** *vb.*

cirrhosis disease of the liver marked by fibrosis and hardening.

cirsectomy surgical removal of a varicose vein.

cirsodesis the tying off or ligation of varicose veins.

cirsoid varicose.

cirsotome a surgical instrument for removing varicose veins.

clamp a device designed to constrict a vessel or to provide a secure hold on a structure.

clap (colloquial) gonorrhea.

claudication the condition of being lame; limping.

claustrophobia an abnormal fear of being in narrow orenclosed spaces.

clavicle a bone of the shoulder; collarbone.

cleft palate fissure of the roof of the mouth occurring congenitally.

climacteric 1. menopause. 2. a period in the male corresponding to the menopause in the female and marked by reduced sexual interest and activity.

climatotherapy treatment of a disease or disorder by moving to a different climate, as to a warm and dry climate in treating bronchitis.

clinic 1. medical instruction based on the examination and discussion of patients. 2. a medical facility supplementary to a hospital and specializing in the treatment of outpatients. 3. a group practice of several physicians working cooperatively. —**clinical** *adj.*

clinician a physician, psychiatrist, or psychologist specializing in clinical practice rather than in laboratory or research work.

clitoris a small organ homologous to the penis and located at the upper part of the vulva.

clitorism a rare, painful condition in which the clitoris remains erect for prolonged periods.

clonus a sequence of muscular spasms in which rigidity is followed by relaxation. —**clonic** *adj.*

club foot talipes; a deformed foot twisted out of normal position: a congenital defect.

coagulate to cause to become or to become thickened into a coherent mass; clot; curdle. —**coagulation** *n.*

coarctotomy surgical division of a stricture.

cobalt a hard, gray metallic element related to nickel and iron.

cocaine an alkaloid from coca leaves that is used as a local anesthetic and can become addictive.

coccus *pl.* **cocci** a spherical bacterium.

coccygeal of or relating to the coccyx.

coccygectomy surgical removal of the coccyx.

coccygodynia pain in the coccyx.

coccyx the terminal bone of the spinal column formed by the fusion of four rudimentary vertebrae.

cochlea the spiral cavity of the internal ear that is the seat of the hearing organ. —**cochlear** *adj.*

coconsciousness two streams of consciousness existing simultaneously.

codeine a morphine derivative that is found in opium and is used as an analgesic and in cough suppressant remedies.

coil a type of intrauterine device.

coition sexual intercourse.

coitus sexual intercourse.

cold *or* **common cold** an infection of the upper respiratory tract, caused by a virus.

colectasia distention of the colon.

colectomy surgical removal of a section of the colon or (rarely) its complete removal.

coleocele a vaginal hernia.

colic severe abdominal pains resulting from spasms of a hollow organ and chiefly affecting infants. —**colicky** *adj.*

colitis inflammation of the colon.

collagen an insoluble fibrous protein forming the major part of intercellular connective tissue.

collapse a state of acute prostration and physical depression.

collarbone clavicle.

colliculus any small anatomical elevation.

collodion a liquid that forms a protective film when applied and is used as a surgical dressing.

colloid a mucinous or gelatinous substance found in the thyroid and in certain other tissues. —**colloidal** *adj.*

collyrium a fluid for cleansing the eyes; eyewash.

colon the part of the large intestine between the cecum and the rectum. —**colonic** *adj.*

coloproctitis inflammation of both the colon and rectum.

color blindness inability to perceive or distinguish one or more colors. —**color-blind** *adj.*

colostomy surgical formation of an artificial anus.

colostrum milk, rich in protein and antibodies, secreted from the breasts directly after parturition.

colotomy surgical incision into the colon.

colpalgia vaginal pain.

coma a state of profound unconsciousness, as from injury, poison, or disease. —**comatose** *adj.*

combat fatigue a usually temporary mental disorder resulting from exhaustion, stress, and other causes brought about by combat.

comedo *pl.* **comedones** a small plug of sebum blocking a sebaceous gland esp. on the face, chest, or back; blackhead.

comminuted (of a fractured bone) broken into several small fragments.

common cold cold.

commotio cerebri brain concussion.

communicable (of a disease) contagious.

compensation correction of an organic defect or loss by inceased functioning of another organ or part.

complement the substance in normal blood serum and plasma that combines with antibodies to combat bacteria and other antigens.

complex a group of repressed desires and memories that exert a powerful influence on a personality.

complex fracture a bone fracture in which the surrounding tissue is badly damaged.

complication a secondary disorder or disease developing in consequence of a primary disease or injury.

compos mentis of sound mind, understanding, and memory.

compound a substance formed by the chemical union of two or more elements in strict proportion by weight.

compound fracture open fracture.

compress a folded pad or cloth, as of gauze, for applying local pressure to a bodily part.

computerized axial tomography *or* **CAT** a procedure in which a computer-driven x-ray scan is taken of the tissues of the brain.

conceive to become pregnant.

conception the act of becoming pregnant; the impregnation of an ovum.

concha *pl.* **conchae** 1. the largest and deepest cavity of the outer ear. 2. one of three thin bones in the nasal cavity.

concretion a hardened mass; calculus.

concussion a jarring injury to the brain that temporarily or permanently impairs its normal functioning.

condition a state of the body or mind at a particular time.

condom a thin rubber sheath worn over the penis to prevent conception or venereal disease during sexual intercourse.

condyle a rounded prominence at the end of a bone.

condyloma a warty growth in the area of the anus and genitals.

cone a cell in the retina that enables color distinction.

confabulation the invention of events esp. to compensate for episodes of memory loss, as in chronic alcoholism.

confinement the state of preparing for childbirth; lying-in.

congenital existing at the time of birth: *congenital deformity.*

congestion an abnormal accumulation of blood in a bodily part.

conjunctiva *pl.* **conjunctivas** *or* **conjunctivae** the mucous membrane lining the inside of the eyelid and the forepart of the eyeball.

conjunctivitis inflammation of the conjunctiva.

connective tissue tissue that supports and binds together other tissues and forms ligaments and tendons.

consolidation an alteration in lung tissue in pneumonia in which air spaces become filled with exudate.

constipation abnormally delayed or difficult passage of feces.

consumption tuberculosis. —**consumptive** *adj.*

contact a person who has been exposed to or transmits an infectious disease.

contact dermatitis a skin condition caused by direct exposure to an irritating medium.

contact lens a thin lens fitted over the cornea of the eye.

contagion the transmission of a disease by contact.

contagious communicable by direct or indirect contact; catching: *contagious disease.*

contraception the voluntary prevention of impregnation or conception.

contraceptive 1. relating to or used for contraception. 2. a contraceptive device or agent.

contraction a tightening of the muscles in the upper part of the uterus during childbirth.

contraindication a caution against the advisability of using a particular medication or medical treatment. —**contraindicate** *vb.* —**contraindicative** *adj.*

contusion bruise. —**contuse** *vb.*

convalesce to regain one's health at a gradual pace. —**convalescence** *n.*

convolution any of the irregular ridges on the surface of the brain; gyrus.

convulsion an abnormal, violent muscular contraction or series of contractions. —**convulse** *vb.* —**convulsive** *adj.*

coprolalia a rare condition in which obscene or vulgar words are uttered involuntarily.

copulation sexual intercourse.

cordate heart-shaped.

cordectomy surgical removal of a cord.

corditis inflammation of the spermatic cord.

corium the layer of skin under the epidermis.

corn a localized hardening and thickening of the skin, as on a toe, from pressure or friction.

cornea the transparent part of the eyeball coat that covers the pupil and iris and admits light.

coronary bypass surgery in which a blockage in a coronary artery is bypassed by connecting a blood vessel directly between the end of the artery and the ascending aorta.

coronary occlusion a blockage in a coronary artery.

coronary vessel any of the arteries and veins that carry the blood supply of the heart muscle.

corpulence *also* **corpulency** the state of being extremely fat. —**corpulent** *adj.*

corpuscle a cell, esp. a red or white blood cell.

corpus luteum a spherical growth on the surface of the ovary, forming after every ovulation and secreting hormones.

cortex the outer layer of an organ or bodily structure. —**cortical** *adj.*

corticipetal (of nerve fibers) conveying nerve impulses toward the cerebral cortex.

corticosteroid a hormone of the adrenal cortex that controls important bodily processes.

corticothalamic relating to nerve fibers that connect the cerebral cortex with specific areas of the thalamus.

coryza an upper respiratory infection, esp. the common cold.

costal of or relating to the ribs.

costive affected with or causing constipation; constipated. —**costiveness** *n.*

costotome a surgical instrument for cutting through a rib.

costotomy surgical division of a rib.

cotyledon a nodule of the placenta.

counterdepressant 1. relating to the action of any drug or agent that prevents or inhibits the potential depressant action of another drug. 2. a drug or agent with this effect.

counterirritant an agent producing localized, superficial inflammation in order to reduce inflammation in adjacent, deeper structures or tissues. —**counterirritation** *n.*

courses menses.

couvercle a blood clot that forms outside of a vessel.

Cowper's gland either of two small glands that discharge into the male urethra.

cowpox a mild infection, transmitted by infected cattle, that usually makes one immune to smallpox.

coxa the hip joint.

coxalgia pain or inflammation involving the hip joint.

coxotomy surgical incision into the hip joint.

Coxsackie virus any of various viruses associated with human diseases.

c.p. *abbr.* chemically pure.

c.p.s. *abbr.* cycles per second; counts per second.

crab louse a louse that infests the pubic region of humans.

crabs infestation with crab lice.

cradle cap dermatitis of the scalp, common in infants.

cramp 1. a painful, spasmodic contraction of a muscle. 2. usually **cramps,** sharp abdominal pain.

crani- *or* **cranio-** *prefix* skull; cranial.

cranial of or relating to the skull.

cranial index the ratio of the maximum breadth of the skull to its maximum height, multiplied by 100.

cranialis toward the head; cranial; superior (in humans); anterior (in quadrupeds).

cranial nerve any of the twelve pairs of nerves arising from the brain to the periphery of the body.

craniectomy surgical removal of a piece of the skull, as in preparation for a brain operation.

craniology a science dealing with the variations in size and shape of the skulls of different races.

craniomalacia abnormal softening of the bones of the skull.

craniomeningocele the protrusion of the covering membranes of the brain (meninges) through a defect in the bones of the skull.

craniometry a science dealing with the measurement of skulls.

craniopathy any disease or disorder of the skull.

cranioplasty surgical repair of a skull defect or deformity.

craniopuncture surgical puncture of the skull.

craniosclerosis an abnormal thickening of the bones of the skull.

craniotomy surgery involving cutting through the skull.

cranium the skull, esp. the part enclosing the brain.

crapulent *also* **crapulous** drunk; intoxicated with alcohol.

crater the depressed central portion of something, such as the recessed portion of an ulcer.

crateriform having a depressed center; hollowed.

c.r.d. *abbr.* chronic respiratory disease.

creatine a nitrogenous, energy-storing substance found in muscles.

crena a cleft or notch.

crena ani the cleft between the buttocks.

crenate *also* **crenated** indented or notched.

crepitant (of a sound heard from the lungs in pneumonia or certain other pulmonary diseases) crackling.

crepitation *also* **crepitus** 1. the fine grating sound heard when two ends of a broken bone rub together. 2. the crackling chest sound heard in pneumonia and other lung infections.

crest a bony ridge or prominence.

cretinism a congenital, abnormal condition caused by thyroid deficiency and marked by mental retardation and small stature. —**cretin** *n.* —**cretinous** *adj.*

cribriform pierced with small holes.

crisis the turning point in a disease or fever after which the patient either improves or declines rapidly.

Crohn's disease chronic, painful inflammation of the small intestine, colon, or both.

croup inflammation of the larynx, esp. in infants, marked by periods of difficult breathing and hoarse cough. —**croupous** *adj.* —**croupy** *adj.*

crural relating to the thigh; femoral.

cry- *or* **cryo-** *prefix* cold; freezing.

cryalgesia pain caused by exposure to cold.

cryanesthesia the inability to sense or perceive cold.

cryesthesia the sensation of cold or the state of being especially sensitive to low temperatures.

cryohypophysectomy the surgical destruction of all or part of the pituitary gland (hypophysis cerebri) by cold.

cryosurgery surgical removal of diseased tissue by freezing.

cryotherapy the therapeutic use of cold, as that produced by liquid nitrogen.

crystalline lens the lens of the eye.

crystalluria the presence of crystals in the urine.

cuneiform wedge-shaped: *cuneiform bone.*

cunnilingus *or* **cunnilinctus** oral stimulation of the vulva and clitoris. —**cunnilingual** *adj.*

cupula a cuplike or dome-shaped structure or part.

curare an extract of a vine used by South American Indians as an arrow poison and in medicine (in very small amounts) as a muscle relaxant.

curettage surgical cleaning or scraping using a curette.

curette *or* **curet** a surgical loop or scoop used in performing curettage. —**curette** *or* **curet** *vb.*

curie a unit of radioactive quantity.

cutaneous relating to or affecting the skin.

cuticle 1. the horny outer layer of the skin, esp. at the margins of the nail beds. 2. epidermis.

cyanocobalamin vitamin B_{12}.

cyanosis a bluish discoloration of the skin resulting from inadequate oxygenation of the blood.

cyclamate an artificially prepared sodium or calcium salt used as a sweetener.

cyst a fluid-filled, membranous sac developing abnormally in a bodily cavity or structure.

cystic fibrosis a hereditary disease of infants, children, and young adults that is attributable to dysfunction of the exocrine glands and is marked by pancreatic deficiency, respiratory problems, and loss of salt in the sweat.

cystine an amino acid that is a metabolic source of sulfur.

cystitis inflammation of the urinary bladder.

cystolith a calculus in the urinary bladder.

cystoscope an instrument for visual examination of the bladder and the introduction of exploratory instruments.

cyt- *or* **cyto-** *prefix* 1. cell: *cytology*. 2. cytoplasm.

cytochrome any of several iron-containing proteins that play an important role in cell oxidations.

cytogenetics the branch of biology dealing with the study of heredity (genetics) in relation to that of cells (cytology).

cytology the biological study of the structure, function, and life history of cells.

cytolysis the disintegration of cells.

cytomegalovirus any of a number of herpesviruses that cause serious diseases.

cytoplasm the protoplasm of a cell excluding the nucleus.

cytotoxin a substance having a toxic effect on cells. —**cytotoxic** *adj.* —**cytotoxicity** *n.*

cytotropic attracted to cells.

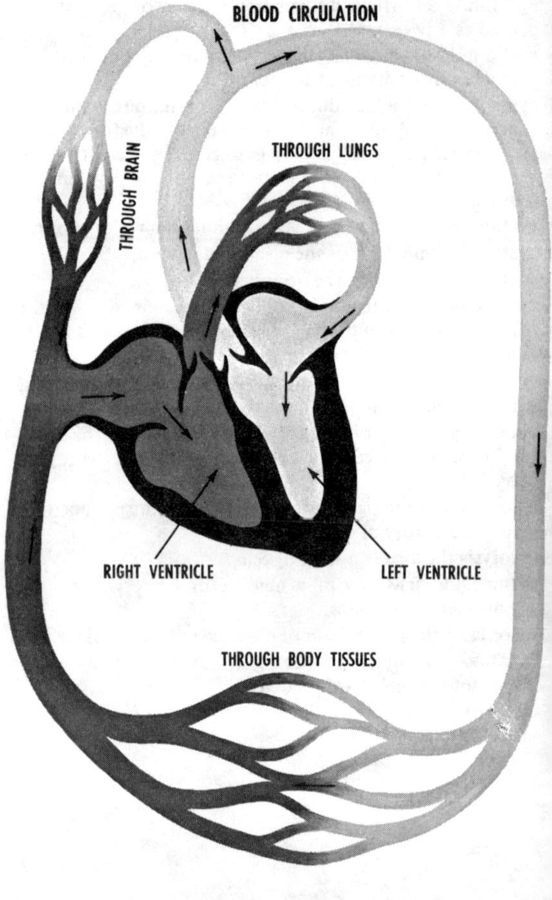
BLOOD CIRCULATION
THROUGH BRAIN
THROUGH LUNGS
RIGHT VENTRICLE
LEFT VENTRICLE
THROUGH BODY TISSUES

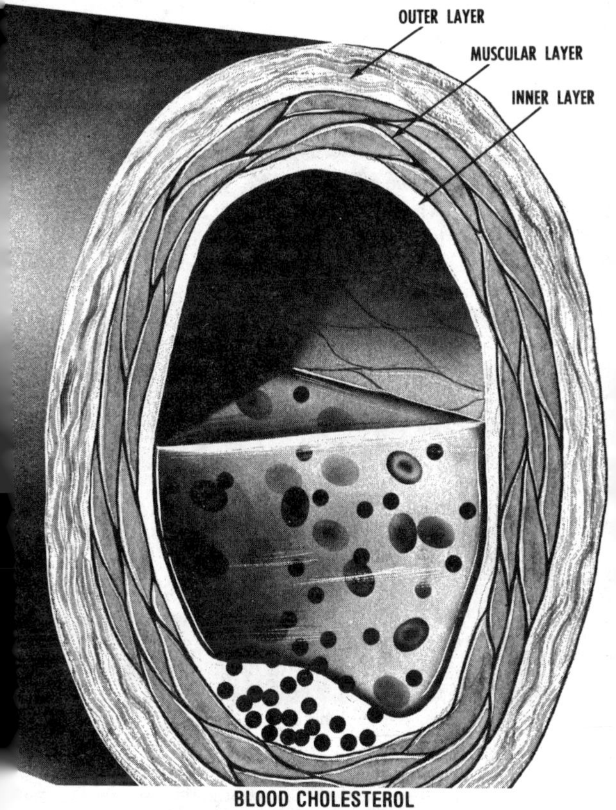

BLOOD CHOLESTEROL

This is a cross section of a blood vessel showing the cholesterol (fat) particles invading the inner wall. A hard yellowish plaque forms which may eventually impede the blood flow.

D

D&C See **dilatation and curettage.**

dacryocystitis inflammation of the tear sac.

dacryocystotome a small knife for making incisions in the tear sac.

dacryolith a calculus in the tear duct.

dacryops the chronic presence of an accumulation of tears in the eye.

dacryopyorrhea the discharge of pus from the tear duct.

dacryopyosis the formation of pus in the tear sac or duct.

dacryorrhea the excessive flow of tears.

dactyl a finger or toe.

dactylalgia pain in a finger or toe.

dactyledema edema of the finger.

dactylology the science or practice of using the finger alphabet in communicating.

dactylomegaly abnormal enlargement of one or more fingers.

daltonism color blindness, esp. involving the color red.

dandruff small whitish flakes of desquamated cells forming chiefly on the scalp; scurf.

Darvon trade name for the painkiller propoxyphene hydrochloride.

Darwinism a theory of the origin and evolution of new species of animals and plants stressing that natural selection favors the survival of some offspring over others; biological evolution.

DDT *abbr.* dichlorodiphenyltrichloroethane: a very powerful insecticide which can be poisonous if ingested with DDT-sprayed food that has not been properly washed.

deaf-mute a person who can neither hear nor speak.

deallergize desensitize.

deaminate to remove the amino group from (a compound). **—deamination** *n.*

deaquation dehydration.

death *Law.* the cessation of any and all activity of the central nervous, cardiovascular, and respiratory systems as stated by a qualified medical doctor.

debilitate to impair the strength of; enfeeble. **—debilitation** *n.*

debility loss of strength; feebleness; weakness.

debridement the surgical removal and cleansing of damaged or contaminated tissue.

decaffeinate to remove the caffeine from.

decalcify to remove calcium or calcium compounds from. **—decalcification** *n.*

decalvant making bald; removing the hair.

decapitate to sever the head of; behead. **—decapitation** *n.* **—decapitator** *n.*

decerebrate 1. having the cerebrum removed or rendered inactive. 2. to remove the cerebrum of or make incapable of cerebral activity.

decerebrize to remove the brain of.

dechloridation removal of salt (sodium chloride) from the body fluids and tissues by restricting the dietary intake of salt.

decidua *pl.* **deciduae** the mucous membrane lining the uterus that thickens and becomes modified in preparation for pregnancy and is cast off during parturition and menstruation. **—decidual** *adj.*

deciduitis inflammation of the decidua.

deciduoma a tumor of the uterus believed to arise from decidual tissue left behind following a miscarriage or abortion.

deciduous falling off or out at a certain stage in the life cycle: *deciduous teeth.*

deciliter one tenth of a liter.

decimeter one tenth of a meter.

decinormal (denoting the strength of a solution) one tenth that of normal or standard values.

decipara a woman who has given birth to ten children.

declinator a surgical instrument for retracting certain parts out of the immediate operative field.

decompensation failure of compensation, esp. inability of the heart to maintain adequate circulation.

decompose to undergo breakdown by hydrolytic enzymes; rot; putrify. **—decomposability** *n.* **—decomposable** *adj.* **—decomposition** *n.*

decompression the relieving of pressure or compression, esp. surgery to release internal bodily pressure. **—decompression** *n.*

decompression sickness caisson disease.

decongestant a drug or agent that relieves congested blood vessels, esp. those of the mucous membrane of the nose.

decorticate to remove the outer covering or cortex from (an organ). **—decortication** *n.* **—decorticator** *n.*

decrudescence the lessening or easing of the symptoms of a disease or illness.

decubitus ulcer an ulcer formed by constant pressure on the skin over a bony prominence while lying in bed; bedsore; pressure sore.

decussate to intersect; cross, as nerve fibers. **—decussation** *n.*

defecation the discharge of feces from the bowels. **—defecate** *vb.*

defemination the loss of secondary sexual characteristics or femininity, esp. as the result of a hormonal disorder.

deferens a duct that conveys spermatozoa from each testicle; vas deferens; ductus deferens.

deferent downward; away from; carrying away.

deferentectomy vasectomy.

deferential relating to the vas deferens or ductus deferens.

deferentitis inflammation of the vas deferens.

defervescence the falling or lessening of a fever or the period during which this occurs.

defibrillate to restore the normal rhythm of (a fibrillating heart) with electrical shocks. —**defibrillation** *n.* —**defibrillator** *n.* —**defibrillatory** *adj.*

deficiency disease a disease, as rickets, beriberi, scurvy, resulting from a dietary deficiency, as of an essential vitamin or mineral.

deflorescence the disappearance of a skin eruption or the period during which a skin rash begins to abate.

defluxio sudden loss of hair.

deformity any abnormal shape or proportion of the body resulting from injury, disease, or birth defect.

deganglionate to deprive of ganglia.

degeneration progressive deterioration in the structure or function of organs or tissues. —**degenerate** *vb.*

deglutition the act or process of swallowing.

degustation the sense of taste; tasting.

dehiscence the bursting open of the edges of a wound, esp. after they have been sutured or sewn together.

dehydration loss of water; an abnormal depletion of body fluids. —**dehydrate** *vb.* —**dehydrator** *n.*

déjà vu the illusion of remembering events and scenes actually being experienced for the first time; paramnesia.

deleterious harmful; injurious.

deliquesce (of certain salts) to become liquid or damp as the result of atmospheric water absorption. **—deliquescence** *n.*

delirifacient 1. causing delirium. 2. a toxic agent capable of causing delirium.

delirium a mental condition characterized by hallucinations, disordered speech, and extreme confusion.

delirium tremens a violent psychotic delirium with tremors and hallucinations that is induced by prolonged and excessive use of alcohol. Also called *D.T.'s.*

delivery parturition; childbirth.

delomorphous of definite shape and form.

deltoid a large triangular muscle covering the shoulder joint and serving to raise and lower the arm laterally.

delusion a false conviction about the self, other persons, or the environment that persists despite the demonstrable facts. **—delusional** *adj.*

dementia a condition of impaired or deteriorated mentality; insanity; madness.

dementia praecox an obsolete term for schizophrenia.

Demerol trade name for the narcotic painkiller meperidine.

demilune a small body shaped like a crescent or half-moon, such as certain cells.

demineralization a loss or progressive diminution of mineral constituents, esp. of calcium from bone.

demorphinization 1. the process or technique of removing morphine from an opiate drug. 2. a method of curing morphine addiction by the gradual withdrawal of the drug.

demulcent a substance capable of soothing or protecting an irritated mucous membrane.

demyelination loss or destruction of the fatty insulating sheath (myelin) that surrounds most nerve fibers.

denarcotize to deprive an opitate drug of its narcotic properties; to remove narcotic properties from.

denature 1. to alter the structure of a protein molecule by physical or chemical action. 2. to make (alcohol) unfit for drinking without otherwise impairing its usefulness. —**denaturation** *n.*

dendriform branching out; tree-shaped.

dendrite any of the branching processes of a nerve cell that conveys impulses toward the cell body. —**dendritic** *adj.*

dendroid branching; like a tree.

dendron dendrite.

denematize deworm; free from infestation with nematodes.

denervate to deprive of a nerve supply. —**denervation** *n.*

dengue an acute viral disease chiefly of the tropics characterized by fever, headache, joint pains, and rash.

denitrify to remove nitrogen from. —**denitrification** *n.*

dens 1. a tooth. 2. a toothlike structure or part.

densimeter an instrument for measuring the density of a liquid.

dental of, relating to, affecting, or used for the teeth.

dentalgia toothache.

dentate notched; having teeth or cogs.

dentes teeth.

denticle 1. a small toothlike projection from a surface. 2. a small tooth.

denticulate notched; having fine teeth; serrated.

dentiform shaped like a tooth.

dentifrice any preparation used to clean the teeth, including toothpaste, tooth powder and special washes.

dentigerous having or containing teeth.

dentilabial relating to both the teeth and lips.

dentilingual relating to both the teeth and tongue.

dentinalgia pain or tenderness of the dentine.

dentine *or* **dentin** the calcareous substance that forms the body of a tooth.

dentiparous bearing teeth.

dentition 1. the development and cutting of teeth. 2. the form and arrangement of the teeth in the mouth.

dentoalveolar relating to the bony sockets surrounding the teeth.

dentulous containing teeth.

denture a partial or complete set of false teeth.

denucleated deprived of a nucleus.

deodorant a preparation that ameliorates or disguises unpleasant odors.

deodorize to eliminate or mask the unpleasant odor of.

deossification the removal of minerals from bone.

deoxidize to remove the oxygen from. —**deoxidation** *n.*

deoxyribonucleic acid a nucleic acid localized chiefly in cell nuclei that is the hereditary material of many organisms; DNA.

depigmentation partial or total loss of pigment or color.

depilate to remove hair. —**depilation** *n.*

depilatory 1. an agent for removing body hair. 2. able to remove hair.

deplumation loss or falling out of the eyelashes as the result of disease.

deprecusis loss of the ability to hear external sounds while eating, as the result of otosclerosis.

depressant an agent that reduces functional bodily activity esp. by inducing muscular relaxation.

depressed marked by or suffering from depression.

depression a condition marked by pessimism, inactivity, dejection, lack of concentration, and often insomnia.

depressomotor 1. inhibiting motor activity. 2. an agent that inhibits or slows motor activity.

depuration purification; removal of waste products.

deradenitis inflammation of the lymph nodes in the neck; cervical adenitis.

derma dermis.

dermabrasion a method for removing scars, tattoos, and other skin blemishes by means of a wire brush or sandpaper under local anesthetic.

dermatalgia pain restricted to the skin.

dermatitis any of various forms of inflammation of the skin.

dermatochalasis loose skin.

dermatoconiosis inflammation of the skin caused by the irritant effects of dust, usually affecting those who work in certain environments where an unusual amount of dust is generated.

dermatodynia pain restricted to the skin; dermatalgia.

dermatoid resembling skin.

dermatology a branch of medicine dealing with the structure, functions, and diseases of the skin. **—dermatologic, dermatological** *adj.* **—dermatologist** *n.*

dermatolysis a congenital defect in which the skin is abnormally loose.

dermatoma an overgrowth or thickening of the skin in a circumscribed area.

dermatome an instrument for removing very thin sections of skin, as in skin grafting.

dermatomegaly a congenital defect in which the skin hangs in heavy folds.

dermatoneurosis any skin eruption caused by emotional stimuli.

dermatopathology the microscopic study of skin lesions.

dermatopathy any disease or disorder of the skin.

dermatophobia an abnormal fear of skin diseases.

dermatophyte a fungus that is parasitic on the skin, hair, or nails. —**dermatophytic** *adj.*

dermatoplasty surgical repair of skin defects; skin grafting.

dermatosis any disease of the skin.

dermatozoon any skin parasite of the animal kingdom.

dermatozoonosis any skin eruption caused by an animal parasite.

dermatrophia *also* **dermatrophy** an abnormal wasting away or thinning of the skin.

dermis the inner mesodermic layer of the skin.

dermitis dermatitis; inflammation of the skin.

dermoid *or* **dermoidal** resembling or made up of skin.

dermoidectomy the surgical removal of a cyst on the skin.

dermology dermatology.

dermotropic attracted to or entering through the skin.

descending aorta the chief part of the aorta that supplies blood to the ribs, stomach, and other parts.

desensitize to render (a hypersensitive individual) insensitive to an aggravating agent. —**densensitization** *n.*

desiccant an agent that absorbs or dries, such as one placed in a bottle of tablets to prevent them from deteriorating in environmental moisture.

desiccate to dry up. —**desiccation** *n.* —**desiccative** *adj.*

desmitis inflammation of a ligament.

desmoenzymes enzymes that exist within cells; intracellular enzymes.

desmology the branch of anatomy concerned with the ligaments.

desmopathy any disease or disorder of the ligaments.

desmotomy the surgical separation of a ligament.

desquamate to peel off in scales. —**desquamation** *n.*

detoxicate detoxify.

detoxify to remove a poison or toxin or the effects of a poison or toxin from. —**detoxification** *n.*

deuteranopia color blindness limited to the inability to perceive green hues.

deviated septum a congenital or acquired (as by injury) deflection of the cartilaginous separation between the nostrils.

Dexedrine trade name for the stimulant for the central nervous system dextroamphetamine sulfate.

dexter relating to or located on the right.

dextroamphetamine amphetamine.

dextromethorphan hydrobromide a cough-suppressing drug.

dextrose a glucose used esp. as an intravenously supplied nutrient replenisher.

dhobie itch a fungal skin infection.

diabetes any of various diseases marked esp. by excessive excretion of urine; (commonly) short for diabetes mellitus.

diabetes insipidus a metabolic disorder of the pituitary gland marked by intense thirst and the passage of large quantities of urine.

diabetes mellitus a metabolic disorder marked by insufficient secretion or utilization of insulin, polyuria, large amounts of sugar in the urine and blood, and by weight loss, thirst, and hunger.

diabetic 1. of, relating to, or affected with diabetes. 2. a person suffering from diabetes.

diabetic coma a serious condition in diabetics, resulting from failure to take insulin as prescribed or from an experience that increases the need for insulin which is inadequate in supply.

diacid an acid with two acid hydrogen atoms. —**diacid** *or* **diacidic** *adj.*

diagnosis the skill or act of identifying a disease from its symptoms and signs. —**diagnose** *vb.*

diagnostic of or relating to diagnosis.

diagnostics the branch of medicine dealing with the diagnosis of disease. —**diagnostician** *n.*

dialysis *pl.* **dialyses** the separation of substances in solution by means of their unequal diffusion through a semipermeable membrane.

dialyze to undergo dialysis. —**dialyzability** *n.* —**dialyzable** *adj.* —**dialyzer** *n.*

diapedesis the passage of blood or blood cells through vessel walls into the tissues. —**diapedetic** *adj.*

diaper rash a skin irritation caused by moisture and heat and especially by the continued wearing of soiled diapers.

diaphanometer an instrument for measuring the relative transparency of fluids.

diaphoresis perspiration, esp. when profuse.

diaphoretic an agent that promotes diaphoresis.

diaphragm 1. the muscular partition separating the chest from the abdomen. 2. a circular cap usually of thin flexible rubber fitted over the cervix of the uterus as a barrier to conception.

diaphragmatic hernia a hernia in which part of the stomach protrudes through an opening in the diaphragm.

diaphysectomy surgical removal of part of the shaft of a long bone.

diaphysis the shaft of a long bone.

diapiresis diapedesis.

diapyesis the formation of pus; suppuration.

diapyetic 1. relating to or causing suppuration. 2. anything that causes the production of pus.

diarrhea *also* **diarrhoea** frequent loose emptying of the bowels.

diarthric relating to two joints.

diarthrosis a joint that permits free movement, such as a ball-and-socket joint.

diastase an enzyme in plant cells and in digestive juice which acts in the conversion of starch into sugar.

diastasis *pl.* **diastases** 1. the rest period of the cardiac cycle occurring before systole. 2. separation of the epiphysis from the shaft of a long bone, as through injury.

diastole the dilation of the heart cavities during which they become filled with blood. —**diastolic** *adj.*

diathermy the therapeutic generation of heat in tissues by means of electric currents. —**diathermic** *adj.*

diathesis a constitutional predisposition toward a particular disease or abnormality.

diatomic having two atoms in the molecule.

diazepam a tranquilizer drug.

dibromide a bromide (such as calcium bromide) that contains two bromine atoms in each molecule.

dichromasia a form of color blindness in which only two of the three primary colors are perceived, those usually perceived being red and blue or blue and green.

dichromat a person affected with dichromasia.

Dick test a test for susceptibility or immunity to scarlet fever by injection of scarlet fever toxin.

dicrotic of or relating to a pulse that beats twice for each single beat of the heart. —**dicrotism** *n.*

dicumarol an anticoagulant drug used in circulatory disorders.

didelphic relating to or having a double uterus.

didymalgia pain in the testicles; orchialgia.

didymitis inflammation of the testicles; orchitis.

diencephalon the part of the brain that includes the thalamus, hypothalamus and related structures; between-brain.

dietetics the science of applying the principles of nutrition to balanced feeding.

diethylstilbestrol a synthetic preparation that is more powerful than natural estrogens, used to treat estrogen deficiencies and menopausal problems; stilbestrol.

dietician *or* **dietitian** a specialist in dietetics.

digest to convert (food) into absorbable form. —**digestibility** *n.* —**digestible** *adj.* —**digestion** *n.*

digestant 1. relating to or stimulating digestion. 2. something that aids or promotes digestion.

digestive 1. relating to or promoting digestion. 2. an agent that aids in or stimulates digestion.

digit a finger or toe. —**digital** *adj.*

digitalis the dried leaf of the common foxglove that when ground to powder acts as a powerful cardiac stimulant.

diiodide a compound that has two atoms of iodine in each molecule.

dilatation the condition of being stretched or expanded beyond normal dimensions: *dilatation of the abdomen.*

dilatation and curettage *or* **D&C** dilatation of the cervix of the uterus and curettage, or scraping, of the endometrium.

dilate to enlarge or widen in extent or degree. —**dilation** *n.*

dilator an instrument for enlarging a bodily opening, as the anus or urethra.

dilute to make thinner, more fluid, or less potent by addition of another substance. —**dilute** *adj.* —**dilution** *n.*

diopter *also* **dioptre** a unit of measurement of the refractive power of the lens.

dioptometer an instrument for measuring the refractive power of the eyes. —**dioptometry** *n.*

dioptroscopy the use of an ophthalmoscope to determine the degree of refraction.

diose the most simple sugar; glycolaldehyde.

diovulatory releasing two ova during one menstrual cycle.

dioxide an oxide containing two atoms of oxygen in the molecule.

diphtheria an acute infectious bacterial disease characterized by the formation of a false membrane in the throat or larynx.

diplacusis the hearing of two sounds from a single source due to a difference in perception by the two ears, either in pitch or time.

diplegia paralysis affecting both sides of the body in like areas. —**diplegic** *adj.*

diplococcus any of a genus of often pathogenic bacteria occurring chiefly in pairs.

diploë osseous tissue between the two layers of the skull. —**diploic** *adj.* —**diploetic** *adj.*

diploid having the basic (haploid) chromosome number doubled.

diplomyelia the abnormal presence of a longitudinal fissure in the spinal cord which divides it into distinct halves.

diplopia double vision.

dipsogen any agent that stimulates thirst.

dipsomania an uncontrollable craving for alcohol; alcoholism. —**dipsomaniac** *n.* —**dipsomaniacal** *adj.*

disaccharide a sugar that yields two monosaccharide molecules.

disarticulation the condition of being disjointed.

disc disk.

discharge the release of something contained, as of pus from a boil.

dischronation a disturbance in the ability to recognize the passage of time; loss of time sense.

discography X-ray of an intervertebral disk.

discoid resembling or shaped like a disk.

discopathy any disease involving an intervertebral disk.

disease a condition that impairs some function of the body or one of its parts. —**diseased** *adj.*

disinfectant an agent, as a chemical, that destroys certain harmful microorganisms: usually for external use only. —**disinfect** *vb.*

disk *or* **disc** any of various flattened and rounded anatomical structures, as one of the fibro-cartilaginous, articulating plates between vertebrae of the spinal column.

dislocation the displacement of a bone from its normal position in relation to another bone. —**dislocate** *vb.*

disorientation loss of a sense of time, identity, or place.

dispensary a place, as an outpatient clinic, providing medical and dental aid.

dispense to prepare and distribute (medication).

dispermy the penetration of an ovum by two sperm cells.

dissect to cut apart or open for scientific examination. —**dissection** *n.*

distal remote from the point of attachment or origin.

distemper any of certain specific infectious diseases of dogs, cats and horses, caused by infection with a virus (dogs and cats) or bacteria (horses).

districhiasis the growth of two hairs from a single hair follicle.

distrix the splitting of the ends of hairs.

disulfiram a drug, given to alcoholics, that causes severe cramps and nausea if alcohol is drunk.

diuresis an increased secretion of urine.

diuretic 1. relating to or tending to increase the flow of urine. 2. a drug or agent that increases the urinary output.

diurnal daily.

diverticulitis inflammation of a diverticulum.

diverticulosis an intestinal disorder marked by the presence of many diverticula.

diverticulum *pl.* **diverticula** a pouch or sac protruding abnormally from a hollow organ, as the bladder or intestine.

divulsion 1. the forcible dilation of the walls of a bodily cavity or passage. 2. the crude removal of a part by tearing or ripping it out.

divulsor an instrument used to force apart the walls of a bodily cavity or passage such as the urethra.

dizygotic *also* **dizygous** fraternal: *dizygotic twins.*

DNA deoxyribonucleic acid.

dolichocephalic having an unusually long head. —**dolichocephaly** *n.*

dolor pain, one of the signs of inflammation.

dolorific producing or causing pain.

dominant relating to or exerting genetic dominance.

donor a person used as the source of biological material, as for an organ transplant or blood transfusion.

dopa dihydroxyphenylalanine; an amino acid used in treating Parkinson's disease.

doraphobia an abnormal fear of petting animals or of touching their fur or skin.

dorsabdominal relating to both the back and the abdomen.

dorsad toward the back or posterior.

dorsal relating to or located near, on, or at the back.

dorsalgia pain in the back.

dorsiflexion an upward turning of the toes or foot.

dosage 1. the administration of drugs or other therapeutic agents in prescribed amounts. 2. the determination of the correct quantity of a drug to be administered or taken at one time.

dose the exact amount of a drug or therapeutic agent to be administered or taken at one time or at prescribed intervals.

double vision a disorder of vision in which two images of the same object are seen simultaneously because of unequal action of the eye muscles; diplopia.

douche 1. a stream of water, with or without medication or other additives, directed so as to irrigate or cleanse a body cavity. 2. a device for giving a douche. **—douche** *vb.*

Down's syndrome mongolism.

drastic acting quickly and powerfully: *a drastic purgative.*

drip system a device for controlling the flow of solutions in intravenous feeding and therapy.

drop foot the inability to flex the foot upward, often caused by injury to the peroneal nerve.

dropsy the excessive accumulation of clear fluid in body tissues or cavities; edema; ascites.

drug 1. a substance used in diagnosing, curing, mitigating, treating, or preventing disease. 2. a narcotic. **—drug** *vb.*

druggist a pharmacist.

D.T.'s delirium tremens.

duct a tube or vessel of the body esp. for the passage of secretions or excretions.

ductless gland a gland that secretes directly into an organ, as an endocrine gland, and has no excretory duct.

duodenum the first part of the small intestine extending from the pylorus to the jejunum. —**duodenal** *adj.*

dura mater the tough outer membrane enveloping the brain and spinal cord.

dwarf a person of unusually or abnormally small stature. —**dwarfish** *adj.* —**dwarfism** *n.*

dys- *prefix* abnormal; difficult.

dysarthria poor articulation of speech, often owing to nerve damage.

dyscrasia an abnormal condition of the body: *blood dyscrasia.*

dysentery a disease that is characterized by intestinal inflammation, abdominal pain, and the passage of mucus and bloody stools and is caused by bacteria or protozoa.

dysfunction abnormal or impaired functioning. —**dysfunctional** *adj.*

dyskinesia inability to perform normal movements of the body.

dyslexia a disturbance in the ability to read; word blindness. —**dyslexic** *adj.*

dysmenorrhea difficult or painful menstruation. —**dysmenorrheal** *adj.* —**dysmenorrheic** *adj.*

dysmetria inability to judge distance.

dyspareunia painful sexual intercourse, an abnormal condition of women.

dyspepsia indigestion. —**dispeptic** *adj.*

dysphagia difficulty in swallowing. —**dysphagic** *adj.*

dysphasia impairment of the ability to use or understand spoken language coherently owing to injury or brain disease. —**dysphasic** *adj.*

dysplasia abnormality of development, as of organs or cells. —**dysplasic** *adj.*

dyspnea difficult or labored respiration. **—dyspneic** *adj.* **—dystrophic** *adj.*

dysuria difficult or painful urination.

E

ear the organ of hearing and equilibrium, consisting of a sound-collecting outer ear separated by a membranous drum (tympanic membrane) from a sound-transmitting middle ear that is itself separated by a membranous fenestra from a sensory inner ear.

earache pain in the ear that may be caused by a disorder in the teeth, oral cavity, jaws, nose, sinuses, etc.

eardrum tympanic membrane.

earlobe the pendent part of the outer ear.

ebonation removal of bony fragments from a wound.

ebrietas *also* **ebriety** the state of being intoxicated with alcohol; drunkenness.

ebullism the formation at high altitudes of bubbles of water vapor in the tissues.

ebur tissue resembling ivory in appearance or consistency.

eburnation a degenerative change in bone in which it becomes hard and dense like ivory.

eburneous resembling ivory; having the color of ivory.

ecaudate without a tail; tailless.

ecbolic 1. hastening childbirth or accelerating the termination of pregnancy. 2. any agent that speeds up delivery or produces abortion; oxytocic.

eccdemic (of a disease) brought into a region or community; not epidemic or endemic.

eccentropiesis pressure exerted outwards.

ecchondroma a tumor formed as an outgrowth of cartilaginous tissue and usually protruding from the surface of a bone within a joint.

ecchymoma a small mass of clotted blood formed as the result of a bruise.

ecchymosis a bruise appearing on the skin or mucous membrane and resulting from the escape of blood into the tissues from ruptured blood vessels. —**ecchymotic** *adj.*

eccoprotic having the properties of a laxative; cathartic.

eccrine exocrine.

eccrisis 1. removal from the body of waste matter. 2. waste matter; excrement.

eccritic 1. acting to expel waste matter. 2. an agent that acts to excrete waste matter.

eccyesis the development of a fertilized ovum outside the uterus; extrauterine pregnancy.

ecdemomania an abnormal desire to wander.

ecdysiasm an abnormal erotic desire or tendency to remove one's clothes in the presence of strangers.

ECG electrocardiogram.

ecgonine an alkaloid derived from cocaine.

echeosis mental suffering and emotional upset caused by prolonged exposure to loud or disturbing noises.

echidnin snake venom.

echidnotoxin a toxic protein in snake venom.

echinococcus *pl.* **echinococci** any of a genus of tapeworms that in the larval stage invade tissues esp. of the liver and constitute a dangerous pathogen.

echinosis an abnormal condition of red blood cells characterized by the loss of their smooth outlines.

echis a highly poisonous snake occurring in parts of Africa and the Middle East; carpet viper.

echoacousia subjective impairment of hearing in which a sound seems to be repeated.

echoencephalography the diagnostic technique of using ultrasound in examining the cranial contents.

echokinesia the involuntary mimicking of a sign or gesture made by another person.

echolalia the often pathological echoing of the words spoken by other people. —**echolalic** *adj.*

echomatism the involuntary and automatic repetition of an observed act.

echophotony the phenomenon of mentally associating a musical tone or tones with a specific color or colors.

echophrasia echolalia.

echopraxia the involuntary repetition or imitation of movements made by someone else; echomatism.

echovirus a virus present in many syndromes but not determined to be a causative agent.

eclabium the eversion of a lip.

eclampsia an attack of convulsions sometimes occurring during pregnancy. —**eclamptic** *adj.*

eclaptogenous convulsive or causing convulsions.

ecmnesia the failure to recall recent events; short-term loss of memory.

ecphoria the ability to remember; recall of memory.

ecphyma a wartlike growth or elevation.

ECT electroconvulsive therapy.

ectacolia dilation of the large intestine.

ectad toward the surface; outward or externally.

ectal outer or external.

ectasia *also* **ectasis** dilation of a tubular passage.

ecthyma a pus-generating bacterial infection of the skin caused by staphylococci or streptococci.

ectiris the outermost layer of the iris.

ecto- *prefix* on the outside; outer.

ectoderm the outermost germ layer of an embryo. —**ectodermal** *adj.* —**ectodermic** *adj.*

ectoglobular not within a red blood cell or other globular body.

ectomorphic having a light, slender body. —**ectomorph** *n.*

-ectomy *suffix* surgical removal: *mastectomy.*

ectoparasite any parasite that lives on the outer surface of the body.

ectoperitonitis inflammation of the layer of peritoneum that lines the abdominal cavity.

ectopic occurring or appearing in an abnormal place, position, or manner.

ectopic pregnancy gestation occurring elsewhere than in the uterus, as a fallopian tube.

ectoplasm the outermost layer of the protoplasm of a living cell.

ectoplastic formed at the outside or periphery.

ectopotomy surgical removal of a fetus developing outside the uterus.

ectopy *also* **ectopia** abnormal displacement of an organ or part.

ectoretina the outermost layer of the retina.

ectosteal relating to the external surface of a bone.

ectotoxemia blood poisoning caused by the introduction of a poison into the body.

ectozoon an animal parasite that lives on the surface of the body.

ectrimma an ulcer caused by constant friction.

ectrogeny the congenital absence of any structure or part.

ectrotic preventing or inhibiting the development of a disease.

eczema inflammation of the skin characterized initially by redness, itching, and oozing vesicles and later by scaling and crusting. —**eczematous** *adj.*

ED effective dose.

ED_{50} a dose which has the desired effect in half of the subjects or laboratory animals.

edeitis inflammation of the external genitals in the female; vulvitis.

edema any condition in which the tissues contain an excessive amount of fluid, such as the result of the inflammatory process, kidney disorders, or increased permeability of the capillary walls.

edematous characterized or marked by edema.

edentate without teeth; toothless.

edulcorate to make sweet or sweeter; sweeten. —**edulcorant** *n.*

EEG electroencephalogram.

effector 1. a muscle or gland that becomes active upon being stimulated. 2. a motor or secretory nerve ending in a muscle or gland.

efferent conveying impulses, blood, etc., outward: *efferent nerves.*

effuse (of the surface appearance of a bacterial culture) widely spreading; thin.

egersis the condition of being unusually alert or attentive; abnormal wakefulness.

egesta any waste matter discharged from the body, esp. feces.

egg the female sex cell; ovum.

eglandulous without glands.

ego (in psychoanalytic theory) the part of the mind or psyche that is conscious and serves to mediate between the id and the superego and react to the outside world.

egotropic self-centered.

egrotogenic (of an illness) induced by the patient.

eidetic 1. relating to or possessing a photographic memory; having total recall of what has been seen before. 2. a person with total recall of what he has seen.

eiloid resembling a loop, coil or roll.

ejaculate 1. to eject (semen) in orgasm. 2. the semen ejaculated in orgasm. —**ejaculation** *n.* —**ejaculatory** *adj.*

ejaculatio precox premature ejaculation of semen; extremely rapid male orgasm at the start of sexual intercourse.

EKG *also* **ECG** electrocardiogram.

elastosis degenerative changes in elastic tissue, esp. the skin.

elbow the joint of the arm between the upper arm and the forearm.

Electra complex the female equivalent of the Oedipus complex; symptoms caused by a daughter's suppressed sexual love for her father.

electroanesthesia anesthesia induced by means of an electric current.

electrobiology the branch of biology concerned with the study of electrical phenomena in living organisms.

electrocardiogram a tracing made by an electrocardiograph.

electrocardiograph an instrument for recording variations in the electrical current of the heartbeat and used esp. to diagnose abnormalities in heart function. —**electrocardiographic** *adj.* —**electrocardiography** *n.*

electrocatalysis the breakdown of compounds or chemical decomposition by means of electricity.

electrocauterization *also* **electrocautery** cauterization by means of an electrically heated wire.

electrochemistry the branch of science concerned with the study of chemical changes brought about by electricity.

electrocoagulation the use of high frequency currents to harden growths and diseased tissues.

electrocontractility the ability of a muscle to contract when stimulated electrically.

electroconvulsive therapy electroshock therapy.

electrode a conductor for establishing electrical contact with a nonmetallic part of a circuit.

electroencephalogram a tracing made by an electroencephalograph.

electroencephalograph an instrument for recording brain waves. **—electroencephalographic** *adj.* **—electroencephalography** *n.*

electrohemostasis the arrest of bleeding by the use of electrocauterization.

electrohysterograph an instrument for recording the electrical activity of the uterus.

electrolysis 1. the destruction of the roots of hair by means of an electric current. 2. chemical change, esp. ionization, of a substance when an electric current is passed through it.

electrolyte a solution or a substance in solution that is decomposed into ions by the passage through it of an electric current, such as certain acids, bases and salts.

electromyograph an instrument for recording the contraction of muscles following their electrical stimulation. **—electromyogram** *n.* **—electromyographic** *adj.* **—electromyography** *n.*

electronarcosis the use of electricity to produce sleep or loss of consciousness.

electroshock therapy the treatment of psychiatric disorders by use of short bursts of an electric current to induce a brief therapeutic coma.

electrosleep therapy the treatment of psychiatric disorders by use of a low electric current to the brain to induce sleep.

electrosurgery the surgical use of electricity.

electrothanasia death by means of electricity; electrocution.

elephantiasis a chronic filarial disease caused by infestation of the lymphatics by nematodes and marked by gross enlargement of the limbs or scrotum and leathery hardening of the skin.

eliminate to expel (waste matter) from the body. —**elimination** *n.* —**eliminative** *adj.*

elinguation the surgical removal of the tongue.

elixir a usually alcohol-containing, sweetened liquid used as a vehicle for a medication, as a cough suppressant.

emaciation the condition of becoming very thin or of wasting away. —**emaciate** *vb.*

emaculation the removal of skin blemishes.

emasculation loss of masculinity by castration of the male. —**emasculate** *vb.*

embolectomy the surgical removal of an embolus.

embolism the sudden obstruction by an embolus of a blood vessel.

embololalia the periodic interjection of nonsense words in a sentence while talking.

embolus an abnormal body, as an air bubble or blood clot, floating in the blood.

embrocate to moisten and massage with a lotion. —**embrocation** *n.*

embryo *pl.* **embryos** the developing human being from the time of fertilization to the end of the eighth week after conception.

embryology the branch of biology dealing with embryos and their development. —**embryologist** *n.*

embryoplastic relating to the formation of an embryo.

emesis *pl.* **emeses** an act or instance of vomiting.

emetic an agent that induces vomiting. —**emetic** *adj.*

emetine hydrochloride a drug used in the treatment of amoebiasis.

emetology the scientific study of the causes and mechanisms responsible for vomiting.

EMF electromotive force; voltage.

EMG electromyogram.

-emia *suffix* blood.

emission a discharge of semen esp. when involuntary.

emmenagogic causing or increasing menstrual flow.

emmenia menses. —**emmenic** *adj.*

emmenology the branch of medical science concerned with the study of normal and disordered menstruation.

emmetropia normal vision.

emolient something that is soft and soothing to the skin or mucous membranes.

emotiovascular relating to vascular changes such as blushing and pallor induced by emotional stimuli.

emphysema a condition marked by air-filled expansion of tissues of the body esp. those of the lungs. —**emphysematous** *adj.*

empyema *pl.* **empyemata** the collection of pus in a body cavity. —**empyemic** *adj.*

emulsion a suspension of minute globules of one fluid within another. —**emulsive** *adj.*

enamel the hard thin calcareous substance forming the outer layer of a tooth.

enanthesis the skin eruption or rash associated with a specific internal disease, such as typhoid fever.

enarthrosis the ball-and-socket articulation of a joint in which the rounded extremity of one bone fits into the cuplike cavity of the other to permit movement in any direction.

encanthis a tiny growth at the inner angle of the eye.

encapsulated surrounded by a membranous capsule or sheath.

encarditis endocarditis; inflammation of the membrane that lines the chambers of the heart.

enceinte pregnant.

encelitis *also* **enceliitis** inflammation of any abdominal organ.

encephal- *or* **encephalo-** *prefix* brain: *encephalitis.*

encephalalgia headache.

encephalatrophy a wasting away of brain tissue; atrophy of the brain.

encephalic lying or situated within the cranial cavity.

encephalitis inflammation of the brain. —**encephalitic** *adj.*

encephalodialysis abnormal softening of the brain.

encephalodynia headache.

encephalogram an X-ray picture of the brain.

encephalography X-ray photography of the brain, esp. after air has been introduced into the lateral ventricles by lumbar puncture or directly into an area at the base of the brain.

encephalolith a calculus within the brain or one of its ventricles.

encephalomalacia softening of the brain.

encephalomeningitis inflammation of the brain and its covering membranes (meninges).

encephalomyelitis inflammation of the brain and spinal cord simultaneously.

encephalomyelopathy any disease involving both the brain and spinal cord.

encephalomyocarditis an acute febrile disease marked by inflammation, degeneration, and lesions of the skeletal and cardiac muscles and the central nervous system.

encephalon the brain of a vertebrate.

encephalopathy disease of the brain. —**encephalopathic** *adj.*

encephalospinal cerebrospinal.

encephalothlipsis brain compression.

encyst to form or become enclosed in a cyst. —**encystation** *n.*

end- *or* **endo-** *prefix* inside; within.

Endamoeba a genus of amoebas, usually distinguished from *Entamoeba,* that are parasitic in the intestines of invertebrates but do not affect man.

endangeitis *also* **endangiitis** inflammation of the inner coat of a blood vessel.

endangeitis obliterans inflammation of the inner coat of a blood vessel resulting in obstruction of the vessel.

endangium the inner coat of a blood vessel.

endaortitis inflammation of the inner coat of the aorta (the largest artery in the body).

endarterectomy the surgical removal of fatty deposits from the inner coat of a large artery.

endarterial within an artery or relating to its inner coat.

endarteritis inflammation of the inner coat of an artery.

endarterium the inner coat of an artery.

endaural within the ear.

endemia any endemic disease.

endemic peculiar or restricted to a particular area: *endemic diseases.*

endepidermis the inner layer of the epidermis.

endo- *prefix* within; inner.

endoangiitis inflammation of the inner coat of a blood vessel.

endocarditis inflammation of the lining of the heart.

endocardium *pl.* **endocardia** the thin membrane lining the inside of the heart.

endoceliac within a body cavity.

endocervicitis inflammation of the mucous membrane that lines the neck of the womb (cervix of the uterus).

endocolpitis inflammation of the mucous membrane that lines the vagina.

endocrine gland a gland, as the thyroid, producing secretions (hormones) that are circulated through the body in the bloodstream.

endocrinology a science dealing with endocrine glands and the hormones they secrete. —**endocrinologic** *or* **endocrinological** *adj.*

endocystitis inflammation of the mucous membrane that lines the urinary bladder.

endoderm the innermost layer of cells of an embryo. —**endodermal** *adj.*

endodontology the branch of dentistry concerned with the diagnosis and treatment of diseases that affect the dental pulp.

endoenteritis inflammation of the mucous membrane that lines the intestines.

endoenzyme any enzyme that is active within a cell.

endoesophagitis inflammation of the mucous membrane that lines the esophagus.

endogenous *or* **endogenic** growing from or produced within the body.

endolymph the fluid in the membranous labyrinth of the ear. —**endolymphatic** *adj.*

endometrial polyp a common, usually benign polyp in the

lining of the womb, frequently treated by dilatation and curettage.

endometriosis growth of the tissues of the lining of the womb outside of the womb.

endometritis inflammation of the lining of the womb caused by bacterial infection.

endometrium *pl.* **endometria** the mucous membrane lining the uterus.

endomorphic having a heavy rounded body with a tendency to become fat. —**endomorph** *n.*

end organ a structure forming the end of a neural path.

endorphin a secretion associated with the pituitary gland that reduces pain by acting on the central and peripheral nervous systems.

endoscope an instrument for viewing the inside of a hollow bodily organ. —**endoscopic** *adj.* —**endoscopy** *n.*

endothelium *pl.* **endothelia** the membrane lining blood vessels, serous cavities, and lymphatics.

endotracheal placed within or applied through the trachea.

enema introduction of a fluid into the rectum by way of the anus to help evacuate the lower bowel, introduce medicine, etc.

enervate 1. to lessen the strength or vitality of. 2. to remove or cut through a nerve.

engorge to congest with blood. —**engorgement** *n.*

engram (in the theory of memory mechanisms) a trace left in the brain following any experience, which is activated in the recall of that experience.

enkephalin a natural amino acid that reduces pain by acting on the neurons in the body.

Entamoeba a genus of amoebas parasitic in the human digestive tract one species of which (*Entamoeba* histolytica)is responsible for causing amoebic dysentery. Compare *Endamoeba.*

enter- *or* **entero-** *prefix* intestine: *enterocolitis.*

enteralgia severe abdominal pain and cramps.

enterectasis dilation of the small intestine.

enterelcosis ulceration of the intestine.

enteric of or relating to the intestines.

enteric-coated (of tablets) having a coating unaffected by the digestive juices of the stomach but which dissolves to release the medication beneath on reaching the small intestine.

enteritis inflammation of the intestines, esp. of the small intestine.

enterobiasis infestation with pinworms (*Enterobius vermicularis*).

enterococcus streptococcus present normally in the intestine.

enterocolitis inflammation of both the large and small intestine.

enterohepatitis inflammation of both the intestine and liver.

enteromycosis any fungal disease of the intestines.

enteron the alimentary canal system esp. of the human embryo.

enteropathy any disease of the intestine. —**enteropathic** *adj.*

enterorrhagia bleeding into or from the intestines.

enterostomy surgical formation of an artificial opening into the intestine through the abdominal wall.

enterozoon any animal parasite inhabiting the intestine.

entoptic within the eyeball.

enuresis involuntary release of urine, esp. during sleep. —**enuretic** *adj. & n.*

enzyme a complex protein produced by living cells and capable of inducing chemical changes without itself being changed or destroyed in the process. **—enzymatic** *or* **enzymic** *adj.* **—enzymology** *n.*

enzymology the branch of science concerned with the study of the structure and function of enzymes.

eosin a red acid dye used for staining.

ephedrine an alkaloid used in the form of a salt to relieve asthma, hay fever, and nasal congestion.

epicanthic fold either of the extended folds of the skin of the upper eyelids over the inner or both angles of the eyes. Also called *Mongolian fold.*

epicardium the inner layer of the pericardium.

epicondylitis severe, painful inflammation of the elbow. Also **tennis elbow.**

epicranium the muscles and skin that cover the cranium; the scalp.

epidemic affecting many individuals of the same community, region, or population simultaneously. **—epidemic** *n.* **—epidemical** *adj.*

epidemiology the scientific study of the distribution and occurrence of diseases. **—epidemiological** *or* **epidemiologic** *adj.* **—epidemiologist** *n.*

epidermis the outermost layer of the skin. **—epidermal** *adj.*

epidermitis inflammation of the outer layers of the skin.

epididymectomy surgical removal of the epididymis.

epididymis *pl.* **epididymides** an extended, convoluted mass of efferent tubes through which the sperm pass from the testis to the vas deferens. **—epididymal** *adj.*

epididymitis inflammation of the epididymis.

epigastric lying upon or over the stomach.

epiglottis the thin cartilaginous plate that folds back and protects the glottis during swallowing. **—epiglottal** *adj.*

epilepsy any of various diseases distinguished by disturbance of the electrical rhythms of the central nervous system with characteristic convulsive episodes and clouding of consciousness. **—epileptic** *n. & adj.*

epinephrine *or* **epinephrin** an adrenal hormone used medicinally as a bronchiole relaxant, heart stimulant, and vasoconstrictor. Also called *adrenaline.*

epiphysis *pl.* **epiphyses** the end of a long bone developing separately from the shaft (from which it is originally separated by an area of cartilage) with which it eventually unites.

episioplasty plastic surgery involving the vulva.

episiorrhagia bleeding from the vulva.

episiotomy surgical incision of the perineum to facilitate childbirth.

epispadias a congenital defect of the penis in which the urethra opens on the back surface.

epistaxis *pl.* **epistaxes** nosebleed.

epithelium *pl.* **epithelia** a membranous, protective tissue forming the outermost layer of the skin and lining tubes, cavities, and other free surfaces of the body. **—epithelial** *adj.*

equine encephalitis a sometimes fatal infection causing inflammation of the tissues of the brain.

erectile tissue tissue that becomes rigid when filled with blood, such as the penis, clitoris and nipples.

erection the condition of being rigid and elevated, as the penis or clitoris when filled with blood.

eremophobia the abnormal fear of being alone; fear of solitude.

ereuthophobia the abnormal fear of blushing.

ergasiophobia the abnormal fear of working or of work.

ergot 1. the dried sclerotium of a fungus replacing the seeds of a grass, as rye. 2. a disease of rye and other grasses caused by ergot fungus. 3. a derivative alkaloid of ergot used medicinally for its contractile action on smooth muscle.

ergotamine an alkaloid derivative from ergot, used esp. in treating migraine.

ergotism a toxic condition produced chiefly by eating grain or grain products infected with ergot fungus.

erogenous *also* **erogenic** producing or gratifying feelings of sexual excitement: *erogenous zones of the body.*

erosion the wearing away of the surface of a structure or part.

erotic of or arousing sexual desire.

erotophobia the abnormal fear of sexual intercourse or of physical contact associated with sexual arousal.

eruct to release stomach gas through the mouth; belch. **—eructation** *n.*

eruption the breaking out of a skin inflammation; rash. **—erupt** *vb.*

erysipelas an acute streptococcal inflammatory disease of the skin.

erythema acute, abnormal redness of the skin. **—erythematous** *adj.*

erythralgia a condition in which the skin is red and painful.

erythroblast an immature red blood cell.

erythroblastosis the abnormal presence in the bloodstream of large numbers of immature red blood cells.

erythrocyte a mature red blood cell.

erythrocytosis an abnormal increase in the number of circulating red blood cells; polycythemia.

erythromycin a drug used as an antibiotic in bacterial infections.

erythropoiesis the production of red blood cells.

eschar a slough formed esp. after a burn.

esophagitis inflammation of the esophagus.

esophagus the part of the digestive tract between the pharynx and the stomach; gullet.

estrinase a liver enzyme that inactivates estrogens.

estrogen any of the female sex hormones, produced by the ovaries or prepared synthetically.

estrus the receptive phase of the sexual cycle of female animals; heat.

ethical describing a drug that is available only by prescription.

ethyl alcohol alcohol.

etiolate to make or become pale from lack of light. **—etiolation** *n.*

etiology the study of the causes of disease or the cause of a specific disease or abnormal condition. **—etiologic** *or* **etiological** *adj.*

eugenics a science dealing with methods to improve the hereditary qualities of a race or breed. **—eugeneticist** *n.* **—eugenic** *adj.*

eunuch a man or boy deprived of the testes; castrated male. **—eunuchoid** *adj.*

euphoria an exaggerated sense of elation and general well-being. **—euphoric** *adj.*

Eustachian tube the tube connecting the throat to the ear and serving to equalize air pressure on both sides of the eardrum.

eustachitis inflammation of the mucous membrane that lines a Eustachian tube.

euthanasia the act or practice of killing individuals considered hopelessly sick or injured or permitting them to die for reasons of mercy.

evacuate to discharge (waste products) from the body. **—evacuation** *n.*

evert to turn or fold outward or inside out. —**eversible** *adj.* —**eversion** *n.*

eviscerate to remove the bowels or entrails of. —**evisceration** *n.*

exacerbation an increase in the severity of a disease or an aggravation of its signs and symptoms.

exanthem any skin eruption associated with a general disease, such as measles.

exarteritis inflammation of the outer coat of an artery.

excipient an inert substance that is used as a vehicle for a drug.

excision the act of removing something by cutting; surgical removal. —**excise** *vb.*

excoriate to remove the skin of; abrade. —**excoriation** *n.*

excrement waste matter discharged from the alimentary canal; fecal matter.

excrescent forming an abnormal or useless outgrowth or enlargement. —**excrescence** *n.*

excreta waste matter.

excrete to discharge (waste matter) from the body. —**excretion** *n.*

exfoliate to cast off in flakes or scales. —**exfoliation** *n.*

exhale to breathe out.

exhibitionism an abnormal urge to expose one's body and genitals to others without warning. —**exhibitionist** *n.* —**exhibitionistic** *adj.*

exhumation disinterment of a dead body. —**exhume** *vb.*

exobiology the branch of science concerned with examining evidence and investigating the possibility of life on other planets.

exocrine gland a gland that secretes outside of the body, as a sweat gland.

exogenous originating from or due to external causes.

exophthalmos *also* **exophthalmus** protrusion of the eyeballs, esp. as a consequence of overactivity of the thyroid gland (hyperthyroidism or thyrotoxicosis).

expectorant an agent that promotes the discharge of mucus from the respiratory tract. —**expectorant** *adj.*

expectorate to eject from the throat or lungs esp. by coughing; spit. —**expectoration** *n.*

exteroceptor an external sensory nerve ending that responds to stimuli outside of the body.

extrasystole premature contraction of the heart.

extravasation the passage of a fluid, esp. blood, from its proper channel or vessels into surrounding tissues. —**extravasate** *vb.*

extravert *or* **extrovert** one whose interests are directed primarily outside the self. —**extraverted** *or* **extroverted** *adj.* —**extraversion** *or* **extroversion** *n.*

extremity a limb of the body; an arm or leg.

extrinsic originating or being on the outside; external.

extrovert extravert.

exudate 1. to exude matter; ooze. 2. matter exudated. —**exudation** *n.*

eye the organ of sight, consisting of a round structure with a clear outer covering (cornea) and a biconvex transparent lens to focus incoming light through the central gelatinous substance (vitreous humor) and onto the back light-sensitive surface (retina), situated as one of a pair in bony frontal orbits of the skull.

eyeball the approximately globular capsule of the vertebrate eye.

eyebrow the bony arch separating the eye from the forehead.

eyelid a movable lid of skin and muscle that can be lowered over the eye.

eyestrain fatigue or discomfort of vision esp. from overuse of the eyes.

THE EYE
(CROSS SECTION)

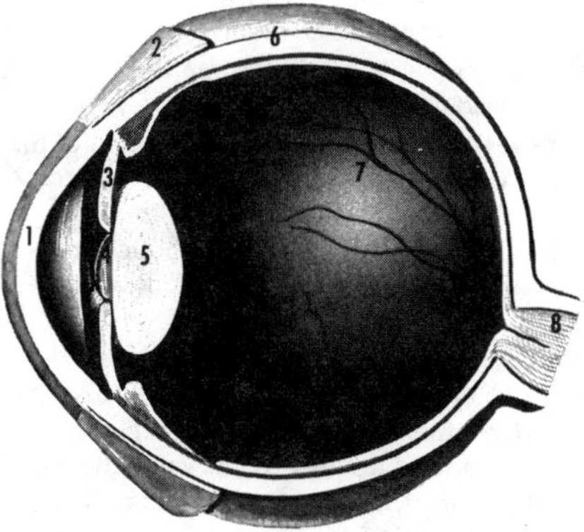

1	CORNEA	5	LENS
2	CONJUNCTIVA	6	SCLERA
3	IRIS	7	RETINA
4	PUPIL	8	OPTIC NERVE

F

face the front part of the human head that includes the forehead, eyes, nose, cheeks, mouth, and chin.

facial relating to the face or situated on the lower anterior part of the head.

facies *pl.* **facies** 1. an appearance or expression of the face indicating a particular condition; countenance. 2. the surface of a structure or part.

faciobrachial relating to or involving both the face and arm, as in the manifestations of juvenile muscular dystrophy.

faciocephalalgia pain in the face and head along the course of one or more nerves; neuralgia of this region.

faciocervical relating to or involving both the face and neck, as in a form of progressive muscular dystrophy.

faciolingual relating to or involving both the face and the tongue, as in a certain form of paralysis.

facioplasty plastic surgery involving the soft tissues of the face.

facioplegia palsy or paralysis of the facial muscles, usually with a loss of sensation in the skin of the face.

factitious fever fever produced artificially, as to fake an illness.

factor one of the thirteen substances present in the blood that affect its coagulation.

faecal fecal.

faeces feces.

falcate *also* **falciform** shaped like a crescent or sickle.

falcial relating to a falx.

falciparum malaria the most serious form of malaria.

fallacia an optical illusion or hallucination.

fallectomy surgical removal of a section of a fallopian tube; salpingectomy.

falling sickness a former popular term for epilepsy or an epileptic condition.

falling womb protrusion of the body of the uterus into the vagina.

fallopian tube either of a pair of tubes through which an ovum, released during ovulation, travels from the ovary to the uterus.

fallostomy surgical opening of a fallopian tube; salpingostomy.

fallotomy surgical separation of a fallopian tube; salpingotomy.

false-negative relating to the results of a test which incorrectly suggest that a disease or specific condition is not present.

false-positive relating to the results of a test that incorrectly suggest that a disease or specific condition is present.

false ribs the lower five pairs of ribs, which are not connected directly with the breastbone (sternum).

falx any structure or part shaped like a sickle.

falx cerebelli a fold or short process of the outermost of the meninges (dura mater) which forms a vertical partition between the two halves of the cerebellum.

falx cerebri a fold of dura mater that dips into the longitudinal fissure between the two halves of the cerebrum.

fames hunger.

familial affecting more members of a family than can be attributed to chance: *familial illnesses.*

family 1. parents and their children. 2. close blood relatives. 3. (in biologic classification) a division between order and genus.

fantasy mental images created in response to psychological need: *sexual fantasies of adolescence.*

faradic relating to induced electricity.

faradism the therapeutic use of an induced electric current. —**faradize** *vb.*

farinaceous starchy.

farsightedness the inability to focus on objects relatively close to the eye; hypermetropia; hyperopia.

fascia *pl.* **fasciae** a sheath of connective tissue enclosing muscle.

fascial relating to or resembling fascia.

fascicle fasciculus.

fascicular arranged in a bundle or rodlike collection.

fasciculation 1. the formation of fasciculi. 2. the involuntary twitching of groups of muscle fibers.

fasciculus *pl.* **fasciculi** a small bundle of fibers, esp. of muscles or nerves.

fasciectomy the surgical removal of strips of fascia.

fasciola a small group of fibers.

Fasciola a genus of flukes.

fasciolopsiasis a common intestinal infection of the Far East caused by eating contaminated water plants.

fascioplasty plastic surgery involving fascia.

fasciotomy surgical incision and separation of fascia.

fat animal tissue composed of cells enlarged with greasy or oily matter. —**fatty** *adj.*

fatigue 1. physical or emotional exhaustion. 2. to weary with labor or exertion.

fat metabolism the breaking down of fats by the cells of the body.

fauces the passage between the soft palate and the base of the tongue that links the mouth and the pharynx.

faucitis inflammation of the fauces.

faveolus a small depression, esp. on the skin.

favus a contagious fungal disease of the skin, esp. of the scalp, characterized by the formation of round cup-shaped yellow crusts having a musty odor.

febrifacient causing or producing fever.

febrile of or relating to fever; feverish.

febrious conducive to the development of fever.

fecal *also* **faecal** of, relating to, or constituting feces.

feces *also* **faeces** solid waste matter formed in the large intestine and expelled through the anus.

fecund fruitful in offspring; prolific. —**fecundity** *n.*

feebleminded mentally incapable or deficient. —**feeblemindedly** *adv.* —**feeblemindedness** *n.*

fellatio *also* **fellation** oral stimulation of the penis.

felo de se 1. a person who commits suicide. 2. the act of suicide.

felon a whitlow.

feminism the abnormal development or condition in a male of feminine characteristics, usually as the result of a hormonal disorder.

femorotibial relating to both the femur and tibia.

femur *pl.* **femurs** *or* **femora** the bone extending from the pelvis to the knee; thighbone. —**femoral** *adj.*

fenestra *pl.* **fenestrae** an anatomical aperture, frequently one closed by a membrane.

fenestrated having openings suggestive of or resembling windows.

fenestration the presence of window-like openings in a structure or part.

ferment 1. to decompose or undergo fermentation. 2. a substance capable of bringing about fermentation.

fermentation the breakdown of complex substances by means of certain enzymes (ferments) produced by microorganisms such as bacteria, molds and yeasts, as in the production of alcohol.

fermentative causing or able to cause fermentation.

ferrous relating to iron or a salt containing iron (such as ferrous sulfate).

ferruginous relating to or containing iron.

fertile producing or capable of producing young; fecund. **—fertility** *n.*

fertilize to cause (a human egg) to become impregnated. **—fertilization** *n.*

fester to become inflamed and produce pus.

fetal *also* **foetal** of or relating to a fetus.

fetal position a resting position in which the body is curved with the legs drawn up, the arms are bent around the chest, and the head is inclined forward.

feticide the destruction of the fetus in induced abortion.

fetid having an offensive smell.

fetish *or* **fetich** an object or body part that becomes psychologically necessary for sexual gratification and may interfere with normal or complete sexual gratification.

fetishism *also* **fetichism** the pathological displacement of erotic interest to a fetish. **—fetishist** *n.*

fetology the study of the unborn fetus, including its disorders. **—fetologist,** *n.*

fetor an extremely foul odor.

fetus *also* **foetus** a developing human being usually from three months after conception to birth.

fever an abnormal rise in body temperature. **—feverish** *adj.* **—feverishness** *n.*

fever blister cold sore.

fiber *or* **fibre** a threadlike structure, esp. a strand of nerve or muscle tissue. —**fibrous** *adj.* —**fibrousness** *n.*

fiberscope an instrument for examining body cavities and passages and composed of flexible bundles of glass fibers through which light is transmitted.

fibr- *or* **fibro-** *prefix* fiber; fibrous.

fibril a very small fiber.

fibrillation 1. irregular and uncoordinated contractions of the heart. 2. muscular twitching resulting from the spontaneous contraction of muscle fibers.

fibrin an insoluble component of blood, created by chemical conversion from fibrinogen, that forms the matrix of blood clots.

fibrinogen a clotting factor in solution in the bloodstream from which fibrin is made.

fibroadenoma a benign breast tumor occurring usually in young women.

fibroblast a cell forming connective tissue. —**fibroblastic** *adj.*

fibrocystic disease cysts in the breasts, benign but predisposing the patient to greater risk of breast cancer.

fibroid 1. resembling or constituting fibrous tissue. 2. a benign tumor esp. when occurring in the uterine wall.

fibroma any fibrous tumor of connective tissue.

fibromatosis a condition characterized by the formation of many fibromas.

fibromyositis any of several disorders characterized by pain or stiffness in the joints.

fibrosarcoma a malignant tumor derived from fibrous connective tissue.

fibrosis the reactive formation of fibrous tissue, as in the healing of a wound.

fibrositis rheumatic inflammation of fibrous tissue.

fibrotic relating to or characterized by fibrosis.

fibrous composed of or containing fibers.

fibula a slender bone that extends from the knee to the ankle on the outer side of the leg.

ficin an enzyme isolated from figs that is capable of dissolving proteins, used in the treatment of worm infestation.

field of vision visual field.

filaria *pl.* **filariae** any of various parasitic nematodes that infest the blood and tissues of mammals.

filariasis disease caused by infestation with filariae.

filariform resembling small threadlike worms or filariae.

filioparental relating to the relationships between parents and their children.

filterable virus a virus of such minute size that a fluid in which it is contained remains virulent even when passed through the pores of a special filter which can trap bacteria and the larger viruses.

filtrate the fluid that has been passed through a filter.

filtration the act or process of passing a fluid through a filter.

filum a threadlike structure; filament.

fimbria *pl.* **fimbriae** any structure or part resembling a fringe or having fringelike attachments, such as the upper part of the fallopian tubes nearest the ovaries.

fimbriate *also* **fimbriated** having fimbriae.

finger a digit of the hand, esp. any of the four digits of the hand other than the thumb.

first aid emergency care and treatment of a person in an accident or suddenly taken ill before a physician can be summoned or hospitalization can occur.

fissure a cleft between two structures or parts; sulcus.

fissure of Rolando the central fissure of the cerebrum, dividing the parietal from the frontal lobe in each hemisphere; central sulcus.

fissure of Sylvius the lateral fissure of the cerebrum, dividing the temporal lobe from the frontal and parietal lobes in each hemisphere.

fistula *pl.* **fistulas** *or* **fistulae** an abnormal passage from an abscess to the surface of the body or from one organ to another. —**fistulous** *adj.*

flaccid lacking in firmness; soft; limp. —**flaccidity** *n.* —**flaccidly** *adv.*

flagellum *pl.* **flagella** a long, slender, tapering process providing the means of locomotion for certain cells, as spermatozoa and some protozoa.

flatfoot a condition of the feet in which the arches of the insteps are flattened so that the soles rest entirely on the ground.

flatulent marked by, affected with, or likely to cause gas within the stomach or intestinal tract. —**flatulence** *n.* —**flatulency** *n.*

flatus gas generated in the bowels or stomach.

flavedo yellowness of the skin; jaundice.

fletcherism a dietary system characterized by eating very small quantities of food each day which is to be excessively chewed before swallowing.

fletcherize to practice the dietary system (fletcherism) devised by the American dietician Horace Fletcher (1849-1919).

flexion 1. a bending of a joint between adjacent bones. 2. the condition or state of being bent.

flexor a muscle that produces flexion.

floater a spot or pattern of spots in the field of vision that may, if they appear suddenly or are reddish, be symptomatic of a disorder.

flooding profuse bleeding from the uterus, esp. following childbirth or in severe menstrual disorders.

fluke any of various species of parasitic flatworms (trematodes) which can infest the liver, blood, intestines or lungs.

fluor albus leukorrhea.

fluorescein a yellow or red dye that produces a vivid green fluorescence in solution, used in the diagnosis of disorders of the cornea and in intravenous injections for studying the rate of blood flow (circulation time).

fluorescent having the ability to become luminous when exposed to light rays, X-rays, or other forms of radiant energy.

fluoridate to add a fluoride to (as drinking water). **—fluoridation** *n.*

fluoride a compound of fluorine.

fluorine a nonmetallic, gaseous, halogenic element.

fluoroscope a device with a fluorescent screen for examining the movement and condition of deep structures of the body by means of X-rays. **—fluoroscopic** *adj.* **—fluoroscopy** *n.*

fluorosis a condition mainly characterized by discoloration of the teeth, caused by the chronic intake of excessive amounts of fluorine in the drinking water.

flush 1. a reddening of the face and neck, as in blushing. 2. a feeling of sudden increase of heat.

flutter 1. abnormal, spasmodic, muscular movement of a part of the body. 2. to move in irregular spasms. **—fluttery** *adj.*

focus *pl.* **focuses** *or* **foci** a point at which rays, as of light, converge.

folic acid a crystalline acid of the B complex found naturally in liver, yeast and green leafy vegetables and used in synthetic form to treat nutritional anemias and sprue.

folie à deux a condition in which two persons in an intimate relationship share the same delusional ideas.

follicle a small narrow-mouthed cavity or depression. —**follicular** *adj.* —**folliculate** *also* **folliculated** *adj.*

follicle-stimulating hormone a hormone from the anterior pituitary gland that acts in the growth of the Graafian follicles in the ovary and in spermatogenesis. Also, **FSH.**

fomentation the application of a moist, hot substance to the skin to ease pain.

fomites articles, as items of clothing, that have been in contact with a person having a contagious disease and may themselves be agents of transmission.

fontanelle *or* **fontanel** a soft membrane-covered space at the top of an infant's skull before the bones have completely merged.

food poisoning acute gastrointestinal distress caused by ingestion of food containing toxic bacteria or chemical residues.

foot *pl.* **feet** the terminal part of a vertebrate leg that serves as support for standing; the part of the leg below the ankle.

foot-and-mouth disease an acute, contagious, febrile disease of viral origin affecting chiefly cloven-footed animals and marked by ulcerating vesicles in the mouth and about the hoofs. Also called *hoof-and-mouth disease.*

foramen *pl.* **foramina** a natural opening or hole, esp. in bone, for the passage of nerves, blood vessels, etc.

foramen magnum the large opening at the base of the skull for the passage of the spinal cord.

forceps *pl.* **forceps** any of various instruments used esp. in surgery for lifting, grasping, or holding.

forcipate resembling or shaped like forceps.

forebrain the part of the embryonic brain that develops into the cerebrum and closely related structures.

forensic medicine the branch of medicine concerned with

the application of medical information to legal problems, as in proving criminal responsibility in a sudden death or death under unusual circumstances.

foreskin a retractable fold of skin that covers the glans of the penis; prepuce.

formaldehyde a pungent gas used in solution as a disinfectant and tissue preservative for anatomical specimens.

formalin an aqueous solution containing 37 per cent formaldehyde.

formication an abnormal sensation of insects creeping over the skin.

formula *pl.* **formulas** *or* **formulae** 1. prescription. 2. a nutritive mixture for feeding an infant. 3. the symbolic or alphanumeric representation of a chemical molecule.

formulary any collection of chemical formulas for compounding or listing the constituents of medicinal preparations.

fornix an arch.

fossa *pl.* **fossae** an anatomical pit or depression.

fovea a small pit or cuplike depression; minute fossa.

foxglove digitalis.

fracture the breaking of hard tissue, as bone. —**fracture** *vb.*

freckle a harmless spot on the skin darker than the surrounding area.

fremitus vibration of the chest wall.

frenulum *pl.* **frenula** a membranous fold of tissue, as that under the tongue, serving as a support or restraint; frenum.

frenum *pl.* **frenums** *or* **frena** frenulum.

friable easily broken or reduced to powder; dry and brittle.

frigidity sexual unresponsiveness or indifference on the part of a woman. —**frigid** *adj.*

frontal 1. anterior. 2. relating to or situated on or near the forehead.

frostbite tissue damage resulting from freezing of a part of the body, esp. parts such as the ears, nose, fingers and toes.

frottage sexual arousal generated by rubbing against someone.

frotteur a person who obtains sexual pleasure by means of the sense of touch, esp. by rubbing against someone.

fructose a sugar occurring in honey and in many fruits.

FSH follicle-stimulating hormone.

fugue long- or short-term amnesia in which the person, unable to cope with a stressful situation, escapes from it mentally and, often, physically, e.g., by leaving his home.

full-term (of a fetus) retained in the uterus for the entire normal duration of pregnancy.

fulminating sudden and severe in onset: *fulminating infections.*

fundus *pl.* **fundi** the part or section of a hollow organ furthest from the natural opening.

fungicide an agent that destroys fungi. —**fungicidal** *adj.*

fungiform (of a structure or part) having a narrow base and a broad or branched upper free area; shaped like a mushroom.

fungus *pl.* **fungi** any of various primitive forms of plant life (including the mushrooms, molds and mildews) characterized by the absence of chlorophyll and living off organic matter.

funiculus any structure shaped like a cord; cordlike.

furuncle a swollen inflammation of the skin; boil.

furunculosis skin disease characterized by the presence of boils.

fusiform spindle-shaped.

G

gag 1. a surgical device for holding the mouth open. 2. to hold (the mouth) open with a gag. 3. to retch.

gait a characteristic manner or style of walking.

galact- *or* **galacto-** *prefix* milk: *galactopoiesis.*

galactacrasia an abnormal composition of breast milk.

galactemia an abnormal condition in which the blood appears milky or cloudy.

galactophagous subsisting on milk.

galactophore a milk duct.

galactophoritis inflammation of a milk duct.

galactopoiesis the production and secretion of milk. —**galactopoietic** *adj.*

galactorrhea the excessive flow of milk.

galactoschesis the retention or inhibition of milk secretion.

galactostasis 1. the inhibition or suppression of milk secretion. 2. an abnormal accumulation of milk within the breast.

galacturia whiteness or milkiness of the urine due to the abnormal presence of chyle or lymph.

galea any structure or part shaped like or resembling a helmet.

galenical 1. relating to or resembling the philosophy and medical teaching of the Greek physician Galen (2nd century A.D.). 2. any therapeutic preparation derived from plants.

galeophilia the abnormal and excessive love of cats.

galeophobia the abnormal fear of cats.

gall secretion of the liver; bile.

gallbladder a pear-shaped membranous sac in which bile from the liver is stored until its release into the small intestine.

gallery the subcutaneous burrow occupied by some metazoan parasites.

galloping consumption a form of tuberculosis that has a rapid course ending in death.

gallop rhythm a sequence of three sounds heard on auscultation of the heart, usually caused by an excessively fast rate of contraction of the ventricles.

gallstone a calculus formed in the gallbladder or in a bile duct.

galvanic relating to or caused by galvanism.

galvanic battery a battery that produces electricity by means of chemical action.

galvanic current the direct current produced by a galvanic battery.

galvanism the therapeutic use of direct current produced by chemical energy in a galvanic battery. —**galvanization** *n.* —**galvanize** *vb.*

galvano- *prefix* direct current electricity.

galvanocautery electrocautery.

galvanochemical electrochemical.

galvanocontractility the ability of a muscle to contract when stimulated by a galvanic current.

galvanolysis electrolysis.

gamete a male or female reproductive cell; spermatozoon or ovum. —**gametic** *adj.*

gametogenesis the production of sperm or ova.

-gamic *suffix* relating to or resulting from sexual union.

gammacism a speech disorder characterized by difficulty

in pronouncing correctly words or syllables that contain the letter *g*.

gamma globulin a globulin of serum or plasma that is involved in antibody production.

gamogenesis sexual reproduction.

gamophobia an abnormal fear of marriage.

gangliectomy *also* **ganglionectomy** the surgical removal of a ganglion or of ganglia.

gangliform resembling a ganglion; having the appearence or form of a ganglion or of ganglia.

ganglion *pl.* **ganglia** a mass of nerve tissue esp. if located outside the spinal cord or the brain. 2. a cystic swelling or tumor on a tendon. —**ganglial** *adj.* —**gangliate** *adj.*

ganglioneure a cell in a nerve ganglion.

ganglionitis inflammation of a ganglion or of ganglia.

gangrene necrosis of soft tissues of the body resulting from loss of blood supply.

gargle 1. a liquid for clearing or soothing the throat. 2. to rinse the throat with a gargle.

gas a basic state of matter characterized by free movement of its molecules, which permits it to expand indefinitely or to occupy the entire volume of a container holding it, or to be compressed until it assumes a liquid or eventually solid state.

gaseous relating to or having the properties or nature of gas.

gastr- *or* **gastro-** *or* **gastri-** *prefix* stomach; belly: *gastrectomy.*

gastralgia pain in the stomach; stomach ache.

gastrectomy surgical removal of part or all of the stomach, as in the treatment of severe gastric ulcers.

gastric of, relating to, or affecting the stomach.

gastric ulcer a peptic ulcer of the stomach.

gastritis inflammation of the mucous lining of the stomach.

gastroatonia loss of normal muscle tone in the stomach.

gastrocardiac relating to or involving both the stomach and the heart.

gastrocele a hernia of the stomach.

gastrocnemius the calf muscle.

gastrocolitis inflammation of both the stomach and the colon.

gastrocolostomy the surgical formation of an artificial opening between the stomach and the colon.

gastrocolotomy surgical incision into the stomach and the colon.

gastroduodenal relating to or involving both the stomach and duodenum.

gastroenteritis inflammation of the stomach and intestines.

gastroenterology the branch of medical science concerned with the study and treatment of diseases of the stomach and intestines. —**gastroenterologist** *n.*

gastrointestinal of, relating to, or affecting the stomach and intestines.

gastrology the branch of medical science concerned with the study and treatment of diseases of the stomach (a part of gastroenterology).

gastromalacia abnormal softening of the walls of the stomach.

gastroscope an instrument for viewing and examining the interior of the stomach. —**gastroscopist** *n.* —**gastroscopy** *n.*

gastrosplenic relating to or involving both the stomach and the spleen.

gastrostomy the surgical formation of an artificial opening through the wall of the stomach.

gather (of a boil or furuncle) to form or ooze pus; come to a head.

gathering 1. the formation and accumulation of pus in a boil or abscess. 2. a localized collection of pus in a boil or abscess.

gauss a unit of the intensity of a magnetic field.

gauze a loosely woven fabric used for dressing wounds.

gavage feeding by means of a tube inserted through the nose and into the stomach; direct gastric feeding.

Gelusil trade name for a combination of antacids and an antiflatulent.

gene a tiny particle usually occurring in pairs on a chromosome and responsible for transmitting hereditary traits and characteristics from one generation to the next.

general anesthesia anesthesia in which a person is totally unconscious, as for major surgery.

generic drug a drug sold under its chemical name rather than a trade name.

genetic *also* **genetical** of or relating to genetics.

genetic code information imbedded in molecules of DNA.

genetic engineering the design and production of artificial changes in DNA molecules in order to modify or control the characteristics of a species.

genetics the branch of science concerned with the various aspects of heredity and the natural development of an organism. —**geneticist** *n.*

geniculate *also* **geniculated** (of a structure or part) bent like a knee.

geniculum any small structure bent like a knee or having a knotlike appearance.

genioplasty plastic surgery involving the chin or cheek.

genital relating to reproduction or the organs of reproduction: *genital organs.*

genitalia the reproductive organs; genitals.

genitals the reproductive organs: the penis and testes in the male and the vulva (external genitals), vagina, uterus, fallopian tubes and ovaries in the female.

genitourinary relating to reproduction and urination or to the organs responsible for these functions; urogenital.

genu 1. the knee. 2. any structure or part resembling a bent knee.

genus *pl.* **genera** a group of related species, the distinct members of which are not usually able to interbreed.

genu valgum knock knee (knees that bend inward).

genu varum bowleg (knees that bend outward).

geopathology the study of diseases in relation to different geographical characteristics, such as climate and terrain.

geriatric relating to old age or to the elderly.

geriatrician a physician who specializes in the practice of geriatrics.

geriatrics the branch of medical science concerned with the study and treatment of diseases in the elderly.

germ any microorganism, esp. one capable of causing disease; microbe.

German measles a viral infection common in children and accompanied by a typical skin eruption, milder than true measles (morbilli) but potentially dangerous to the developing fetus of a pregnant woman not previously exposed to the disease. Compare *measles.*

germ cell an ovum or spermatozoon.

germicide an agent capable of destroying germs. **—germicidal** *adj.*

gerontology the branch of medical science concerned with the study of the process of aging and the social and health problems of the elderly.

gestation the developmental period within the womb from conception (fertilization of the ovum) until birth, averaging 266 days. Also called *gestation period.*

gigantism enlargement of the entire body or a limb as the result of overproduction of growth hormone by the pituitary gland before puberty, rarely producing a human giant up to eight feet tall. Compare *acromegaly*.

gingiva the gums.

gingivectomy surgical removal of some of the tissues of the gums, as in the management of severe infection (pyorrhea).

gingivitis inflammation of the gums.

gland a cell or collection of cells that produces specialized substances (secretions) from materials in the blood which are either used by the body or eliminated as waste matter.

glandular fever an acute infectious disease caused by a virus. Also called *infectious mononucleosis*.

glans *pl.* **glandes** the bulbous, vascular extremity of the penis or the clitoris.

glaucoma an eye disease marked by increased pressure within the eyeball and gradual loss of vision.

glioma one of the major varieties of brain tumors.

globulin any of a group of simple proteins occurring in animal and plant tissue, the best known of which is gamma globulin (important in the production of antibodies).

glomerulonephritis a disease affecting the glomerulus of the kidney.

glomerulus a group of nerve fibers or blood vessels.

glossal of or relating to the tongue.

glossitis inflammation of the tongue.

glossodynia pain in the tongue, usually caused by an ulcer, infection, etc.

glossolalia "speaking in tongues," the rapid speech in an unknown language by a person in an excited state, in religious contexts often taken to be a message from a supreme being.

glossopharyngeal involving or relating to the tongue and the pharynx.

glottis the two vocal cords and the space between them, concerned with sound production.

glucagon a hormone secreted by the islands of Langerhans that controls hypoglycemia.

glucocorticoid one of three hormones secreted by the adrenocortex, as hydrocortisone.

glucose a colorless, soluble sugar that occurs widely in nature and is produced naturally in the body by the breakdown of dietary starch.

glucosuria presence of glucose in the urine, as in nephrosis, diabetes mellitus, and other diseases.

gluteal of or relating to the buttocks or the gluteus muscles.

gluten a protein substance in cereals, responsible for a digestive disease (celiac disease) in children who are hypersensitive to it.

gluteus muscle any of the large muscles forming the buttocks.

glycerin *also* **glycerol** a sweet syrupy alcohol produced by the saponification of fats and used esp. as a solvent.

glycogen the carbohydrate that provides the body with a reserve of energy and heat, stored in the liver and converted into glucose on demand by active muscles.

glycosuria the abnormal presence of sugar in the urine, one sign of diabetes mellitus.

goiter *also* **goitre** abnormal enlargement of the thyroid gland.

gomphosis the fitting of a structure or process into a bony socket, as a tooth root into a jawbone.

gonad one of the sex glands; an ovary or testis. —**gonadal** *adj.*

gonadotrophin any of several hormones that stimulate the ovaries or testes.

gonococcus a bacterium that causes gonorrhea. —**gonococcal** *or* **gonococcic** *adj.*

gonorrhea a contagious bacterial disease typically characterized by inflammation of the urethra, urinary frequency, a burning sensation during urination and a discharge of pus from the penis or vagina, transmitted mainly during sexual intercourse with an infected partner (venereal disease). Also called *clap.*

gout a metabolic disorder characterized by excessive deposits of crystals of uric acid (urate) in the tissues and marked by painful swelling of the joints, esp. of the big toe. Also called *gouty arthritis.* —**gouty** *adj.*

Graafian follicle a small sac in an ovary that contains an ovum, one follicle rupturing each month during menstruation to release a mature ovum.

graft the transfer of a tissue or organ from one person to another or from one place on a person to another on the same person.

grand mal the most severe form of epilepsy.

granuloma a nodule or mass of chronically inflamed tissue.

granulomatosis any condition in which granulomas are present.

graphospasm writer's cramp.

gravel a mass of small concretions in the kidneys or bladder.

gravid pregnant.

gray matter *or* **grey matter** unmyelinated nerve cells and fibers of the brain and spinal cord, having a grayish color.

greenstick fracture a bone fracture in which the bone is partially fractured and partially bent.

grippe influenza. —**grippy** *adj.*

groin the area of the lower abdomen at the juncture of the legs with the trunk.

growing pains nonspecific pains often occurring in the legs of children.

gullet esophagus.

gumboil an abscess of the gums caused by tooth decay, injury, or infection.

gumma a rubbery tumor that can appear anywhere on the body during the third stage of syphilis.

gut intestine.

gynecology the branch of medical science concerned with the diagnosis and treatment of diseases that affect women, esp. those involving the female reproductive system. —**gynecologist** *n.* —**gynecological** *adj.*

gynecomastia abnormal enlargement of the male breasts.

gyrus a convolution of the brain.

H

habena *pl.* **habenae** a restricting fibrous band. —**habenular** *adj.*

habit an act or response that has become virtually automatic and is thus difficult to break or interrupt. —**habitual** *adj.*

habituation a psychological dependence, esp. on drugs for which the user has an abnormal or compulsive craving or desire.

habitus the physical characteristics of an individual that are thought to play a role in the tendency to be affected by certain diseases or disorders.

hacking cough a short, frequent and usually dry (nonproductive) cough.

haem- *or* **haemo-** *prefix* hem-.

hagiotherapy therapy that depends on religious convictions, as when a sick person submits to religious rituals, goes on pilgrimages, touches sacred relics, etc.

hairball trichobezoar.

halation blurring of vision by strong light coming directly in front of or behind the viewed object or scene.

halethazole an antiseptic agent that is also effective against some species of fungus.

half-life the period of time taken for a radioactive isotope to lose half of its activity through disintegration.

half-way house a center or institution for housing patients who no longer require intensive medical or psychiatric care but who are not yet ready to resume normal social activities or employment within the community.

halide a salt or compound of a halogen.

haliphagia the ingestion of abnormally large quantities of a salt or salts, esp. of sodium chloride (common table salt) or sodium bicarbonate (a common antacid).

halisteresis a deficiency of calcium in the bones; osteomalacia. —**halisteretic** *adj.*

halitosis a condition of having foul breath.

halitus an expired breath; exhaled vapor.

hallex hallux.

hallucination 1. the perception of objects or sounds having no basis in reality and commonly arising from a nervous disorder, fatigue, or the use of a drug. 2. the objects or sounds so perceived. —**hallucinate** *vb.* —**hallucinatory** *adj.*

hallucinogen a drug, as LSD, inducing hallucinations. —**hallucinogenic** *adj.*

hallucinosis a severe mental disorder characterized by persistent or recurring hallucinations.

hallux *pl.* **halluces** the great toe; first digit of the foot. —**hallucal** *adj.*

hallux valgus a deformity of the big toe in which it bends over or beneath the adjacent toe.

hallux varus a deformity of the big toe in which it bends toward the inner side of the foot away from the adjacent toe.

haloderma a skin disorder caused by the ingestion of halides such as iodides and bromides.

halogen any of the elements fluorine, chlorine, bromine and iodine that combine with metals to form salts and with hydrogen to form acids. —**halogenous** *adj.*

halogenation the altering of the physical and therapeutic properties of a molecule by the incorporation of halogen atoms in its structure.

haloid resembling salt or a halogen.

halophil *also* **halophile** any microorganism that needs a high concentration of salt for enhanced growth. —**halophilic** *adj.*

haloprogin an antifungal agent.

halothane a general anesthetic developed by British chemists in the 1950s for its nonirritant and nonflammable properties.

ham the buttock and posterior part of the thigh.

hamartophobia an abnormal fear of error or of committing a sin.

hamate having a hook; hooked.

hammer malleus; one of the three small conducting bones of the middle ear.

hammertoe a deformity of a toe characterized by permanent angular flexion.

hamstring either of two groups of tendons at the back of the knee.

hamstring muscle any of the three muscles at the back of the thigh that extend the thigh when the leg is flexed.

hamular having the shape of a hook; hook-shaped.

hamulus any hooklike structure or part.

hangnail a small piece of partially detached skin at the base of a nail, esp. of a fingernail.

Hansen's disease leprosy.

hapalonychia lack of firmness or rigidity of the nails.

haphalgesia abnormal sensitivity of the skin to pain when touched lightly.

haphephobia abnormal dislike or fear of being touched by another person.

haplopia normal, single vision. Compare *diplopia*.

hapten *also* **haptene** an incomplete antigen capable of stimulating antibody formation only when covalently linked to protein.

haptodysphoria an unpleasant tactile sensation.

haptometer an instrument for measuring a person's sensitivity to touch.

hard palate the roof of the mouth between the alveolar ridge and the soft palate.

harelip a congenital deformity in which the center of the upper lip is marked by a vertical fissure like that of a hare, often associated with cleft palate.

Hashimoto's disease chronic inflammation of the thyroid gland.

hashish resin obtained from the flowering tops of the female hemp plant (*Cannabis sativa*) and chewed or smoked for its hallucinogenic effect. Also called *charas, hash*.

haustus a medicinal potion.

hay fever acute allergic rhinitis and sometimes conjunctivitis caused typically by exposure of a hypersensitive person to pollens and dust.

headache pain or aching in the head. —**headachy** *adj.*

headshrinker *Slang* psychiatrist; psychoanalyst.

heal to make or become sound and whole.

health the condition of being sound in body and mind; freedom from pain or illness. —**healthy** *adj.*

health officer an official responsible for health and sanitation laws.

heart a hollow muscular organ that acts by rhythmic contraction to pump the blood through the circulatory system of the body.

heart attack an acute episode of dysfunctioning of the heart.

heart block irregularity in the rhythm of the heart resulting in decreased cardiac output.

heartburn a burning sensation at the lower end of the esophagus; pyrosis.

heart failure a condition in which the heart cannot pump blood at an adequate rate or in adequate volume to sustain life.

heart-lung machine a machine used for maintenance of oxygenation and circulation of the blood while the heart is stopped during heart surgery.

heart murmur an abnormal murmuring sound heard through the chest wall.

heat exhaustion a condition marked by nausea, weakness, dizziness, and sweating that results from exertion in a very warm climate and from the loss of sodium chloride from the body.

heat prostration heat exhaustion.

heat rash inflammation of the skin, usually in a protected area, as the groin, resulting from hot and humid conditions.

heatstroke heat exhaustion.

hebephrenia schizophrenia marked chiefly by childish behavior, hallucinations, and regressive response. **—hebephreniac** *n.* **—hebephrenic** *adj.*

hebetic relating to youth.

hebetude emotional disinterest; lethargy.

hebosteotomy surgical enlargement of the opening of the bony pelvis to facilitate childbirth.

hederiform (of specific sensory nerve endings in the skin) ivy-shaped.

hedonophobia an abnormal fear of pleasure or of having fun.

hedrocele prolapse of part of the intestine through the anus; proctocele.

Heimlich maneuver an emergency technique for dislodging a gob of food from the windpipe by grasping the victim from behind, clasping one hand over the other just under the sternum, and pulling upward abruptly and firmly.

helcoid resembling an ulcer.

helcoplasty the repair of ulcers by the use of skin grafts, being a form of dermatoplasty.

helcosis the development of an ulcer; ulceration.

helicine relating to a coil or helix; spiral.

helicoid resembling a helix or spiral.

heliencephalitis inflammation of the brain as a consequence of sunstroke.

helioaerotherapy treatment involving exposure to sunlight and fresh air.

heliopathy any injury incurred as a result of exposure to sunlight.

heliophobia an abnormal fear of being exposed to the rays of the sun.

heliosis sunstroke.

heliotherapy treatment by exposure to sunlight.

helix *pl.* **helices** *also* **helixes** 1. the inward-curving rim of the outer ear. 2. one of the two coiled strands forming the structure of DNA.

helminth a parasitic worm esp. of the intestine. —**helminthic** *adj.*

helminthiasis infestation with parasitic worms.

helminthoid wormlike.

helminthology the study of parasitic worms.

heloma a corn.

helosis the condition of having corns on the feet or toes.

helotomy the surgical removal of a corn or corns.

hem- *or* **hemo-** *or* **haem-** *or* **haemo-** *prefix* blood.

hema- *or* **haema-** *prefix* blood.

hemachrosis unusual redness of the blood.

hemadostenosis a narrowing or contraction of the arteries.

hemagglutinate to cause agglutination of red blood cells. —**hemagglutination** *n.*

hemagglutinin an agent that causes hemagglutination.

hemagogue 1. promoting or enhancing the flow of blood. 2. an agent that promotes the flow of blood.

hemal relating to, involving, or affecting the blood or blood vessels.

hemanalysis laboratory examination or analysis of a sample of blood.

hemangio- *prefix* relating to or involving the blood vessels.

hemangioma a benign tumor made up of blood vessels.

hemangiosarcoma a malignant tumor made up of blood vessels.

hemarthrosis the abnormal presence of blood in a joint.

hematemesis the vomiting of blood or food mixed with blood.

hemathermal *also* **hemathermous** warm blooded.

hemathidrosis *also* **hematidrosis** an abnormal condition in which a person's sweat contains traces of blood.

hematic 1. relating to the blood. 2. any drug used in the treatment of anemia.

hematimeter a device used to count the number of blood cells in one cubic millimeter of blood.

hematin the portion of the hemoglobin molecule containing iron in the ferric state.

hematinemia the presence of heme in the circulating blood.

hematinic 1. relating to the blood. 2. any agent that

increases the concentration of hemoglobin or the number of red blood cells in the circulating blood, used in the treatment of anemia.

hematinuria the abnormal presence of heme in the urine.

hematischesis the control or arrest of bleeding.

hematobium any parasite that lives in the blood.

hematoblast an immature or primitive cell from which all blood cells are derived. Also called *hemocytoblast.*

hematocele 1. a blood cyst. 2. the abnormal accumulation of blood within a bodily canal or cavity. 3. swelling caused by effusion of blood into the sheath surrounding a testicle.

hematocelia bleeding into the peritoneal cavity.

hematochezia the passage of feces containing blood.

hematochyluria the abnormal presence of both blood and chyle in the urine.

hematocolpometra the accumulation of menstrual blood in the uterus and vagina, usually due to an obstruction of normal outflow by an intact hymen.

hematocrit 1. a centrifuge for separating the solid constituents of a blood sample from the plasma. 2. the percentage (by volume) of red blood cells in a sample of blood that has been centrifuged (which causes the cells to become packed in one end of the test tube or other container).

hematocystis an abnormal effusion of blood into the urinary bladder.

hematocyturia the presence of red blood cells (rather than just hemoglobin) in the urine. Compare *hemoglobinuria.*

hematogenesis the production of blood cells; hemopoiesis. —**hematogenic** *adj.* —**hematogenous** *adj.*

hematoglobin *also* **hematoglobulin** hemoglobin.

hematoid resembling blood; bloody; sanguineous.

hematology the study of the structure, functions, and diseases of blood and blood-forming tissues. —**hematologist** *n.*

hematoma *pl.* **hematomas** *or* **hematomata** a swelling or tumor composed of clotted blood.

hematometra an accumulation of blood within the cavity of the uterus.

hematomyelia bleeding into the substance of the spinal cord, usually as a response to injury.

hematopenia a deficiency in the size or number of the blood cells.

hematophagia 1. (esp. of leeches or animals such as vampire bats) subsistence on the blood of other animals. 2. the drinking of blood as a supposed means of curing a disease or disorder.

hematophagous (esp. of certain insects) surviving on a diet of blood.

hematopoiesis normal generation of blood cells in bone marrow.

hematopsia bleeding into the eye.

hematorrhachis bleeding of or into the spine; spinal hemorrhage.

hematosalpinx the abnormal accumulation of blood within a bodily tube, esp. a fallopian tube.

hematoscheocele the abnormal accumulation of blood within the cavity of the scrotum.

hematospectroscopy the examination of a sample of blood with the use of a spectroscope.

hematuria the presence of blood or blood cells in the urine.

heme the portion of hemoglobin that carries oxygen and gives the blood its characteristic color.

hemeralopia reduced visual capacity in the presence of bright light.

hemi- *prefix* one half.

hemiopalgia pain in one eye, usually associated with migraine.

hemiplegia paralysis of one side of the body. —**hemiplegic** *adj.*

hemochromatosis an iron metabolism disorder characterized by bronzing of the skin from iron-containing pigments deposited in the tissues.

hemodialysis purification or filtration of the blood, as with an artificial kidney, through dialysis.

hemoglobin an iron-containing respiratory pigment in the red blood cells.

hemoglobinemia the presence of free hemoglobin in the blood plasma.

hemoglobinuria the presence of free hemoglobin in the urine. —**hemoglobinuric** *adj.*

hemolysin a substance causing the breakdown of red blood cells.

hemolysis the breakdown or destruction of red blood cells. —**hemolytic** *adj.*

hemolytic anemia a condition caused by the premature destruction of red blood cells.

hemophilia a hereditary blood defect of males marked by delayed clotting of the blood and a tendency to hemorrhage after the slightest injury. —**hemophiliac** *n. & adj.* —**hemophilic** *adj.*

hemopoiesis the production of blood or blood cells in the body.

hemoptysis the coughing or spitting up of blood or sputum mixed with blood.

hemorrhage a heavy outpouring of blood from the blood vessels. —**hemorrhage** *vb.* —**hemorrhagic** *adj.*

hemorrhoids varicose dilation of veins near or at the anal sphincter. Also called *piles.* —**hemorrhoidal** *adj.*

hemostasis 1. the arresting of bleeding. 2. stagnation of the blood.

hemostat a surgical clamp for compressing a blood vessel that is bleeding.

hemostatic 1. stopping hemorrhage. 2. an agent that stops hemorrhage.

hemotoxin any substance, esp. one of biological origin, that causes destruction of red blood cells.

hemp a plant, *Cannabis sativa,* from which the drugs marijuana and hashish are derived.

heparin a polysaccharide acid ester occurring esp. in the liver and useful in prolonging blood clotting time, as in the treatment of thrombosis and embolism.

hepat- *or* **hepato-** *prefix* 1. liver. 2. hepatic.

hepatalgia pain in the liver.

hepatatrophia *also* **hepatatrophy** a wasting away or atrophy of the liver.

hepatectomy surgical excision of part of the liver. **—hepatectomize** *vb.*

hepatic relating to, resembling, or affecting the liver.

hepatitis inflammation of the liver.

hepatocele herniation of part of the liver through the diaphragm or the abdominal wall.

hepatography X-ray photography of the liver.

hepatolithiasis the presence of calculi in the liver.

hepatologist an expert on the liver and the treatment of diseases that affect it.

hepatology the branch of medical science concerned with the liver and the diagnosis and treatment of diseases that affect it.

hepatoma a tumor of the liver.

hepatomegaly abnormal enlargement of the liver.

hepatopathy any disease of the liver.

hepatosplenomegaly abnormal enlargement of both the liver and spleen.

hepatotoxic capable of causing toxic damage to the liver. **—hepatotoxicity** *n.*

hereditary genetically transmittable or transmitted from generation to generation; inheritable or inherited.

heredity the sum of the genetic characteristics transmitted from one generation to the next chiefly through the chromosomes of the germ cells.

hermaphrodite one having sexual tissues or genitals of both sexes. **—hermaphroditic** *adj.* **—hermaphroditism** *n.*

hernia *pl.* **hernias** *or* **herniae** the protrusion of an organ or part through the wall or cavity within which it is normally contained. Also called rupture. **—hernial** *adj.*

herniate to develop a hernia.

heroin a narcotic drug obtained from morphine, formerly used as an antitussive but now rendered illegal in the U.S. because of its addictive properties and potential for abuse.

herpangina a children's disease, characterized by sore throat, pain, headache, loss of appetite, and other symptoms, usually caused by a coxsackievirus.

herpes any of various inflammatory viral diseases marked by clusters of vesicles. **—herpetic** *adj.*

herpes simplex a viral disease marked by clusters of watery vesicles on the mucous membranes chiefly of the lips, mouth, or genitals.

herpes zoster shingles.

heterosexual relating to relationships with the opposite sex.

hexachlorophene an antibacterial agent used in some soaps and detergents.

hexylresorcinol a broad-spectrum drug used in the treatment of worm infestations.

hiatus any gap, opening or fissure.

hiatus hernia *also* **hiatal hernia** an abnormal condition in which a portion of the top part of the stomach protrudes up through a gap in the diaphragm.

hiccup *also* **hiccough** repeated spasmodic inhalation of the breath accompanied by closure of the glottis and by a characteristic explosive sound. —**hiccup** *or* **hiccough** *vb.*

hidrosis the secretion of sweat; perspiration. —**hidrotic** *adj.*

high *Slang* intoxicated with drugs or alcohol. —**high** *n.*

hindbrain the division of the embryonic brain that develops into the cerebellum, pons, and medulla oblongata.

hip the upper part of the thigh.

hip joint the articulation between the innominate bone and the femur.

Hippocratic oath an oath traditionally taken by those entering medical practice that embraces a code of medical ethics attributed to the Greek physician Hippocrates, born about 460 B.C. and known as the "Father of Medicine".

hirsute 1. having hair; hairy. 2. relating to hirsutism.

hirsutism pronounced or excessive growth of hair esp. on the body.

histamine a compound found esp. in animal tissue and in ergot that causes dilation of the blood vessels in many allergic reactions. —**histaminic** *adj.*

histogenesis the formation and differentiation of animal tissues. —**histogenetic** *adj.*

histology a branch of anatomy dealing with the microscopic study of tissues. —**histological** *adj.*

histolysis the disintegration or degeneration of tissues.

hives urticaria.

Hodgkin's disease a neoplastic disease that is marked chiefly by enlargement of the lymph glands, liver, and spleen and by progressive anemia.

holistic pertaining to treatment directed at the whole person, including psychological, social, emotional, and other factors.

homeopath a practitioner of homeopathy.

homeopathy the treatment of a disease by administering minute doses of a substance or agent that in large doses in a healthy person would produce symptoms of the disease itself. —**homeopathic** *adj.*

homeostasis the automatic self-regulation of bodily functions under environmental variations, resulting in a basic balance or equilibrium of temperature, blood pressure, water content, blood sugar, etc.

homoerotic homosexual. —**homoeroticism** *n.*

homologous having the same relative position, structure, or function.

homosexual relating to or practicing homosexuality —**homosexual** *n.*

homosexuality sexual desire toward or sexual activity practiced with members of one's own sex.

hookworm a parasitic nematode worm that attaches to the intestinal wall of the host and is a serious bloodsucking pest.

hormone a chemical substance secreted directly into the bloodstream by the endocrine glands which has a specific effect on cells remote from its point of origin. —**hormonal** *adj.*

hot flash a temporary feeling of warmth experienced by some women during menopause. The causes are unknown but hot flashes are harmless.

housemaid's knee a swelling of the knee due to enlargement of the bursa in front of the patella and caused typically by prolonged kneeling on a hard surface or substance.

humerus the bone of the upper arm.

Hutchinson's freckle an often malignant, dark patch of skin occurring on one side of the face on an elderly person.

hydantoin an anticonvulsant drug, similar to a barbiturate.

hydatid a fluid-filled cyst, esp. one caused by the dog tapeworm *Echinococcus granulosis.*

hydr- *or* **hydro-** *prefix* water.

hydrocephalus *also* **hydrocephaly** an abnormal increase in the amount of cerebrospinal fluid in the cranium resulting in enlargement of the skull and atrophy of the brain.

hydrochloric acid an important ingredient of gastric juice.

hydrocortisone *or* **cortisol** a natural steroid hormone synthesized for use as an anti-inflammatory agent in drugs.

hydrogen peroxide an anti-infective liquid used to cleanse open wounds, as a mouthwash, etc.

hydrophobia rabies.

hydrotherapy the scientific use of water in treating disease. —**hydrotherapeutic** *adj.*

hygiene the science and practice of maintaining good health. —**hygienic** *adj.*

hymen a membranous fold partially closing the entrance to the vagina; maidenhead. —**hymeneal** *adj.*

hyper- *prefix* excessive; above.

hyperacidity excessively acid. —**hyperacid** *adj.*

hypercalcemia the presence of abnormally large amounts of calcium in the blood.

hypercalciuria the presence of abnormally large amounts of calcium in the urine.

hypercholesterolemia the presence of abnormally large amounts of cholesterol in the blood.

hyperglycemia the presence of abnormally large amounts of glucose in the blood.

hyperkalemia the presence of abnormally large amounts of potassium in the blood.

hypernatremia the presence of abnormally large amounts of sodium in the blood.

hyperopia the condition of being farsighted.

hypersensitive abnormally susceptible to a drug, antigen, or other agent. —**hypersensitivity** *n.*

hypertension blood pressure exceeding normal limits.

hypertrophy enlargement of an organ caused by enlargement of its cells.

hyperventilation excessive respiration caused by asthma, the early stages of emphysema, etc., and resulting in chest pain, dizziness, etc.

hypnosis a state resembling sleep that is induced by a hypnotist and in which the subject readily responds to suggestion. —**hypnotist** *n.* —**hypnotize** *vb.*

hypnotic 1. tending to induce sleep; soporific. 2. an agent that induces sleep.

hypo- *or* **hyp-** *prefix* 1. under; down. 2. less than normal.

hypoacidity a condition caused by the insufficient secretion of hydrochloric acid into the gastric juice.

hypochondria a depressed state of mind often centering on concern for imaginary illnesses. —**hypochondriac** *n. & adj.* —**hypochondriacal** *adj.*

hypochondriasis hypochondria.

hypodermic 1. relating to the parts beneath the skin. 2. adapted for injection beneath the skin: *hypodermic needle.*

hypoglycemia the absence of glucose in the blood in normal amounts, usually caused by insulin imbalance or diet, and possibly fatal if not treated.

hypokalemia the absence of normal amounts of potassium in the blood.

hyponatremia the absence of normal amounts of sodium in the blood.

hypothalamus the portion of the brain that controls the peripheral autonomic nervous system, and endocrine and other functions, as sleep, appetite, body temperature, etc.

hypothermia a dangerous condition in which the body temperature is below 95°F.

hypoxemia the absence of normal amounts of oxygen in the blood of the arteries.

hysterectomy surgical removal of the uterus.

hysteria a psychoneurotic disorder marked by extreme excitability and disturbances of various psychic and physical functions.

I

iatrogenic caused by a treatment, medical personnel, or by exposure in a medical care facility: *iatrogenic disease.*

iatrology medical science.

ibuprofen a substitute for aspirin that acts to reduce pain and fever.

ichthyoid shaped like a fish.

ichthyophagy the habit or practice of subsisting on fish.

ichthyophobia an abnormal fear of fish, whether living or dead.

ichthyosis a dry, scaly skin condition.

ichthyotoxin a toxic substance found in the roe of certain fishes.

ichthyotoxism poisoning caused by eating toxic fish roe, characterized by disorders of the nervous system and gastrointestinal tract.

ICSH *abbr.* interstitial cell-stimulating hormone.

ictal relating to or caused by a seizure or stroke.

icteric relating to or characterized by jaundice (icterus).

ictero- *prefix* relating to jaundice (icterus).

icterogenic causing jaundice.

icterohematuric relating to jaundice associated with blood in the urine.

icterohepatitis inflammation of the liver (hepatitis) marked by jaundice.

icterus jaundice.

id (in Freudian theory of psychoanalysis) one of the three basic divisions of the psyche, considered to be the most primitive part of the personality and accounting for simple drives and instinctive behaviour. Compare *ego, superego.*

identical twins monozygotic twins.

identity crisis a psychiatric disorder in which a person loses his sense of self and of relationship with others.

idiocy a condition of severely marked low intellectual capacity, typically with a functional IQ below 75.

idiopathic relating to any state or condition of unknown cause: *idiopathic disease.*

idiot one marked with idiocy.

idiot savant a severely mentally handicapped person capable of doing complicated arithmetic calculations in his head with great speed.

Ig immunoglobulin.

ileitis inflammation of the ileum.

ileostomy the surgical construction of a communicating passage through the abdominal wall to the ileum.

ileum the distal section of the small intestine.

ilium the upper part of the innominate bone.

imbalance any abnormal quantity of substances in the body that may lead to illness.

imbecility a condition of marked mental incapacity. **—imbecile** *n.*

immune response a normal reaction by the body to produce antibodies that destroy foreign antigens and malignancies.

immunity a condition of resistance to infection.

immunization the procedure or technique of bringing about or increasing a state of immunity in an individual, as by theinjection of a vaccine or other agent into the body or taking an oral substance that provides protection against a specific disease.

immunoglobulin any one of five kinds of antibodies produced by the body to destroy foreign antigens and malignancies.

immunosuppressive 1. relating to any of various drugs that act to suppress the body's natural immune response, used esp. to permit the surgical transplant of a foreign organ or tissue by inhibiting its biological rejection. 2. a drug with this action.

immunotherapy therapy aimed at the production of immunity in the patient.

immunotoxin any antitoxin.

impacted pressed or jammed together or against something else: *impacted teeth.*

impaction the state or condition of being impacted.

impalpable incapable of being detected by means of the sense of touch.

impaludism malaria.

imparidigitate possessing an odd number of toes or fingers.

impatent not open or patent; closed.

imperception the inability to form a mental image of an object subjected to the senses; inadequate or insufficient perception.

imperforate lacking an opening; closed. —**imperforation** *n.*

impermeable not capable of being penetrated; impervious to fluids.

impetigo a contagious skin rash.

implant 1. to graft or insert. 2. the material grafted or inserted. —**implantation** *n.*

impotence *also* **impotency** inability in the male to achieve erection of the penis. —**impotent** *adj.*

impotentia impotence.

impregnate 1. to cause to conceive. 2. to fill or permeate with some other substance; saturate. —**impregnation** *n.*

impressio *pl.* **impressiones** an indentation or impression apparently made by the pressure of one structure or part upon another.

impulsive relating to actions or behavior actuated by an impulse rather than conscious thought or reason.

imus (or a structure or part compared with a similar neighbor) lowermost; being most caudal or inferior.

inanition extreme weakness or lack of strength and drive due to dietary insufficiency or failure of the digestive system to assimilate food.

inappetence absence of craving or desire; lethargy.

inarticulate unable to speak or communicate clearly or intelligibly.

in articulo mortis at the time of death.

incise to cut with a knife or knife-like instrument.

incision 1. a separation or division of soft tissue with a scalpel or other knife-like instrument. 2. a cut or surgical wound.

incisor any one of the eight front teeth, four in each jaw.

incisura incision.

incisure a notch or incision.

incontinence inability of the body to control the elimination of urine (urinary incontinence) or feces (fecal incontinence). —**incontinent** *adj.*

incrustation the formation over a healing wound of a crust or scab.

incubation 1. the technique or practice of maintaining tissue cultures or microorganisms at a controlled temperature that favors their growth or development. 2. care of a premature baby in an incubator. 3. the period of time from exposure to an infecting microorganism to the first appearance of the signs or symptoms of the disease it causes.

incubator 1. an apparatus in which premature babies are placed and maintained at the optimum temperature and humidity. 2. any container or receptacle for the incubation of tissue cultures or microorganisms.

incubus a nightmare.

incus one of the three tiny conducting bones of the middle ear; anvil.

indigestion difficulty in digesting food or imperfect digestion, characterized by a burning sensation in the stomach or lower part of the esophagus (heartburn) and the formation of gas in the stomach, usually relieved by taking antacids; dyspepsia. —**indigestible** *adj.*

indomethacin a powerful anti-inflammatory drug used in the treatment of rheumatoid arthritis and other forms of joint inflammation.

induce to cause deliberately: *induced fever.*

indurated (of the normally soft tissues of the body) hardened; becoming firm or firmer. —**indurative** *adj.*

inebriant 1. intoxicating. 2. a drug or agent able to cause intoxication or drunkenness. —**inebriation** *n.*

inebriety the chronic consumption of excessive amounts of alcoholic beverages.

inert 1. slow; sluggish. 2. not active. 3. having no therapeutic or pharmacologic properties or action: *an inert chemical.*

in extremis at the point of death.

infant a baby, esp. one less than a year old. —**infancy** *n.*

infanticide the murder of a child.

infantile paralysis poliomyelitis.

infarct a necrotic area in an organ or tissue resulting from circulatory blockage. —**infarction** *n.* —**infarcted** *adj.*

infection invasion of the body by pathogenic organisms or the clinical signs and symptoms of such an invasion. **—infectious** *adj.*

infectious hepatitis an acute viral inflammation of the liver marked by fever, jaundice, and nausea.

infectious mononucleosis an acute infectious viral disease primarily affecting the lymph glands, which become swollen and tender. Also called *glandular fever.*

infecundity the inability of a woman to conceive; female sterility or barrenness.

inferior (of a structure or part) situated lower or below another structure or part; caudal.

inferiority complex acute feelings of lack of personal worth typically manifested in timidity or in overagressiveness resulting from overcompensation.

infertility the inability to conceive or father offspring. **—infertile** *adj.*

infirm weak or feeble, esp. as the result of old age or a debilitating illness. **—infirmity** *n.*

infirmary a small hospital or medical center for the care and treatment of the ill or infirm, esp. one attached to a school or college.

inflammation the changes that take place in tissues in response to local damage, typically characterized by pain, heat, swelling, reddening and an interruption of function in the affected area.

inflammatory relating to or characterized by inflammation: *inflammatory disease.*

influenza an acute contagious viral disease affecting esp. the respiratory tract. **—influenzal** *adj.*

infraction *also* **infracture** a fracture, esp. one in which the broken bones are not displaced.

infrahyoid (of certain muscles) situated below the hyoid bone.

infundibulum any funnel-shaped structure or part, esp.

the stalk-like extension by which the pituitary gland is attached to the base of the brain.

infuse 1. to administer a drug, nutrient, etc., into a vein or between the tissues. 2. to brew or steep an herb in water.

ingest to introduce food or drink into the stomach through the mouth. —**ingestion** *n.* —**ingestive** *adj.*

ingrown hair a hair that has become imbedded in the skin because of a blocked follicle, etc.

ingrown toenail a condition in which a sliver of nail growing along the side of a nail, has begun to grow into the tissue at the side.

inguinal relating to or located near the groin.

inhalation therapy the therapeutic use of a nebulized solution of drugs or other therapeutic agents which the patient breathes in.

inhale to breathe in; take air or gas into the lungs. —**inhalation** *n.*

inject to introduce (fluid) into the body by means of a syringe. —**injection** *n.*

inner ear labyrinth.

innervate to supply with nerves. —**innervation** *n.*

inoculate any method for introducing an immunizing substance through the skin, as by injection, scarification, etc.

inquest a judicial inquiry into the causes of a death.

insanity a deranged state of the mind; madness. —**insane** *adj.*

insecticide an insect-killer.

inseminate to introduce semen into the vagina or uterus of a female.

insemination the deposition of semen within the vagina during sexual intercourse or introduced artificially (artificial insemination).

insensible 1. not appreciable by the senses. 2. not conscious.

insidious developing for a period before being detected: *insidious disease.*

in situ in a natural or original position.

insomnia inability to fall or stay asleep. —**insomniac** *n.*

inspiration the act of inhaling; inhalation.

insufflate to blow a medication into a bodily cavity or to distend it, by blowing, for examination.

insulin a hormone secrcted by the islets of Langerhans in the pancreas and crucial to the metabolism of carbohydrates, also used in the treatment and control of diabetes mellitus.

insulinemia the presence of an abnormally large amount of insulin in the circulating blood.

insulin shock coma resulting from excessive amounts of insulin in the system.

insuloma a tumor of the islets of Langerhans of the pancreas (an adenoma).

integument an enveloping membrane or skin.

intelligence quotient a number indicating the apparent intelligence level of a person and arrived at by dividing the mental age by the chronological age and multiplying by 100. Also called *IQ.*

intensive care unit a department of a hospital specializing in the treatment and close monitoring of patients with the most serious life-threatening afflictions.

inter- *prefix* between; among.

intercostal between the ribs.

intergyral between the convolutions (gyri) of the cerebral cortex.

intermittent fever a fever that comes and goes, as in malaria.

intern a recent graduate of a medical school undergoing

training at a hospital, usually for a period of one year, before becoming fully qualified to practice.

internal ear labyrinth.

internal medicine a branch of medicine dealing with the diagnosis and treatment of diseases not requiring surgery, esp. those involving the internal organs of the chest and abdomen.

internist a physician specializing in internal medicine.

internuncial (of a neuron) connecting two other neurons.

interstitial situated between the cellular components of an organ or part.

interstitial between the tissues: *interstitial emphysema.*

intervertebral disk disk.

intestinal relating to, affecting, or occurring in the intestine.

intestinal flu gastroenteritis caused by a virus in the intestinal tract.

intestine the tubular section of the alimentary canal extending from the stomach to the anus.

intima *pl.* **intimae** *or* **intimas** the innermost coat of an organ or artery.

intimitis inflammation of an intima.

intolerance exceptional sensitivity, as to a drug or medication.

intra- *prefix* 1. between. 2. during. 3. inward; within.

intracardiac occurring or existing within the heart.

intracranial occurring or existing within the cranium.

intradermal occurring, accomplished, or situated within the layers of the skin.

intramuscular characterizing an injection into a muscle.

intraocular pressure the pressure of the aqueous humor within the eye.

intrauterine device a device, as a metal or plastic coil or loop, inserted and left in the uterus to prevent conception. Also called *intrauterine contraceptive device; IUCD; IUD.*

intravenous within a vein: *intravenous injection.*

introvert one whose interests and concerns center primarily on the self. **—introverted** *adj.* **—introversion** *n.*

intubation the insertion of a tube into a hollow organ, as the trachea. **—intubate** *vb.*

intussusception the abnormal infolding of one segment of the intestine within another segment. **—intussusceptive** *adj.*

in utero within the uterus.

involution 1. a turning inward or rolling over of a rim. 2. any backward or retrograde change. 3. the shrinking back to normal size of the uterus after childbirth. 4. a physical decline in bodily vigor, as that associated with menopause in women.

iodide a compound, as a salt, of iodine.

iodinate to combine or treat with iodine.

iodine a nonmetallic element of the halogen group, essential in minute amounts in the diet (as in iodized table salt) for the proper development and functioning of the thyroid gland.

iodize to impregnate or treat with iodine.

ion an atom or atom group containing a positive or negative charge of electricity.

ipecac an emetic drug.

IQ intelligence quotient.

iridectomy surgical removal of part of the iris of the eye.

iridemia bleeding from the iris.

iris the pigmented diaphragm surrounding the pupil of the eye.

iritis inflammation of the iris of the eye.

iron a metallic element essential in the diet for the prevention of iron-deficiency anemia, the production of hemoglobin, and as an essential component of certain enzymes.

irradiation exposure to radiant energy, esp. to x ray in therapy.

irrigation the washing out or cleansing of a structure or part with water or other fluid. —**irrigate** *vb.*

irritant 1. tending to produce physical irritation. 2. something that irritates.

irritation a state of soreness or inflammation or irritability or overexcitation.

ischemia *also* **ischaemia** inadequate blood supply to an organ or part due to obstruction or constriction of the blood vessels. —**ischemic** *adj.*

ischium *pl.* **ischia** the posterior dorsal bone of the pelvis.

islets of Langerhans any of the groups of endocrine cells within the pancreas that secrete insulin.

isometrics a system of exercises stressing the contraction of opposing muscles in such a way that shortening is minimal but the increase in muscle fiber tone is great.

isopropyl alcohol the main ingredient of rubbing alcohol.

isthmus a contracted or restricted anatomical part connecting two larger bodily parts.

itching a persistent irritation of the cutaneous tissues that causes an urge to scratch and that is often held to result from mild stimulation of pain receptors. —**itch** *vb. & n.*

IUCD intrauterine contraceptive device.

IUD intrauterine device.

I.V. intravenous.

J

jactitation extreme restlessness; tossing from one side to the other.

jargon terms or expressions peculiar to a specific activity or field of interest: *medical jargon.*

jaundice yellowing of the skin, body fluids, and tissues resulting from the deposit of bile pigments. —**jaundiced** *adj.*

jaw either of the two bony structures within the mouth into which the teeth are set, forming an upper and immovable structure (maxilla) and a lower movable structure (mandible).

jejunectomy surgical removal of all or part of the jejunum.

jejunitis inflammation of the jejunum.

jejuno- *also* **jejun-** *prefix* relating to the jejunum.

jejunocolostomy the surgical formation of an artificial opening between the jejunum and the colon.

jejunoileal relating to both the jejunum and the ileum.

jejunoileitis inflammation of both the jejunum and the ileum; inflammation of the small intestine.

jejunojejunostomy the surgical formation of an artificial junction between two portions of the jejunum, as to bypass a diseased or permanently obstructed area.

jejunostomy the surgical formation of an artificial opening between the jejunum and the wall of the abdomen.

jejunotomy surgical incision into the jejunum.

jejunum the part of the small intestine between the duodenum and the ileum. —**jejunal** *adj.*

jet lag a sluggish, exhausted feeling experienced by airplane travelers who pass through several time zones. It is marked by irregular bowel movements, insomnia, and other symptoms which soon pass.

jogger's heel a painful condition caused by calcaneal spurs, bruising, bursitis, and other results of jogging and long-distance running.

joint a point of articulation between two or more bones.

jugular 1. of or relating to the throat or the neck. 2. a jugular vein.

jugular vein either of two large veins in the neck that return blood from the head.

jugulum the neck or throat.

jugum *pl.* **juga** 1. a ridge connecting two points. 2. a type of surgical forceps.

junctura a joint; articulation.

K

kabure a form of schistosomiasis occurring in Asia, esp. in Japan.

kainophobia an abnormal fear of things unfamiliar or new; neophobia.

kala-azar a tropical or subtropical infectious disease caused by a species of protozoa (*Leishmania donovani*) and transmitted by the bite of infected sandflies (*Phlebotomus* species).

kaliemia the presence of potassium in the blood.

kaolin a fine clay used as an absorbent in drugs to relieve diarrhea, usually combined with pectin.

karyogenesis the formation and development of the nucleus of a cell.

karyokinesis equal division of the nucleus during cell division. —**karyokinetic** *adj.*

karyology a branch of cytology that studies chromosomes and the nuclei of cells.

karyolysis the dissolution or destruction of the nucleus of a cell or its loss of ability to be stained by basic dyes. —**karyolytic** *adj.*

karyomitosis changes in the nucleus of a cell during cell division or mitosis.

karyomorphism the shape or form of the nucleus of a cell.

karyophage a parasitic protozoan within a cell that destroys its nucleus.

katabolism catabolism.

kathisophobia an abnormal fear of sitting down and remaining still.

kation cation.

keloid a dense scar resulting from growth of connective tissue.

kenophobia an abnormal fear of empty spaces.

keratectomy surgical removal of a portion of the cornea of the eye.

keratiasis the formation on the skin of horny warts.

keratic relating to horn or horny substances.

keratin a sulfur-containing fibrous protein constituting the basis of horny epidermal material, including the hair.

keratinize (of tissues) to make or become horny or hard.

keratitis inflammation of the cornea of the eye.

kerato- *also* **kerat-** *prefix* 1. the cornea. 2. a horny substance.

keratodermatitis inflammation of the horny layer of the skin.

keratogenous producing or causing the development of horny tissue.

keratohelcosis ulceration of the cornea.

keratoiritis inflammation of both the cornea and the iris.

keratolysis 1. periodic shedding of the skin. 2. a loosening of the skin's horny layer. —**keratolytic** *adj.*

keratoma a callus or horny growth.

keratomalacia a result of vitamin A deficiency of early childhood characterized by a softening of the cornea of the eye. Also called *xerotic keratitis.*

keratome a surgical knife for making incisions into the cornea of the eye.

keratometer a special instrument for measuring the curves of the cornea of the eye.

keratomycosis a fungal infection involving the cornea of the eye.

keratonyxis surgical puncture of the cornea.

keratoplasty surgical repair of the cornea.

keratosis any disorder characterized by overgrowth of horny material on the skin. —**keratotic** *adj.*

ketogenesis the generation of ketone bodies, as in diabetes.

ketone an organic compound having a carbonyl group linking two carbon atoms. —**ketonic** *adj.*

ketone body one of the three compounds, acetoacetic acid, beta-hydroxybutyric acid, and acetone found in the urine and blood esp. in diabetes mellitus.

ketosis an abnormal increase of ketone bodies, as in diabetes mellitus.

ketosteroid a steroid containing a ketone group.

kg *abbr.* kilogram.

kidney *pl.* **kidneys** either of a pair of bean-shaped organs, located near the spinal column behind the peritoneum, that excrete waste products of metabolism in the form of urine.

kilo- *prefix* one thousand.

kilogram one thousand grams. Abbr. *kg.*

kinaesthesia *or* **kinaesthesis** kinesthesia.

kinesia motion sickness.

kinesialgia pain caused by muscular activity.

kinesiology the branch of science concerned with the study of muscles, muscle groups, and muscular activity.

kinesioneurosis any functional disorder characterized by muscular spasms or tics.

-kinesis *suffix* movement.

kinesthesia *or* **kinesthesis** sensory awareness of bodily movements, as of muscles. —**kinesthetic** *adj.*

Klebsiella a genus of gram-negative bacteria associated with infections of the respiratory tract.

kleptomania a neurotic compulsion to steal without any economic need. —**kleptomaniac** *n.*

klieg eyes a condition of the eyes characterized by conjunctivitis and excessive watering and caused by prolonged exposure to very bright light.

knee a joint in the mid-part of the leg that connects the femur, tibia, and patella.

kneecap patella.

knee jerk an involuntary forward kick of the lower leg that results normally when the tendon below the patella is tapped lightly.

knock-knee a condition in which the legs turn inward at the knee. —**knock-kneed** *adj.*

knuckle a rounded prominence formed at the joining of two adjacent bones, esp. of a finger.

Koplik's spots a diagnostic sign of measles consisting of the development of tiny white spots on a red base on the inner surface of the cheeks, typically seen just before the appearance of the characteristic skin rash.

Korsakoff's syndrome *or* **Korsakoff's psychosis** an abnormal mental condition that is usually induced by chronic alcoholism and is marked chiefly by disorientation, hallucinations, and amnesia compensated for by confabulation.

kwashiorkor acute malnutrition in the young as the result of a diet low in protein and high in carbohydrates.

kyphosis abnormal curvature of the spine in a backward direction. —**kyphotic** *adj.*

L

labia *pl. of* labium.

labial of or relating to the lips or the labia.

labia majora the two fleshy, fatty outer lips that form the boundaries of the vulva.

labia minora the inner vascular lips of the vulva.

labio- *prefix* relating to lips.

labiochorea a chronic spasm of the lips, frequently presenting difficulty in producing clear speech sounds.

labioclination abnormal inclination of a tooth toward the lips.

labioglossolaryngeal relating to a paralysis affecting the lips, tongue and larynx.

labiomental relating to the lower lip and the extremity of the chin.

labiomycosis any fungal infection involving the lips.

labiopalatine relating to both the lips and the palate or roof of the mouth.

labioplacement (of a tooth or teeth) abnormal positioning toward the lips.

labor 1. the physiological activities that take place in the process of giving birth. 2. the period during which this takes place.

labrum *pl.* **labra** a lip or any structure or part shaped like or resembling a lip or lips.

labyrinth the bony and membranous structures that constitute the inner ear.

labyrinthectomy surgical removal of the labyrinth of the inner ear.

labyrinthitis inflammation of the labyrinth of the inner ear.

labyrinthotomy surgical incision into the labyrinth of the inner ear.

lacerate to tear roughly or jaggedly.

laceration a ragged, torn wound.

lacertus 1. any band of muscles or fibers. 2. the muscular part of the arm.

lachrymal *or* **lacrimal** of or relating to tears or to the glands that produce tears.

lacrimation the excessive formation and secretion of tears.

lacrimator any agent or substance that produces tears by its irritant effects on the eyes, such as tear gas.

lacrimatory causing the production of tears.

lacrimotomy surgical incision into the glands that produce tears.

lact- *or* **lacti-** *or* **lacto-** *prefix* milk.

lactate to secrete milk. —**lactation** *n.*

lacteal 1. relating to or like milk; milky. 2. a lymphatic vessel in which chyle is conveyed from the intestine.

lactescent resembling milk; milky.

lactic relating to milk.

lactiferous conveying or secreting milk: *lactiferous ducts.*

lactifuge any agent that arrests the flow of milk from the mammary glands.

lactigenous producing milk.

lactogen an agent that stimulates the production or secretion of milk.

lactogenesis milk production. —**lactogenic** *adj.*

lactovegetarian a vegetarian who includes dairy products in his diet, such as milk and cheese, as well as eggs.

lacus *pl.* **lacus** any very small collection or accumulation of fluid.

lacus lacrimalis a small space at the medial angle of the eye where tears collect after bathing the surface of the eyeball.

lagneia 1. sexual intercourse; coitus. 2. lust; sexual urge.

lagnesis *also* **lagnosis** excessive and persistent sexual desire in a man or woman; nymphomania or satyriasis.

lagophthalmos a neurological or muscular disorder in which the eye does not close completely.

lake (of blood in hemolysis) to change so that the hemoglobin is dissolved in the plasma.

-lalia *suffix* speech disorder.

laliophobia an abnormal fear of speaking or stuttering.

lallation a speech defect characterized by difficulty in enunciation of words that contain the letter *l*.

lalochezia psychological or emotional relief obtained by swearing or speaking obscene or vulgar words.

lalognosis the understanding of speech or spoken communication.

lalopathology a branch of science concerned with disorders of speech production and their treatment.

lalopathy any type of speech defect.

laloplegia paralysis of the muscles required in the production of speech sounds.

lalorrhea an excessive flow of words and phrases.

Lamaze method a method of natural childbirth.

lambdacism 1. difficulty in or inability to pronounce or articulate the letter *l*. 2. pronunciation of the letter *l* as the letter *r*.

lamella *pl.* **lamellae** any thin layer or sheet. **—lamellar** *adj.*

lamina *pl.* **laminae** 1. any flat layer or thin plate. 2. the flattened part on either side of a vertebral arch. **—laminar** *adj.*

laminectomy surgical removal of a vertebral lamina, esp. the posterior arch of a vertebra.

laminitis inflammation of a lamina.

laminotomy surgical incision into a vertebral lamina.

lance 1. to incise an abscess, boil, etc., as to permit the release of pus. 2. a lancet.

lancet a small, pointed, two-edged knife used in surgery.

lancinating (of pain) piercing, cutting, or extremely sharp; tearing.

Landsteiner's classification the system of ABO blood classification.

Langerhans' islets islets of Langerhans.

laniary (of the canine teeth) adapted for tearing.

lanolin wool grease refined esp. for use as the base of various ointments.

lanosterol a sterol found in wool fat.

lanthanides the rare earth elements.

lanthionine an amino acid obtained from wool.

lanuginous covered with soft hair; downy.

lanugo soft, downy hair covering the body.

lapactic laxative; purgative.

laparocele an abdominal hernia.

laparocolostomy the surgical formation of an artificial anus by creating a permanent opening between the colon and the abdominal wall.

laparocolotomy surgical incision through the abdominal wall to the colon; colotomy.

laparocystectomy surgical removal of an ovarian cyst or cystlike tumor through an incision made in the abdominal wall.

laparocystotomy removal of the contents of an ovarian

cyst or cystlike tumor by means of a surgical incision in the abdominal wall.

laparoenterostomy surgical formation of an artificial anus by means of an incision into the loin.

laparohepatotomy surgical incision into the liver from the side.

laparohysterectomy surgical removal of the uterus (hysterectomy) by means of an abdominal incision.

laparomyositis inflammation of the lateral muscles of the abdominal wall.

laparonephrectomy surgical removal of the kidney by means of an incision in the loin.

laparosalpingectomy surgical removal of a fallopian tube by means of an abdominal incision.

laparoscopy examination of the peritoneal cavity through the abdominal wall by means of a laparoscope, a lighted tube with optical devices.

laparosplenectomy surgical removal of the spleen by means of an incision in the abdominal wall.

laparosplenotomy surgical incision into the spleen through the abdominal wall.

laparotomize to subject (a patient) to laparotomy.

laparotomy *pl.* **laparotomies** surgical section of the abdominal wall.

large intestine a part of the digestive tract between the cecum and the rectum.

laryngeal of or relating to the larynx.

laryngectomy *pl.* **laryngectomies** surgical removal of all or part of the larynx.

laryngitic relating to or caused by inflammation of the larynx.

laryngitis inflammation of the larynx.

laryngo- *also* **laryng-** *prefix* relating to the larynx.

laryngograph an instrument for measuring the movements of the larynx by means of a tracing (laryngogram).

laryngology a branch of medicine dealing with diseases of the larynx and nasopharynx.

laryngomalacia an abnormal softening of the cartilages of the larynx.

laryngoparalysis paralysis of the muscles of the larynx.

laryngopathy any disease or disorder affecting the larynx.

laryngopharyngectomy surgical removal of part of the larynx and pharynx, as in the treatment of cancer.

laryngopharyngitis inflammation of both the larynx and pharynx.

laryngoscope an instrument for visual examination of the larynx. **—laryngoscopic** *adj.* **—laryngoscopist** *n.* **—laryngoscopy** *n.*

laryngostenosis abnormal narrowing or stricture of the lumen of the larynx.

laryngostomy the surgical formation of a permanent opening from the neck into the larynx.

laryngotome a surgical knife for making incisions into the larynx.

larynx *pl.* **larynges** the upper part of the trachea that contains the vocal cords.

laser a device that produces a beam of coherent light, used in surgery.

Lassa fever a viral disease first noted in Nigeria in 1969, characterized by high fever, headache, facial flushes, vomiting and bleeding from the skin and mucous membranes, thought to be transmitted by a species of rat.

lassitude a feeling of profound weakness; fatigue.

latent present but not active or visible: *latent infection.* **—latency** *n.*

lateral relating to, situated on, or coming from the side. **—laterally** *adv.*

lateralis lateral; at the side.

latissimus dorsi a large, triangular muscle of the back, extending on each side from the spine upward and outward with its apex under the arm.

laudanum a tincture that contains opium, formerly widely used as a pain killer.

laughing gas nitrous oxide.

lavage the therapeutic irrigation of a hollow organ, such as the stomach or lower intestine.

laxative any agent serving to relieve constipation; cathartic.

LD lethal dose.

L-dopa levodopa.

L.E. *abbr.* 1. left eye. 2. lupus erythematosus.

lead poisoning chronic poisoning that is the result of ingestion or absorption of lead and is characterized by colic, a dark line along the gums, and muscular paralysis.

Leboyer method a method of childbirth aimed at reducing the birth trauma for the infant.

leg either of the lower limbs, used for standing and moving.

Legionnaire's disease a sometimes fatal form of bacterial pneumonia with the symptoms of influenza.

leiodermia the condition of having abnormally smooth or glossy skin.

leiomyoma a benign tumor derived from smooth or nonstriated muscle.

leiomyomatosis the condition of having several leiomyomas in different parts of the body.

leiomyosarcoma a malignant tumor derived from smooth or nonstriated muscle.

leiotrichous having hair that is straight; straight-haired.

Leishmania a genus of parasitic protozoa.

leishmaniasis infection with protozoa of the genus *Leishmania,* one species of which causes the disease kala-azar.

leishmaniosis leishmaniasis.

leishmanoid any pathological condition that resembles the signs of leishmaniasis.

lemic relating to any epidemic disease, esp. the plague.

lens a transparent, nearly spherical body in the eye that focuses light rays upon the retina.

lenticular having the shape of or resembling a lens.

lenticulopapular (of a skin eruption) having papules that are shaped like a tiny dome or convex lens.

lentiform lenticular; shaped like a lens.

lentigo a benign, freckle-like colored spot on the skin.

leprology the branch of medical science concerned with the study and treatment of leprosy.

leprosy a chronic, communicable disease that is caused by a bacillus and is marked by the formation of granules on the skin that enlarge and spread, eventual paralysis of muscle, and the development of deformities. —**leprous** *adj.*

-lepsy *suffix* seizure: *catalepsy.*

lepto- *prefix* thin, slender or light; frail.

leptocephalous having an abnormally small head. —**leptocephalus** *n.*

leptochroa the condition of having skin that is abnormally delicate.

leptodermic characterized by or having abnormally thin skin.

leptomeninges the two inner membranes that envelop the brain and spinal cord; pia mater and arachnoid (as distinguished from the dura mater).

leptomeningitis inflammation of the pia mater and arachnoid; inflammation of the leptomeninges.

leptophonia the condition of having an abnormally weak voice. —**leptophonic** *adj.*

leptopodia the condition of having unusually narrow or slender feet.

leptoprosopia the condition of having an unusually narrow face.

leptospirosis an infectious disease caused by a spirochete transmitted in the urine of animals, esp. rats and dogs.

Lesbian *or* **lesbian** a female homosexual. —**lesbianism** *n.*

lesion an abnormal change in a part or tissue resulting from disease or injury.

lethal relating to or causing death; deadly; fatal. —**lethality** *n.* —**lethally** *adv.*

lethal dose the amount of anything, esp. a drug, that can cause death.

lethargy abnormal drowsiness, fatigue, or indifference. —**lethargic** *adj.*

lethe loss of memory; amnesia. —**letheral** *adj.*

leuk- *or* **leuko-** *or* **leuc-** *or* **leuco-** *prefix* white; colorless: *leukocyte.*

leukemia *also* **leukaemia** a malignant, progressive disease marked by an abnormal increase in the number of white blood cells in the tissues and in the blood. —**leukemic** *adj.*

leukocyte *or* **leucocyte** a white blood cell. —**leukocytic** *adj.*

leukocytoblast any immature cell that eventually develops into one of the white blood cells (leukocytes).

leukocytogenesis the formation and development of white blood cells; leukocytopoiesis.

leukocytoid resembling a white blood cell.

leukocytolysin any of various substances that cause the destruction or dissolution of white blood cells.

leukocytolysis the destruction or dissolution of white blood cells. —**leukocytolytic** *adj.*

leukocytoma the local accumulation of white blood cells in a dense mass.

leukocytopoiesis the formation and development of white blood cells; leukocytogenesis.

leukocytosis *or* **leucocytosis** an increased number of white blood cells in the circulating blood. —**leukocytotic** *adj.*

leukocytotoxin any toxic substance that causes the degeneration or destruction of white blood cells.

leukocyturia the presence of white blood cells in the urine.

leukoderma a partial or total absence of pigment in the skin. —**leukodermatous** *adj.*

leukodontia the desirable condition of having white teeth.

leukodystrophy the degeneration or destruction of the white matter of the brain, thought to be caused by a disorder of fat metabolism.

leukoencephalitis the inflammation of the white matter of the brain.

leukoma *or* **leucoma** a dense white opacity of the cornea of the eye.

leukopenia a condition in which there is an abnormally small number of white blood cells in the bloodstream. Also called *leukocytopenia.*

leukorrhea a whitish discharge from the vagina resulting from inflammation of its mucous membranes. —**leukorrheal** *adj.*

leukotomy the surgical division of nerve fiber tracts in the white matter of the frontal lobe of the cerebrum.

leukotrichia the state or condition of having white hair.

levallorphan tartrate a drug used to combat some of the effects of narcotics.

levator a muscle that raises a body part.

levodopa *or* **L-dopa** a drug prescribed in the treatment of Parkinson's and other diseases.

levulose fructose; fruit sugar.

Leydig's cells cells that produce testosterone in the testes.

libido, emotional or psychic energy, esp. sexual drive. —**libidinal** *adj.* —**libidinous** *adj.*

Librium a trade name for a tranquilizer.

lichen any of various skin diseases marked by patches of small, firm papules.

lid eyelid.

lidocaine hydrochloride a local anesthetic.

life-span 1. an individual's duration of existence. 2. the average duration of existence of the members of a particular species.

ligament a tough band of tissue that connects bones together at the joints or supports an organ in place. —**ligamentary** *adj.* —**ligamentous** *adj.*

ligation ligature.

ligature any of various threads or wires used in surgery to tie off or constrict a vessel or part.

light adaptation adaptation of the eye to intensified light through contraction of the pupil and a decrease in visual purple.

limbus the region forming a margin between the cornea and sclera of the eye.

liminal of or relating to a sensory threshold; barely perceptible.

limitrophic (of the sympathetic nervous system) governing or controlling nutrition.

limosis abnormal and persistent hunger.

lindane a drug applied topically against scabies and louse infestation.

linea any long, narrow strip or mark anatomically distinguished from the surrounding areas by its elevation, color or texture.

lingua *pl.* **linguae** the tongue or a structure or part that resembles the tongue.

lingual of, relating to, or lying near the tongue.

lingually in the direction of the tongue; toward the tongue.

linguo- *prefix* relating to the tongue.

liniment a liquid preparation used for soothing irritated skin or as a counterirritant or cleansing agent.

linolenic acid a liquid, fatty acid held to be essential to nutrition.

lip 1. either of the two fleshy folds forming the margins

lip- *or* **lipo-** *prefix* fat; fatty. of the mouth. 2. labium.

lipase any of various enzymes that dissolve or split fat.

lipectomy the surgical removal of fatty tissue.

lipemia the presence in the bloodstream of an abnormally large amount of fatty material.

lipid any type of fat (such as fatty acids) or fatlike substance (such as cholesterol).

lipidosis any disorder of fat metabolism.

lipoarthritis inflammation of the fatty tissues of joints.

lipoblast an immature fat cell.

lipoblastoma a tumor of fatty tissue; lipoma.

lipocardiac 1. relating to fatty degeneration of the heart. 2. a person who suffers from fatty degeneration of the heart.

lipochondroma a tumor that contains both fat and cartilage.

lipoclasis lipolysis; the splitting up of fat.

lipocyte a fat cell.

lipodystrophy a disorder of metabolism of fat that affects chiefly women and is marked by obesity of the buttocks and legs.

lipofibroma a fatty tumor that contains a relatively large amount of fibrous tissue. Also called *fibrolipoma.*

lipogenesis the formation and development of fats or fatty tissue. **—lipogenetic** *adj.*

lipogenic fat producing; lipogenetic.

lipogenous producing fat.

lipoid 1. resembling fat. 2. a lipid.

lipoidemia the presence in the bloodstream of an abnormally large quantity of lipids; lipemia.

lipoiduria lipids in the urine.

lipolysis the decomposition or dissolution of fat. **—lipolytic** *adj.*

lipoma *pl.* **lipomas** *or* **lipomata** a tumor of fatty tissue. **—lipomatous** *adj.*

lipomatosis a condition characterized by the excessive deposition of fat in the tissues.

lipoprotein a protein, produced mainly by the liver, which contains lipids.

liposarcoma a malignant cancer in fat cells.

lipostomy congenital absence of the mouth.

Lippes loop an S-shaped plastic intrauterine device.

liquor an aqueous solution of a drug.

lithiasis *pl.* **lithiases** the formation of stony concretions in the body.

lithium a metallic element compounds of which are used in drugs for the treatment of manic phases in manic-depressive disorders.

lithotomy *pl.* **lithotomies** surgical incision into the bladder to remove a stone.

lithotrite a device for crushing a stone in the urinary bladder so it can be passed in the urine.

liver a large vascular organ in the upper right part of the abdomen that secretes bile, maintains the composition of the blood, and regulates many important metabolic processes.

liver spot a darkish spot on the skin that occurs in older people.

lobar of or relating to a lobe.

lobar pneumonia infection of a lobe of the lung.

lobe a rounded protuberance of a bodily part or organ.

lobectomy surgical removal of a lobe of the lung.

lobotomize to perform a lobotomy on.

lobotomy *pl.* **lobotomies** surgical incision of some or all of the fibers of a lobe of the brain performed for the relief of some mental disorders.

lobule a small lobe or a subsection of a lobe. —**lobular** *adj.*

local anesthetic an anesthetic affecting only a part of the body.

localized restricted to a limited region or spot.

lockjaw 1. an initial symptom of tetanus in which spasms of the jaw muscles prevents opening of the jaws. 2. tetanus.

locomotor ataxia impairment in the coordination of bodily movements and irregularity of gait often occurring as a late symptom of syphilis.

locum tenens a person who substitutes for another, esp. a physician who temporarily takes over the responsibilities of another physician.

loin 1. the section on each side of the spinal column between the hipbone and the false ribs. 2. *pl.* the abdominal region about the hips including the pubic region. 3. *pl.* genitals.

Lomotil trade name for an anti-diarrheal drug.

long bone any of the large, elongated bones supporting a limb.

longevity a long duration of individual life.

lorazepam a tranquilizer.

lordosis abnormal curvature of the spine in a forward direction. —**lordotic** *adj.*

lotion a liquid preparation for cosmetic use or medicinal soothing of the skin.

Lou Gehrig's disease amyotrophic lateral sclerosis.

louse *pl.* **lice** any of several small wingless insects that are parasitic on warm-blooded animals.

lower respiratory tract the organs and areas involved in respiration consisting of the bronchi and the lungs. See also **upper respiratory tract.**

LSD lysergic acid diethylamide; an organic compound sometimes used experimentally in treating mental disorders and often having as side effects hallucinating and psychotic behavior.

lucid having full command of one's faculties; sane.

lues syphilis.

lumbago painful muscular rheumatism of the lumbar region.

lumbar of or relating to the loins or to the region of the back between the hipbone and the false ribs.

lumen *pl.* **lumina** *or* **lumens** the cavity within the tube of an organ or vessel.

Luminal trade name for phenobarbital.

lung either of two thoracic organs that are the chief functional organs of respiration.

lunule a crescent-shaped part of the body, as the light-colored area at the base of a nail.

lupus any of various diseases marked by skin lesions, as lupus erythematosus.

lupus erythematosus *or* **systemic lupus erythematosus** chronic inflammation of various systems of the body, including lesions of the skin and nervous system.

luteinizing hormone a hormone, produced by the anterior

pituitary, that induces the production of testosterone; in women, it stimulates the production of estrogen.

luxate to throw out of joint; dislocate. —**luxation** *n.*

lying-in the state or period attending childbirth; confinement.

Lyme arthritis an arthritis-like disease caused by the bite of a tick.

lymph a transparent, slightly yellowish liquid occurring in the lymphatic vessels, bathing the tissues, and carrying away wastes.

lymphadenitis inflammation of the lymphatic glands.

lymphangioma a benign skin tumor.

lymphangitis inflammation of a lymphatic vessel.

lymphatic pertaining to or involving lymph or a vessel transporting lymph.

lymph node *or* **gland** an oval structure in the lymphatic system that performs various functions.

lymphocyte either of two kinds of leukocytes that develop in bone marrow and constitute one quarter of the number of white blood cells.

lymphocytopenia a disorder resulting from an abnormally small number of lymphocytes.

lymphoma cancer of lymph tissue.

lysergide LSD.

lytic cocktail *Informal.* a drug mixture used as an anesthetic.

THE LACRIMAL APPARATUS

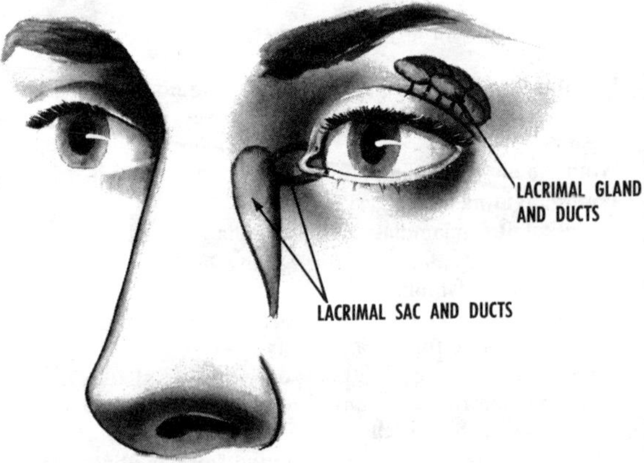

The lacrimal gland secretes tears which are poured over the eyes through small ducts. The tears collect in the inner corner of the eye and pass through two small openings into the lacrimal ducts and into the lacrimal sac. The sac empties into the nose.

THE NASAL CAVITY
(CROSS SECTION)

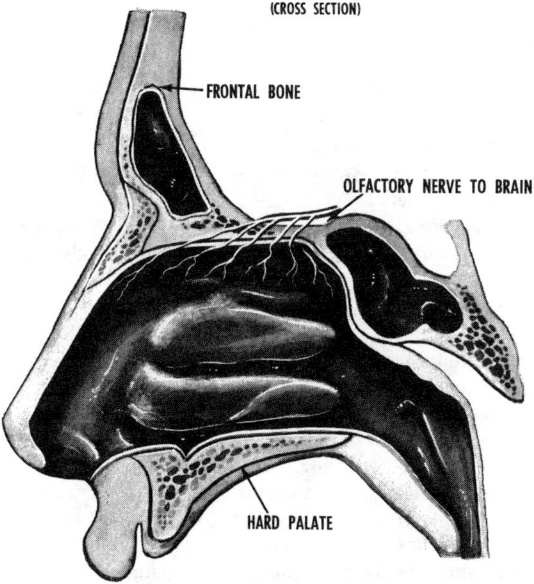

OLFACTORY SENSE

Specialized sensory neurons, capable of being stimulated by airborne odor particles, are located in the roof of the nasal cavity. The neurons collect into numerous small nerves which form the olfactory nerve. The odors most recognized are floral, fruity, herbal or spicy, resinal, and smoky.

M

maceration the softening of a solid by soaking it in a fluid substance. —**macerate** *vb.*

macies emaciation.

macrencephaly *also* **macrencephalia** extensive growth of the brain; the condition of having an unusually large brain.

macro- *or* **macr-** *prefix* large; long.

macrobiosis longevity; an unusually long span of life.

macrobiote any organism that is relatively long-lived.

macrobiotic 1. long-live. 2. tending to extend or prolong life.

macrobiotics the scientific study of factors that influence the prolongation of life.

macroblast a large immature red blood cell (erythroblast).

macroblepharia the state or condition of having unusually large eyelids.

macrobrachia the condition of having unusually long or large arms.

macrocardia the state or condition of having an abnormally enlarged heart. Also called *cardiomegaly.*

macrocardius a person with an abnormally large heart.

macrocephalous *or* **macrocephalic** having an abnormally large head or cranium. —**macrocephaly** *n.*

macrocephalus a fetus with an abnormally large head.

macrocheilia abnormal enlargement of the lips. Also called *macrolabia.*

macrocyte an abnormally large red blood cell occurring in various forms of anemia. —**macrocytic** *adj.*

macroscopic *also* **macroscopical** sufficiently large to be visible to the naked eye.

macula *pl.* **maculae** *or* **maculas** macule. —**macular** *adj.*

macule a discolored but not elevated spot on the skin.

mal any disease or disorder.

mal- *prefix* bad; ill.

malabsorption ineffective or faulty absorption of nutrient materials from the alimentary canal.

malacia an abnormal softening of an organ, structure or part.

-malacia *suffix* abnormal softening.

malaco- *prefix* soft; softening.

malacoma malacia.

malacosis malacia.

malacosteon abnormal softening of the bones; osteomalacia.

malacotic relating to or characterized by an abnormal softening of an organ, structure or part; relating to malacia.

malacotomy surgical incision into soft structures or parts, esp. those of the abdominal wall.

maladie malady; illness; disease.

malady any illness or disease, esp. one of a potentially serious nature.

malaise a general feeling of ill health or torpor often accompanying the onset of a determinable illness.

malar of or relating to the cheek or to the side of the head.

malaria an infectious, febrile protozoal disease transmitted by female *Anopheles* mosquitoes and characterized chiefly by intermittent attacks of chills and fever. —**malarial** *also* **malarian** *adj.*

malariology the branch of medical science concerned with the study and treatment of malaria.

malarious relating to or characterized by the presence or prevalence of malaria.

malassimilation inadequate, incomplete or faulty assimilation of food.

mal comitial epilepsy. See *grand mal* and *petit mal.*

maldigestion inadequate or incomplete digestion.

malemission the failure of semen to be ejaculated from the penis during sexual intercourse.

maleruption imperfect or faulty eruption of a tooth or teeth.

malformation irregular or faulty structure or formation.

malignant tending to produce severe deterioration or death: *malignant disease.* —**malignancy** *n.*

malinger to feign illness so as to avoid duty or work. —**malingerer** *n.* —**malingering** *n.*

malleation a nervous disorder characterized by the repeating hammering or beating of the hands against the thighs.

malleolus *pl.* **malleoli** *or* **malleoluses** a rounded protuberance, as that on either side of the ankle joint.

malleotomy surgical division of the malleus.

malleus the largest of the three conducting bones of the middle ear; hammer.

malnutrition inadequate or faulty nutrition caused by a disorder of assimilation, insufficient dietary intake, or chronic imbalance of the diet.

malocclusion incorrect alignment of the teeth when the jaws are closed, as caused by loss of teeth, imperfect development, or abnormal growth and development of the jaw bones.

maloplasty plastic surgery involving the cheek or cheeks.

malpractice negligent, improper or careless treatment of a patient by physicians, nurses or other qualified medical personnel.

maltase an enzyme active in the hydrolysis of maltose to glucose.

maltose a sugar obtained by the hydrolysis of starch.

malum any disease.

malum caducum epilepsy.

malum cordis heart disease.

malus venereum syphilis.

mamma *pl.* **mammae** a mammary gland; breast. —**mammate** *adj.*

mammal any individual belonging to the class Mammalia, characterized by being warm-blooded vertebrates that suckle their offspring.

mammalogy the branch of biological science concerned with the study of mammals.

mammaplasty *also* **mammoplasty** plastic reconstruction of a breast.

mammary of, relating to, or located near the breasts.

mammary gland either of two large, compound glands situated on the chest of female mammals and modified to secrete milk for the feeding of young.

mammectomy *pl.* **mammectomies** mastectomy; surgical removal of the breast.

mammiform having the shape of a breast; breast-shaped; resembling a breast or mammary gland.

mammill- *or* **mammilli-** *prefix* 1. relating to the nipple or nipples. 2. relating to any small, rounded elevation resembling a nipple.

mammilla *pl.* **mammillae** 1. the nipple. 2. any structure or part that resembles a nipple.

mammillary relating to or resembling a nipple.

mammillated possessing projections or elevations that resemble a nipple.

mammillation 1. the condition of possessing projections or elevations that resemble a nipple. 2. any elevation or projection that resembles a nipple.

mammilliform shaped like a nipple.

mammillitis inflammation of a nipple.

mammitis inflammation of a breast or mammary gland; mastitis.

mammo- *prefix* relating to the breasts or mammary glands.

mammogram an X-ray photograph of the breast or mammary gland.

mammography X-ray examination of the breasts.

mammoplasty mammaplasty.

mammose 1. resembling or shaped like a breast or mammary gland. 2. possessing unusually large breasts.

mammotomy surgical incision into the breast or mammary gland. Also called *mastotomy*.

mammotropic having a direct effect on stimulating the formation, development or growth of the breasts.

mandible the lower jaw.

mandibula *also* **mandibulum** the lower jaw or mandible.

mandibular relating to the lower jaw or mandible.

mandibulectomy surgical removal of part or all of the lower jaw.

mandibulofacial relating to both the lower jaw and the face.

maneuver any specific procedure or movement, esp. in surgery or obstetrics.

mania an abnormal psychic state marked chiefly by elation, disorganized behavior, and physical hyperactivity.

maniac madman; lunatic. —**maniacal** *adj.*

manic affected with or resembling mania.

manic-depressive marked by psychotic alternation

between seizures of mania and depression. —**manic-depressive** *n.*

manifestation (in medicine) the exhibition or development of specific diagnostic signs or symptoms of a disease or disorder.

maniphalanx any bony segment of a finger.

manometer any of various instruments for measuring gas or vapor pressure. —**manometric** *adj.* —**manometry** *n.*

mantle any layer that covers a structure or part.

manubrium *pl.* **manubria** an anatomical part or process shaped like a handle, esp. the upper part of the breastbone.

manus the hand.

manustupration masturbation.

marasmus progressive emaciation, esp. in the very young, resulting from malnutrition. —**marasmic** *adj.*

marcid wasting away or emaciating.

marcor marasmus.

margo margin or border; edge.

marihuana *or* **marijuana** cannabis.

mariposia the ingestion or drinking of sea water.

marmorated (of the skin) having a streaked or marble-like appearance.

marrow the soft, vascular substance that fills the cavities of most bones.

martial relating to or containing iron.

maschaladenitis inflammation of the axillary glands.

maschale axilla.

maschalephidrosis sweating in the armpits (axillae).

maschaloneus a tumor in the armpit or axilla.

maschalyperidrosis excessive sweating in the armpits.

masculine relating to or having male characteristics.

masculinity the sexual characteristics (primary and secondary) of the male.

masculinization the normal or (in women) abnormal development of male characteristics. —**masculinize** *vb.*

masculinus masculine.

masochism a form of sexual deviation in which pleasure is gained through being punished or humiliated. —**masochist** *n.* —**masochistic** *adj.*

masque mask.

massa a lump or mass; an accumulation of coherent material.

massage therapeutic stroking or kneading of the body, esp. to promote circulation of the blood or to relax muscles.

masseter a large, powerful muscle that raises the lower jaw and assists in chewing. —**masseteric** *adj.*

masseur a man skilled in massage and physiotherapy.

masseuse a woman skilled in massage and physiotherapy.

massotherapy the therapeutic use of massage.

mast- *or* **masto-** *prefix* breast; mammary gland.

mastadenitis inflammation of a breast or mammary gland; mastitis.

mastadenoma a benign tumor of the breast.

mastalgia pain in the breast. Also called *mastodynia.*

mastatrophy *also* **mastatrophia** a wasting away or atrophy of breast tissues; degeneration of the mammary glands.

mastauxe excessive growth of breast tissues; hypertrophy of the breasts.

mast cell a large cell occurring in connective tissue.

mastectomy *pl.* **mastectomies** surgical removal of a breast; mammectomy.

masthelcosis the formation of ulcers of the breasts; ulceration of the breast.

mastication the process of moving the jaws in chewing, esp. in preparation for swallowing food. —**masticate** *vb.* —**masticatory** *n.*

masticatus chewed or masticated.

mastitis inflammation of the breast or udder. —**mastitic** *adj.*

masto- *or* **mast-** *prefix* relating to or involving the breast.

mastodynia pain in the breast. Also called *mastalgia.*

mastoid 1. relating to or being a process of the temporal bone behind the ear. 2. resembling or shaped like a breast. —**mastoidal** *adj.*

mastoidectomy *pl.* **mastoidectomies** surgical removal of the mastoid process.

mastoiditis inflammation of the mastoid process.

mastoidotomy surgical incision into the mastoid process.

mastology the branch of medical science concerned with the anatomy, physiology and pathology of the breasts or mammary glands.

mastoncus a swelling or tumor of the breasts.

mastoparietal relating to the suture that unites the mastoid process and the parietal bone of the skull or to the bones themselves.

mastopathy any disease or disorder that involves the breasts or mammary glands.

mastopexy a surgical procedure for correcting excessively sagging breasts.

mastoplasia abnormal or excessive enlargement of the breasts.

mastoplasty any form of plastic surgery that involves the breasts.

mastoptosis a sagging of the breasts.

mastorrhagia bleeding from a breast or mammary gland.

mastosyrinx a fistula of the breast.

mastotomy surgical incision of the breast or mammary gland.

masturbation stimulation of the genitals exclusive of sexual intercourse and typically with the purpose of inducing orgasm. —**masturbate** *vb.* —**masturbatory** *adj.*

mater 1. anything that nourishes or forms. 2. mother.

materia substance; matter.

materia medica the branch of medical science dealing with drugs and medicines.

materies morbi any substance that is the direct cause of a disease.

maternal relating to or coming or derived from a mother.

maternity 1. relating to the obstetrical ward or department of a hospital or medical center. 2. the state or condition of being a mother; motherhood.

matrical relating to a matrix.

matricide 1. the murder of one's mother. 2. one who kills their own mother.

matrix 1. the intercellular substance of a tissue. 2. a mold in which something is cast. 3. the formative portion of a nail or a tooth. 4. the uterus or womb.

matter 1. any substance. 2. pus.

maturate (of a wound) to exude pus; suppurate.

maturation the process of becoming fully developed.

maxilla *pl.* **maxillae** *or* **maxillas** the upper jaw. —**maxillary** *adj.*

maxillitis inflammation of the upper jaw.

maxillodental relating to the upper jaw and the teeth it contains.

maxillofacial relating to the jaws and face.

maxillomandibular relating to both the upper and lower jaws.

maximus (in anatomical nomenclature) greatest.

mayidism pellagra.

MBC *abbr.* maximum breathing capacity.

M.C. *abbr.* 1. Medical Corps. 2. Master of Surgery (*Magister Chirurgiae*).

M.D. *abbr.* Doctor of Medicine (*Medicinae Doctor*).

M.D.S. *abbr.* Master of Dental Surgery.

measles a contagious viral disease, esp. of childhood, marked chiefly by the eruption of red circular spots on the skin and by infection of the respiratory tract.

meato- *prefix* relating to a meatus.

meatotomy surgical incision to enlarge the meatus of the urethra.

meatus *pl.* **meatuses** *or* **meatus** an opening to a body passage or organ. —**meatal** *adj.*

mechanophobia an abnormal fear of machines or machinery.

meconism addiction to or poisoning from the prolonged use of opium.

meconium 1. fecal matter accumulated in the bowel during fetal development and evacuated shortly after birth. 2. opium.

mediad toward the middle line.

medial relating to or located at or near the middle; median.

medialis medial.

median situated in the middle of the body or a part; central; medial.

medianum *or* **medianus** medial.

mediastinitis inflammation of the cellular components of the mediastinum.

mediastinography X-ray photography of the mediastinum.

mediastinum *pl.* **mediastina** a septum or space between two parts, esp. the space between the lungs containing the heart and other thoracic organs.

medic one who is engaged in medicine, esp. an assistant to a physician.

medicable capable of being treated; admitting of treatment and possible cure.

Medicaid a program of medical aid to people of incomes below a certain amount, funded by the federal government and administered by the states.

medical of, relating to, or involving the practice of medicine or physicians.

medical examiner a public official who performs post mortems to determine the cause of death.

medicament a substance or agent used to ease physical discomfort or treat disease.

Medicare a program of medical aid to people over 65 eligible for Social Security or railroad retirement benefits, funded by the federal government and by contributions from those enrolled and administered by the government.

medicate 1. to treat with medicine. 2. to infuse with a medication. —**medicated** *adj.*

medication 1. the process or act of medicating. 2. a substance or agent that promotes healing or soothes pain.

medicinal used to cure disease or relieve pain.

medicine 1. a preparation, substance, or drug used in treating disease. 2. the science of maintaining good health and of the alleviating, preventing, or curing of disease or injury.

medico *pl.* **medicos** a physician or medical student.

medico- *or* **medi-** *prefix* medical.

medicobiologic *also* **medicobiological** relating to the biological aspects of medicine or medical science.

medicochirurgical 1. relating to both medicine and surgery. 2. relating to both physicians and surgeons.

medicolegal relating to or concerning both medicine and the law.

medicomechanical (of therapy) relating to the use of both medical and mechanical measures.

medicus a physician or medical doctor.

mediocarpal relating to the central part of the wrist (carpus).

medulla *pl.* **medullas** *or* **medullae** 1. marrow. 2. the central part of an organ. 3. medulla oblongata.

medulla oblongata the lower portion of the brainstem continuous posteriorly with the spinal cord.

medullary *also* **medullar** of or relating to marrow or to a medulla.

mega- *or* **meg-** *prefix* large; great.

megabacterium a bacterium of unusually large size.

megacardia an abnormally enlarged heart. Also called *cardiomegaly.*

megacephaly the condition of having an abnormally large head.

megacolon a condition in which the colon is abnormally large and dilated.

megacycle one million cycles.

megadactyl having or characterized by unusually large fingers. —**megadactyly** *n.*

megadolichocolon a condition in which the colon is unusually long and dilated.

megakaryocyte a large cell found chiefly in bone marrow and regarded as being the source of blood platelets.

megal- *or* **megalo-** *prefix* large; giant; enormous.

megalgia extremely severe pain.

megalocardia an abnormally enlarged heart; megacardia. Also called *cardiomegaly*.

megaloencephalic relating to a brain of unusually large size. —**megaloencephaly** *n*.

megaloenteron the state or condition of having an unusually large intestine.

megalogastria the state or condition of having an unusually large stomach.

megalomania a delusional disorder marked by infantile convictions of one's own worth, importance, power, or greatness. —**megalomaniac** *n*. —**megalomaniacal** *or* **megalomanic** *adj*.

megalosplenia splenomegaly.

megalourethra a congenital dilation of the urethra.

megarectum extreme dilation of the rectum.

megavolt one million volts.

megohm one million ohms (a measure of electrical resistance).

megrim migraine.

meiosis the process of cell division resulting in the number of chromosomes in gamete-producing cells being reduced to one-half. —**meiotic** *adj*.

melalgia pain in an arm or leg, esp. pain that radiates from the foot to the upper leg or thigh (possibly caused by a disease related to vitamin deficiency).

melan- *or* **melano-** *prefix* dark; black.

melancholia an abnormal mental condition marked by extreme depression, impaired bodily and mental activity, loss of appetite, and insomnia. —**melancholiac** *n*. —**melancholic** *adj*.

melanin the dark brown pigment of the skin and hair.

melanism an excessive amount of dark pigmentation of the skin and hair. —**melanistic** *adj*.

melanocyte a cell that produces melanin.

melanoderma an abnormal deposition of melanin or metallic substances (such as iron or silver) in the skin causing severe darkening.

melanodermatitis the deposit of excessive amounts of melanin in an inflamed area of skin.

melanoid a dark pigment resembling melanin.

melanoma *pl.* **melanomas** *or* **melanomata** a dark-pigmented, usually malignant tumor.

melanomatosis a condition characterized by the widespread occurrence of melanomas.

melanonychia discoloration of the nails with a black pigment.

melanoplakia an abnormal condition characterized by the deposition of pigmented patches on the tongue and the inner surfaces of the cheeks.

melanosis a condition marked by abnormally intense dark pigmentation of the tissues of the body.

melanosity a dark complexion.

melanotic relating to or characterized by melanosis.

melanotrichous possessing black hair.

melanous having a dark complexion; brunette.

melanuria a condition in which the excreted urine has an abnormally dark color, caused by the presence of various pigments and the derivatives of products containing coal tar.

melasma gravidarum the unusual but often temporary discoloration of the skin during pregnancy.

melasma universale a patchy pigmentation of the skin occurring in old age.

melatonin the hormone introduced into the blood stream by the pineal gland.

melena the passage of dark, tarry stools as the result of traces of blood in the intestinal secretions and juices.

membrana *pl.* **membranae** a membrane.

membrana abdominis the peritoneum.

membranaceous membranous.

membrana cordis the pericardium.

membranate resembling a membrane; having the nature of a membrane.

membrane a thin, pliable layer of tissue. —**membranous** *adj.*

membraniform having the characteristics of appearance of a membrane.

membrum *pl.* **membra** a member or limb.

membrum muliebre the clitoris.

membrum virile the penis.

menarche the beginning of menstruation. —**menarcheal** *adj.*

mendelism the body of hereditary and genetic principles derived from Mendel's laws.

Mendel's laws laws of genetics stating that characteristics are determined by pairs of factors (genes); one member of each pair is dominant to the other; the members of each pair separate during gamete formation so that the gametes contain only one factor for each characteristic.

Menière's disease a dysfuntion of the membranous labyrinth of the inner ear marked by attacks of tinnitis, dizziness, and deafness. Also called *Menière's syndrome.*

meningeal of or relating to the meninges.

meninges the three membranes that surround the brain and spinal cord; the pia mater, arachnoid and dura mater.

meningioma *pl.* **meningiomas** *or* **meningiomata** a slow-growing tumor arising from the meninges and often exerting pressure on the brain.

meningism a condition that simulates meningitis but is characterized by irritation rather than true inflammation.

meningitis inflammation of the meninges. —**meningitic** *adj.*

meningo- *or* **mening-** *prefix* relating to the meninges.

meningocele protrusion of the covering membranes of the brain or spinal cord through a gap or defect in the skull or vertebral column.

meningocortical relating to both the meninges of the brain and the cerebral cortex.

meningoencephalitis inflammation of both the brain and its covering membranes (meninges). Also called *cerebromeningitis.*

meningomyelocele protrusion through a defect in the vertebral column of a part of the spinal cord and its covering membranes.

meningopathy any disease or disorder of the covering membranes of the brain or spinal cord.

meningoradiculitis inflammation of both the spinal meninges and the roots of the spinal nerves.

meningorhachidian relating to both the spinal cord and its covering membranes.

meningorrhagia bleeding into or beneath the covering membranes of the brain or spinal cord.

meninx *pl.* **meninges** any of the three membranes surrounding the brain and spinal cord.

meniscectomy surgical removal of a meniscus, esp. one from the knee joint.

meniscotome a knife-like instrument used in the surgical removal of a meniscus.

meniscus any crescent-shaped structure or part, esp. the crescentic cartilage of the knee joint (*meniscus medialis*).

meno- *prefix* relating to menstruation or to the menses.

menolipsis a temporary interruption or cessation of menstruation.

menopause the period, usually occurring between the ages of 45 and 50, during which menstruation ceases. —**menopausal** *adj.*

menorrhagia abnormally heavy menstrual flow. —**menorrhagic** *adj.*

menosepsis a relatively rare form of blood poisoning caused by the absorption of septic material from retained menstrual blood.

menostasis *also* **menostasia** the absence of menstruation. Also called *amenorrhea.*

menostaxis an unusually prolonged flow of menstrual blood.

menothermal relating to hot flushes experienced as one symptom of the menopause.

menouria an abnormal condition in which some of the menstrual blood flows into the urinary bladder as a result of a fistula between the uterus and the bladder.

menoxenia any disorder or abnormality of menstruation.

menses the menstrual flow.

menstruant menstruating.

menstruation a discharge of tissue debris, secretions, and blood from the uterus in nonpregnant females from puberty occurring at approximately monthly intervals. —**menstrual** *adj.* —**menstruate** *vb.*

mental 1. of or relating to the mind. 2. of or relating to the chin.

mental defective one who has mental deficiency.

mental deficiency inadequate mental development usually attributed to a brain disorder or defect and thought to be incurable; feeblemindedness.

meperidine hydrochloride a narcotic pain-killing drug.

meprobamate a mild tranquilizer used in the relief of anxiety states and emotional tension.

meralgia pain in the upper part of the leg or thigh.

mercury poisoning a chronic or acute toxic disorder

resulting from eating or inhaling mercury or mercury compounds.

merisis an enlargement resulting from an increase in the number of cells rather than from their expansion.

mes- *or* **meso-** *prefix* mid; middle; intermediate.

mesaortitis inflammation of the middle coat of the aorta.

mesarteritis inflammation of the middle coat of any artery.

mescaline a poisonous alkaloid derived from the dried tops of the mescal cactus and used as an antispasmodic and as a stimulant and hallucinogen. Also called *peyote.*

mescalism addiction to mescaline or psychological dependence on its effects (exotic or beautiful visions).

mesencephalon the middle part of the brain; midbrain. **—mesencephalic** *adj.*

mesencephalotomy surgical interruption of any of the fiber tracts or section of any of the tissues in the midbrain, as in the relief of intractable pain.

mesenteric of or relating to a mesentery.

mesenteritis inflammation of a mesentery.

mesenterium mesentery.

mesentery a membrane in the form of a double fold serving as attachment for various bodily organs, esp. the peritoneal fold connecting the small intestine to the back wall of the body.

mesmerism hypnotism. **—mesmeric** *adj.*

mesoderm the middle of the three primary germ layers of an embryo that develops into bone, muscle, connective tissue, and other structures. **—mesodermal** *or* **mesodermic** *adj.*

mesomorph one having a husky, muscular body build. **—mesomorphic** *adj.*

mesothelium *pl.* **mesothelia** epithelium derived from the mesoderm and lining serous body cavities. —**mesothelial** *adj.*

metabolism the chemical changes in living cells through which energy is provided for vital activities and processes by the breakdown of molecules and new molecules are synthesized to replace them. —**metabolic** *adj.*

metabolite any product of metabolism, such as an intermediate substance or waste product, esp. as produced during catabolism.

metabolize to subject to or perform metabolism.

metacarpal 1. of or relating to the metacarpus. 2. a bone of the metacarpus.

metacarpus the skeletal part of the hand between the carpus and the phalanges that is made up of the five elongated bones of the palm.

metaplasia the transformation of one kind of tissue into another form of tissue.

metastasis *pl.* **metastases** the transfer of a malignancy or a disease-producing agent from the original site to another part of the body. —**metastatic** *adj.* —**metastasize** *vb.*

metatarsal 1. of or relating to the metatarsus. 2. a bone of the metatarsus.

metatarsus the part of the foot between the tarsus and the phalanges.

methadone a narcotic pain-killing drug used in the treatment of addicts and in detoxification.

methadone hydrochloride a narcotic pain-killing drug given as a heroin substitute in treating drug addicts.

methamphetamine hydrochloride a drug used as a stimulant.

methanol wood alcohol, used as an industrial solvent. Drinking it may cause blindness and death.

methaqualone a drug used as a sedative and hypnotic.

methylcellulose a tasteless powder that swells when mixed with water, used in antiobesity therapy as a bulk substitute in foods.

metopodynia pain in the forehead, or toward the front of the head; frontal headache.

metra the uterus.

metra- *or* **metr-** *prefix* relating to or denoting the uterus.

metralgia pain in the uterus. Also called *hysteralgia.*

metratonia the lack of muscular tone in the walls of the uterus following childbirth.

metritis inflammation of the uterus.

metrocystosis the formation of cysts in the uterus.

metropathy any disease or disorder involving the uterus.

metrorrhagia profuse bleeding from the uterus at times other than during the normal menstrual period. **—metrorrhagic** *adj.*

mg. *abbr.* milligram.

mho the unit of electrical conductivity (the reciprocal of ohm, the unit of electrical resistance).

miasmology the branch of ecology concerned with the study and control of air pollution.

microbe germ; microorganism. **—microbial** *or* **microbic** *adj.*

microbicide any agent that kills microorganisms; an antiseptic.

microbiology a branch of biology concerned with microscopic forms of life. **—microbiological** *also* **microbiologic** *adj.* **—microbiologist** *n.*

microcephalic having an abnormally small head. **—microcephaly** *n.*

micrococcus *pl.* **micrococci** a small, rounded bacterium. **—micrococcal** *adj.*

microcyte a small red blood cell. **—microcytic** *adj.*

micronutrient an organic compound or chemical element minute quantities of which are essential for normal bodily processes.

microorganism an organism of microscopic size.

microscope an optical instrument for viewing minute objects through magnification. —**microscopy** *n.*

microscopic *also* **microscopical** 1. of or relating to a microscope or to the use of a microscope. 2. invisible without the aid of a microscope.

microsome a minute structural part of a cell, consisting of ribosomes associated with endoplasmic reticulum. —**microsomal** *adj.*

microtome a special knife-like instrument for cutting sections of tissue for microscopic examination.

micturition the act or process of urinating; urination. —**micturate** *vb.*

midbrain the part of the vertebrate brain between the forebrain and hindbrain.

middle ear the part of the ear situated between the external ear and the labyrinth.

midgut the central part of the embryonic alimentary canal.

midline the median line or plane of the body or of some part of the body.

midriff the middle section of the human torso, esp. the diaphragm.

midwife a woman who assists another woman in childbirth. —**midwifery** *n.*

migraine severe headache often accompanied by nausea, vomiting, and distortion of vision. —**migrainous** *adj.*

miliaria an eruptive, itching inflammation of the skin, as prickly heat.

miliary consisting of a profusion of projecting lesions or tubercles.

milium *pl.* **milia** a small whitish protrusion of the skin resulting from blockage of the duct of an oil gland.

milk the fluid secreted by the mammary glands of females for the nourishment of their young.

milk tooth any of a set of initial, deciduous teeth replaced by permanent teeth.

Miltown trade name for meprobamate.

mineral an inorganic substance that is important in nutrition.

mineral oil a laxative.

Minimata disease a form of mercury poisoning seen among Japanese who eat seafood taken from polluted Minimata Bay.

miosis *pl.* **mioses** marked smallness or contraction of the eye pupil. —**miotic** *adj.*

miscarriage abortion, esp. when spontaneous.

mite a tiny, eight-legged arachnid (related to ticks and spiders) that burrows under the skin to lay eggs which hatch into larvae that cause discomfort, itching, and various diseases.

mitochondrion *pl.* **mitochondria** a long, slender, membranous intracellular body producing energy for a cell. —**mitochondrial** *adj.*

mitosis *pl.* **mitoses** the process of division of the nucleus of a cell. —**mitotic** *adj.*

mitral valve the valve between the left ventricle and the left atrium of the heart. Also called *bicuspid valve.*

molar a tooth with a flattened or rounded surface adapted for grinding food. —**molar** *adj.*

mole a pigmented protuberance or mark on the human skin.

molecule the smallest particle of a substance, composed of one or more atoms. —**molecular** *adj.*

mongolism *also* **mongolianism** a form of congenital idiocy marked by the formation of a broad, short skull, slanting eyes, and broad, short-fingered hands.

mongoloid *or* **mongolian** of or relating to mongolism.

moniliasis *pl.* **moniliases** thrush.

monocular of, relating to, or affecting a single eye.

monomania abnormally pronounced concentration on a single idea or object. —**monomaniac** *n.* —**monomaniac** *or* **monomaniacal** *adj.*

mononucleosis an acute, infectious, disease marked by fever, inflammation of the mucous membranes, and swelling of the lymph glands. Also called *infectious mononucleosis* and *glandular fever.*

monosaccharide the simplest form of a sugar, as glucose.

monozygotic twin one of two individuals developing originally from a single egg.

mons pubis the rounded, fleshy mound over the female pubic bones. Also called *mons veneris.*

monster one grotesquely malformed during fetal development.

morbid relating to, characteristic of, or affected with disease. —**morbidity** *n.*

morbus disease.

morgue a place where bodies of persons found dead are kept until they are identified or released for burial.

moribund being in a state approaching death; dying. —**moribundity** *n.*

morning sickness nausea and vomiting occurring during the early months of pregnancy, esp. on arising in the morning.

moron a mentally defective adult with a mental age of between 8 and 12 years.

morphine a bitter, addictive narcotic base that is the chief alkaloid of opium and is used as a sedative and painkiller.

morphinism a state of ill health resulting from the habitual use of morphine.

morphocytology the branch of biology concerned with the study of the size, shape, structure and other physical properties of cells.

morphology a branch of science dealing with the structure and shape of organisms. —**morphological** *adj.* —**morphologically** *adv.* —**morphologist** *n.*

mortality the ratio of the number of deaths to the total population; death rate.

mortuary *pl.* **mortuaries** a place in which dead bodies are kept until burial.

morula *pl.* **morulae** a solid mass of cells constituting an early stage of a fertilized ovum. —**morulation** *n.*

mosaic an organism composed of cells of different genetic types, caused by mutation or an anomaly of chromosome division. —**mosaicism** *n.*

motile capable of independent movement. —**motility** *n.*

motion sickness nausea induced by the movements of travel, as by plane, ship, or car.

motor 1. relating to a nerve that transmits impulses from a nerve center to a muscle or gland. 2. of or relating to movement of the muscles.

mountain sickness sickness resulting from insufficient oxygen at high altitudes.

moxibustion the burning of an herb close to the skin to change the function of a bodily system, sometimes used in acupuncture.

mucoid resembling or constituting mucus.

mucous 1. secreting or containing mucus. 2. covered with mucus.

mucous membrane a bodily membrane that secretes and is protected by mucus.

mucus a slippery, viscous, glandular secretion produced by mucous membranes.

multiparous having undergone one or more previous childbirths.

multiple myeloma a disease of the bone marrow marked by many myelomas.

multiple sclerosis a disease affecting the nerve fibers of the brain and spinal cord in which the myelin sheath deteriorates progressively. Also **MS.**

mumps a contagious viral disease marked chiefly by fever and swelling of the parotid glands.

mural relating to the wall of any bodily cavity.

murmur an abnormal sound heard on auscultation of the heart, lungs or blood vessels.

muscae volitantes cells and cell fragments in the vitreous humor and lens of the eye that appear as floating spots.

muscicide any agent that kills flies.

muscle body tissue that consists of long cells and expands or contracts a bodily part when stimulated. **—muscular** *adj.*

muscular dystrophy a complex of inherited diseases in which the skeletal muscles weaken and waste away.

musculature the muscular structure of the body.

musculus *pl.* **musculi** a muscle.

mutation a change in hereditary genetic material or the resulting morphological or organic change transmitted to a subsequent generation.

mute a person who is unable to speak. **—mute** *adj.*

my- *or* **myo-** *prefix* muscle.

myalgia muscular pain. **—myalgic** *adj.*

myasthenia gravis a disease marked by progressive weakening of the muscles without atrophy.

myco-, myc- *prefix* fungus.

mycosis *pl.* **mycoses** disease caused by a fungus. —**mycotic** *adj.*

Mycostatin trade name for nystatin.

mydriasis prolonged or marked dilation of the pupil of the eye.

mydriatic 1. causing dilation of the pupil. 2. an agent with this action.

myelin the fatty white substance sheathing the nerve fibers.

myelitis inflammation of bone marrow or of the spinal cord.

myeloid of or relating to the spinal cord or to bone marrow.

myeloma a bone marrow tumor. —**myelomatous** *adj.*

myelopathy disease of the spinal cord or of the bone marrow. —**myelopathic** *adj.*

myocardial infarction occlusion of a coronary artery; heart failure.

myocardiograph an instrument for making a traced recording of heart-muscle action. —**myocardiographic** *adj.*

myocarditis inflammation of the myocardium.

myocardium the muscular tissue of the heart.

myogenic relating to or originating from muscle tissue.

myoglobin an oxygen-binding protein in muscles, similar to hemoglobin in blood.

myology the study of muscles. —**myologic** *or* **myological** *adj.*

myoma *pl.* **myomas** *or* **myomata** a tumor composed of muscle tissue. —**myomatous** *adj.*

myopathy any abnormal condition of muscle or muscle tissue. —**myopathic** *adj.*

myope one having myopia.

myopia a condition of the eyes in which a visual image is focused in front of the retina, resulting in imperfect perception of distant objects; nearsightedness. **—myopic** *adj.* **—myopically** *adv.*

myosarcoma cancer in muscular tissue.

myositis inflammation of muscular tissue.

myotonia a tonic muscular spasm. **—myotonic** *adj.*

myringectomy surgical removal of the tympanic membrane.

myringitis infection or inflammation of the tympanic membrane.

myringotomy surgical incision of the tympanic membrane.

mysophobia an abnormal dread of dirt.

myxedema a hypothyroid condition marked by dry skin and hair, swelling of tissues, and decline of mental and physical vigor. **—myxedematous** *adj.*

myxoma *pl.* **myxomas** *or* **myxomata** a tumor of connective tissue cells. **—myxomatous** *adj.*

N

NAD *abbr.* no appreciable disease.

nail a horny sheath covering and protecting the outer end of each finger and toe.

nalorphine a drug used in the treatment of some types of overdose with narcotics and, since it induces severe withdrawal symptoms in morphine addicts, as a means of diagnosing morphine addiction.

nanism dwarfism.

nano- *prefix* (in the metric system of measurement) one-billionth (10^{-9}).

nanometer one-billionth of a meter; 10^{-9} meter.

nape the back of the neck.

narcissism 1. erotic interest in and attraction to one's own body. 2. egocentricity; egotism. **—narcissist** *n.* **—narcissistic** *adj.*

narcohypnosis deep sleep or unconsciousness induced by hypnosis.

narcolepsy an abnormal condition marked by frequent, sudden periods of deep sleep. **—narcoleptic** *n. & adj.*

narcomania 1. an intense desire or craving for narcotics. 2. severe mental disability caused by addiction to narcotic drugs.

narcosis a condition of unconsciousness or stupor induced by drugs or chemicals.

narcotic a drug, as opium or morphine, that is used in small amounts to ease pain or cause sleep but that in large amounts may cause addiction and death. —**narcotic** *adj.*

naris *pl.* **nares** either of the openings of the nose; nostril.

nasal of or relating to the nose or the nostrils.

nasogastric involving the nose and the stomach: *nasogastric feeding.*

nasopharynx the nasal passages in continuation with the upper pharynx. —**nasopharyngeal** *adj.*

nates buttocks.

naturopathy therapy involving natural foods, exercise, and avoiding medication.

nausea a sensation of queasiness in the stomach, often associated with an urge to vomit. —**nauseate** *vb.*

navel a small depression in the center of the abdomen marking the former point of attachment of the umbilical cord; umbilicus.

ne- *or* **neo-** *prefix* 1. new; recent. 2. new and different in form.

neck 1. the part of an animal that connects the head with the body. 2. a necklike structure or part; cervix.

necrophilia obsessive and usually erotic interest in dead bodies. —**necrophilic** *adj.*

necrophobia an abnormal fear of dead bodies.

necropsy the detailed examination of a body and its organs and parts after death. Also called *post mortem, autopsy.*

necrosis *pl.* **necroses** the localized death of living tissue. —**necrotic** *adj.*

negative (of a test or sign) absent.

neisseria any of a genus of microorganisms including those causing gonorrhea.

nematode any of various cylindrical parasitic worms; esp. hookworm.

Nembutal a trademark for the sodium salt of pentobarbital.

Neo-Cort-Dome a trademark for a compound of hydrocortisone and neomycin sulfate.

neomycin a broad-spectrum antibiotic.

neomycin sulfate an antibiotic drug used chiefly in the treatment of infections caused by gram-negative organisms.

neonatal relating to or affecting a newborn infant, esp. during the first month after birth.

neonate a newborn child or one less than a month old.

neonatology the study of new-born infants and of their disorders. **—neonatologist** *n.*

neoplasia the formation of tumorous tissues. **—neoplastic** *adj.*

neoplasm new and abnormal tissue having no organic function; tumor. **—neoplastic** *adj.*

neph- *or* **nephro-** *prefix* kidney.

nephrectomy *pl.* **nephrectomies** the surgical removal of a kidney.

nephremorrhagia bleeding into or from the kidney.

nephritic renal; relating to the kidney.

nephritis inflammation of the kidney.

nephrogenic developing in the kidney or produced or originating in kidney tissue. **—nephrogenically** *adv.*

nephrology the study of the kidney and of its diseases. **—nephrologist** *n.*

nephron the functional unit of the kidney which filters the blood of its waste products, numbering approximately one million in each kidney.

nephropathy an abnormal state of the kidney. **—nephropathic** *adj.*

nephrosis *pl.* **nephroses** degeneration of the kidneys without inflammation. **—nephrotic** *adj.*

nerve a filamentous band or bundle of nerve fibers outside the central nervous system that connects the brain and spinal cord with various organs and tissues of the body.

nerve gas a war gas that interrupts normal nerve transmission and induces intense respiratory spasm.

nervous 1. relating to or composed of neurons. 2. relating to or affecting the nerves. 3. easily excited or irritated; edgy.

nervous breakdown 1. neurasthenia, esp. when incapacitating. 2. emotional despair, esp. when intense and severe enough to require medical or psychiatric treatment.

nervous system the central nervous system or autonomic nervous system.

nervus *pl.* **nervi** nerve.

nervy excitable; irritable; nervous. —**nerviness** *n.*

nettle rash urticaria; hives.

neural of, relating to, or affecting the nerves or the nervous system. —**neurally** *adv.*

neuralgia acute pain radiating paroxysmally along the course of one or more nerves. —**neuralgic** *adj.*

neurasthenia a fundamentally neurotic condition marked chiefly by exhaustion, feelings of inadequacy, depression, loss of concentration and of appetite, insomnia, and often gastrointestinal disturbance. —**neurasthenic** *adj.* —**neurasthenically** *adv.*

neuritis *pl.* **neuritides** *or* **neuritises** painful inflammation of a nerve. —**neuritic** *adj.*

neuroblastoma *pl.* **neuroblastomas** *or* **neuroblastomata** a malignant tumor of nerve ganglia.

neurodynia neuralgia.

neuroglia one of the two main types of nerve cells.

neurolepsis a semiconscious condition in which the patient is subdued yet able to respond to commands.

neuroleptanalgesia *or* **neuroleptoanalgesia** the administration of an analgesic agent and a tranquilizing drug jointly, esp. as an adjunct to surgery. —**neuroleptanalgesic** *or* **neuroleptoanalgesic** *adj.*

neuroleptic a drug used to alleviate mental disturbance; tranquilizer.

neuroleptic *or* **neurolept** a person in a state of neurolepsis or a drug that can induce that state.

neurologist a physician specializing in the diagnosis and treatment of disease of the nervous system. —**neurology** *n.* —**neurologically** *adv.*

neuroma *pl.* **neuromas** *or* **neuromata** a tumor or new growth arising from a nerve or from nerve fibers.

neuromuscular relating to or involving the nervous system and muscles jointly.

neuron a nerve cell and its processes (axon and dendrites), being the chief unit of the nervous system. —**neuronal** *adj.* —**neuronic** *adj.*

neuronitis inflammation of a nerve cell.

neuropathy *pl.* **neuropathies** an abnormal and often degenerative condition of the nervous system. —**neuropathic** *adj.* —**neuropathically** *adv.*

neuropharmacology a branch of medicine concerned with the effects of drugs on the nervous system. —**neuropharmacologic** *or* **neuropharmacological** *adj.* —**neuropharmacologist** *n.*

neuroplegia nerve paralysis, as from injury or a neuroleptic drug.

neuropsychiatry a branch of medicine dealing with the relationships of mental and physical aspects of mental disorders. —**neuropsychiatric** *adj.* —**neuropsychiatrically** *adv.* —**neuropsychiatrist** *n.*

neurosis *pl.* **neuroses** any of various emotionally based, disabling, functional nervous disorders lacking a related physical lesion. —**neurotic** *adj. & n.* —**neurotically** *adv.*

neurosurgery surgery involving any part of the spinal cord, brain, or peripheral nerves. —**neurosurgeon** *n.* —**neurosurgical** *adj.* —**neurosurgically** *adv.*

neurotoxin a poisonous protein complex that acts on the nervous system. —**neurotoxic** *adj.*

neutropemia a condition resulting from an abnormal decrease in neutrophils.

neutrophil a white blood cell.

nevus *pl.* **nevi** a pigmented area of the skin; mole; birthmark.

Newcastle disease a viral disease transmittable to humans that involves respiratory and nervous symptoms.

niacin nicotinic acid.

nicotine a poisonous alkaloid that is the active principle of tobacco.

nicotinic acid an acid of the vitamin B complex used in the treatment of pellagra. Also called *niacin.*

nictitate to blink the eyelids; wink. —**nictation** *n.* —**nictitation** *n.*

night blindness impaired visual capacity in faint light or in darkness. Also called *nyctalopia.*

nipple the pigmented protuberance in the center of each breast that in the female serves as the outlet for the secretion of milk in nursing.

nit the egg of a parasitic insect, esp. of a louse.

nitrate a salt of nitric acid.

nitric acid a chemical used as a local caustic agent, the fumes from which can be dangerous to health.

nitroglycerin a highly explosive oily liquid, the main constituent of dynamite, used medically as a vasodilator, esp. in the symptomatic relief of pain caused by angina pectoris.

nitrous oxide a colorless gas used chiefly as an anesthetic in dentistry and often producing laughter and exhilaration before the onset of insensibility. Also called *laughing gas.*

node a thickened or swollen enlargement of a part; a circumscribed mass of tissue: *lymph node.*

nodus *pl.* **nodi** node.

noetic relating to the mental processes.

norepinephrine a hormone, secreted by the adrenal glands, that constricts the blood vessels, thereby increasing blood pressure without affecting the heart. Synthesized, it is used as a drug.

normal average or acceptable in health and bodily functions.

nose the part of the face bearing the nostrils and constituting the chief vehicle for olfactory sensations.

nosology the branch of medical science concerned with the classification or description of diseases. **—nosologic** *adj.*

Novocain a trademark for procaine hydrochloride.

noxious physically harmful to living organisms: *noxious gases.*

nucleic acid an acid composed of sugar or a derivative of a sugar, a base, and phosphoric acid that is found chiefly in cell nuclei.

nucleolus *pl.* **nucleoli** a small spherical body within the nucleus of a cell, being occasionally one of two to five such bodies within a single cell nucleus.

nucleus *pl.* **nuclei** the center of a cell, which controls its functions.

nulliparous describing a female who has never borne offspring.

numb lacking partial or total sensation in a bodily part.

nutation the act of nodding the head, esp. involuntarily.

nyctalopia night blindness.

nymphomania abnormally intense sexual desire on the part of a female, esp. when unresolved by sexual intercourse. **—nymphomaniac** *n. & adj.*

nystagmus an involuntary, rapid oscillation of the eyeballs.

nystatin an antifungal antibiotic drug.

THE ORAL CAVITY

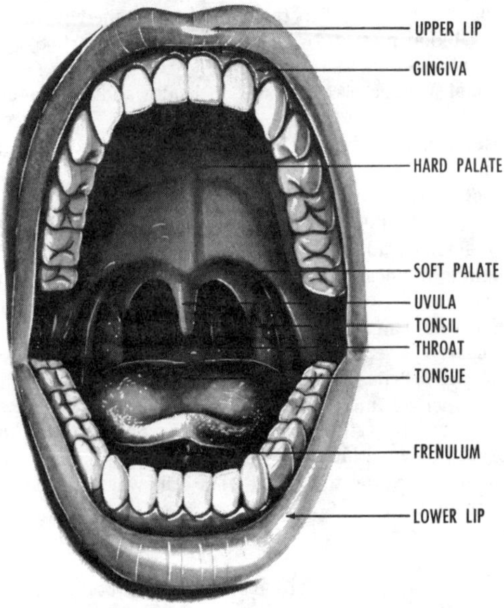

O

obesity a condition of having excessive bodily fat. **—obese** *adj.*

oblique muscles 1. two large muscles of the abdominal wall. 2. two external muscles of the eyeball.

obsession a persistent, often upsetting preoccupation with a particular idea, object, or person. **—obsess** *vb.* **—obsessive** *adj. & n.*

obsessive compulsive neurosis a mental disorder characterized by compulsive behavior known or recognized by the patient himself to be absurd.

obstetric *or* **obstetrical** of, relating to, or dealing with obstetrics.

obstetrics the branch of medicine dealing with birth and its attendant concerns. **—obstetrician** *n.*

occipital lobe a lobe of the cerebral hemisphere, situated near the occiput.

occiput the back of the head. **—occipital** *adj.*

occlusion a closing up; obstruction. **—occlude** *vb.* **—occlusive** *adj.*

occult difficult to see; hidden.

occult blood blood passed in the stools and detectable, because of the very small amounts, only by means of special laboratory tests.

occupational accident an accident arising from one's regular occupation or occurring at one's place of work.

occupational disease disease or disability arising from one's regular occupation.

occupational therapy therapy for a convalescent or handicapped person that involves training in skills that are useful, profitable, and diverting and that provide exercise.

ocular of or relating to the eyes or to sight. —**ocularly** *adv.*

oculomotor nerves the third pair of cranial nerves which act to help move the eyeball.

O.D. the right eye; *abbr.* of *oculus dexter.*

odontalgia toothache.

-odontia *suffix* of the teeth.

odontolith dental tartar; calcareous material deposited on a tooth.

odontology dentistry.

oesophagus esophagus.

ohm the unit of electrical resistance. Compare *mho.*

olfactory of or relating to the sense of smell.

olig- *or* **oligo-** *prefix* few; deficient; a little.

oligemia lack of blood.

oligospermia abnormally few spermatozoa in the semen.

omentum a free fold supporting or connecting structures within the abdominal cavity.

oncology the study of tumors and cancer. —**oncologist** *n.*

onychia inflammation of the matrix of a nail.

onychocryptosis an ingrowing nail.

onychomycosis a fungal infection of the nails or a nail.

oocyte an incompletely developed ovum.

oogenesis *pl.* **oogeneses** the production of ova within the ovary.

oophorectomy the surgical removal of an ovary.

open fracture a bone fracture in which one or more pieces of bone protrude through a break in the skin.

open heart surgery surgery performed within the heart of a living patient.

operation any surgical procedure.

ophthalm- *or* **ophthalmo-** *prefix* eyeball; eye.

ophthalmia inflammation of the eye and usually the conjunctiva.

ophthalmologist a physician or surgeon specializing in diseases of the eye. —**ophthalmological** *adj.* —**ophthalmology** *n.*

ophthalmoscope a small illuminated instrument for examining the interior of the eye, esp. the retina.

opiate any narcotic drug, specifically one containing opium, an opium derivative, or a synthetic compound that acts like opium.

opium a compound containing codeine, morphine, and papaverine, derived from certain varieties of poppy, and used in analgesic and anesthetic drugs.

optic of or relating to the eyes or to sight. —**optically** *adv.*

optic disc the point at which the optic nerve enters the eye.

optician a maker of optical instruments and devices.

optic nerve one of a pair of nerves connecting the eyes with the visual cortex of the brain.

optometry the profession of examining the eyes for defects of structure and refraction and prescribing corrective lenses. —**optometrist** *n.*

O.R. operating room.

oral of, relating to, or affecting the mouth. —**orally** *adv.*

orbit the bony cavity of the skull containing the eyeball.

orchis testicle.

orchitis inflammation of a testicle.

organ a differentiated bodily structure performing specific functions within the body.

organic relating to or affecting the organs of the body: *organic diseases.*

orgasm the climax of sexual excitement, which in the male leads to ejaculation of semen. —**orgasmic** *or* **orgastic** *adj.*

orifice an opening, esp. a natural opening of the body.

orthodontics the dental practice of diagnosing and treating dental irregularities, as by the application of braces, etc. —**orthodontist** *n.*

orthopedics the study of bones, joints, muscles, and the skeleton. —**orthopedist** *n.*

O.S. the left eye; *abbr.* of *oculus sinister.*

os 1. bone. 2. mouth; orifice.

osseous resembling or composed of bone; bony.

ossicle a small bone or bony structure, esp. any of the three sound-conducting bones of the middle ear. —**ossicular** *adj.* —**ossiculate** *adj.*

ossification 1. the formation of bone. 2. the abnormal change into bone, as of connective tissues. —**ossify** *vb.*

oste- *or* **osteo-** *prefix* bone.

osteitis inflammation of bone.

osteoarthritis degenerative arthritis chiefly of the larger joints.

osteoclasis *or* **osteoclasty** the deliberate breaking of a bone to correct a deformity.

osteomyelitis inflammation of bone marrow.

osteopathy medical practice that ascribes the source of many diseases to be loss of structural integrity and uses the manipulation of joints as a healing technique. —**osteopath** *n.* —**osteopathic** *adj.*

osteoporosis weakening and degeneration of bone, usually in postmenopausal women.

otalgia earache.

otitis inflammation of the ear.

otitis externa inflammation of the outer ear.

otitis interna labyrinthitis.

otitis media inflammation of the middle ear.

otology the study of the ear and its diseases. —**otologist** *n.*

otoscope a lighted instrument for examining the external and middle ear.

ovarian relating to or affecting the ovaries.

ovariectomy *pl.* **ovariectomies** the surgical removal of an ovary. —**ovariectomized** *adj.*

ovaritis inflammation of an ovary.

ovary *pl.* **ovaries** either of two female reproductive organs that produce eggs and female sex hormones.

over-the-counter (of a drug) available without a prescription.

ovulation the monthly development and discharge of a mature ovum from an ovary. —**ovulate** *vb.*

ovum *pl.* **ova** a female gamete; egg.

oxygenation to saturate or supply with oxygen. —**oxygenate** *vb.*

P

pacemaker 1. an area in the wall of the heart (sino-atrial node) where the impulse is generated that governs the rhythm of the heart's activity. 2. an electrical device for steadying or stimulating the action of the heart or for re-establishing the action of an arrested heart. Also called *artificial pacemaker.*

pachydermatous having an abnormal thickening of the skin.

pachydermia thickening of the skin.

pachylosis a condition characterized by an abnormally rough, dry and thick skin, esp. of the legs.

pachymeningitis inflammation and thickening of the outermost membrane (dura mater) that covers the brain and spinal cord.

paediatrics pediatrics.

Paget's disease a disease in which the bone deteriorates, commonly afflicting middle-aged people.

pain a usually localized physical suffering associated with a bodily disorder, injury, or disease. **—painful** *adj.* **—painfully** *adv.* **—painfulness** *n.*

painter's colic lead poisoning.

palliative 1. a medicine or method of treatment that eases symptoms of a disease. 2. relating to the relief of symptoms; mitigating.

pallor deficiency of natural color of the skin, esp. of the face; paleness.

palm the flexible surface of the hand between the wrist and the base of the fingers.

palmar relating to or located on the palm.

palpation medical examination by means of the sense of touch. —**palpate** *vb.*

palpebra *pl.* **palpebrae** eyelid.

palpebral relating to an eyelid or to the eyelids.

palpebrate 1. having eyelids. 2. to open and close the eyelids very quickly; wink.

palpebration the act of winking.

palpitation a pronounced throbbing or pulsation of the heart that is perceptible to the patient. —**palpitate** *vb.*

palsy paralysis or partial paralysis; paresis.

paludism malaria.

panacea a remedy that is claimed to cure all ills.

pancreas a large gland that secretes digestive enzymes and insulin. —**pancreatic** *adj.*

pancreatic juice a clear, alkaline fluid produced by the pancreas and important to the digestive process.

pancreatitis, inflammation of the pancreas.

pandemic occurring over a large area and affecting large numbers of people: *pandemic diseases.*

Papanicolaou test a test commonly used to detect cancer of the cervix.

papaverine hydrochloride a relaxant for the smooth muscles, an ingredient of opium.

papilla *pl.* **papillae** a small, nipple-shaped structure.

papilloma a benign tumor composed of epithelial tissue and characterized by one or more outward projections or outgrowths.

Pap test *Informal.* Papanicolaou test.

papule a small, conical elevation of the skin. —**papular** *adj.*

para- *or* **par-** *prefix* 1. alongside. 2. abnormal; faulty.

paracentesis withdrawal of fluid from a bodily cavity by means of surgical puncture and aspiration. —**paracentetic** *adj.*

paradenitis inflammation of the tissues that surround or are adjacent to a gland.

parageusia an impairment of the sense of taste.

paralysis *pl.* **paralyses** loss of function in part of the body, esp. when involving sensation or motion. —**paralytic** *adj.* —**paralyze** *vb.*

paramedian near the middle line of an organ, structure or part.

paramedical supplementing the work of professional medical personnel. —**paramedic** *n. & adj.*

paranoia a psychosis characterized chiefly by delusions of persecution or grandeur. —**paranoiac** *adj. & n.* —**paranoid** *adj. & n.*

paranoid schizophrenia a psychosis characterized by paranoia along with hallucinations and often characterized by mental deterioration.

paraplegia paralysis of the lower half of the torso and of both legs. —**paraplegic** *adj. & n.*

parasite an organism that lives on and gains its nourishment from another organism.

parasympathetic nervous system a part of the autonomic nervous system.

parathyroid glands several small glands, attached to the thyroid gland, that secrete a hormone.

parenteral not by means of or into the digestive tract, as a drug to be injected subcutaneously or intramuscularly, intravenous feeding, etc.

paresis partial or incomplete paralysis.

paresthesia an unaccountable numb, creeping, tingling, or prickling sensation of the skin.

parietal relating to the parietal bone of the skull.

parietal bone either of the two bones that together form the sides and roof of the skull.

Parkinson's disease a progressive disease, esp. of late life, marked by tremors and rigidity of resting muscles and by an shuffling gait when walking. Also called *parkinsonism, Parkinson's syndrome.*

parolfactory related to or associated with the sense of smell or the olfactory system.

parotid gland either of a pair of large salivary glands located below and in front of the ear.

parotitis 1. inflammation of a parotid gland. 2. mumps (properly, *infectious parotitis*).

paroxysm 1. the sudden flare-up of the symptoms of a disease. 2. a fit or convulsion. —**paroxysmal** *adj.*

parrot fever psittacosis.

pars *pl.* **partes** a part.

parturient giving or about to give birth.

parturition the act of giving birth to young; childbirth.

partus parturition; childbirth.

parvus small.

passive immunity immunity to one or more diseases that is passed on to an infant in the mother's womb.

pasteurization exposure of a substance, as milk, to controlled heat to kill certain organisms without altering the chemical structure. —**pasteurize** *vb.*

patch test a test for determining which of a number of allergens affect an individual by placing it on the skin and covering with an adhesive patch. Those areas that are red and swollen upon the removal of the patch are the suspected allergens.

patella *pl.* **patellae** *or* **patellas** a thick, triangular, movable bone at the front of the knee; kneecap.

pathogenic capable of causing disease: *pathogenic bacteria.* —**pathogenesis** *n.*

pathology the branch of medicine dealing with the nature of diseases and the bodily changes they cause. —**pathologic** *or* **pathological** *adj.* —**pathologist** *n.*

pathophobia an abnormal fear of disease.

pavor excessive terror.

pectoral of or relating to the chest or its muscles.

pectoralis major one of a pair of large breast muscles used to move the arm in the shoulder joint.

pediatric of or relating to the treatment of children's diseases.

pediatrician a doctor specializing in the treatment of children's diseases, in monitoring their proper growth and nutrition, etc. —**pediatrics** *n.*

pediculosis the state or condition of being infested with lice.

pellagra a disease resulting from insufficiency of niacin, either from an improper diet high in maize or from a metabolic disorder.

pelvis *pl.* **pelvises** *or* **pelves** 1. the bony cavity outlined by the hips and lower bones of the spine and holding the lower intestine, bladder and (in females) the internal genital organs. 2. any bodily cavity resembling a basin or cup, such as that at the base of the kidney (renal pelvis). —**pelvic** *adj.*

penicillin any of several antibiotics produced by molds or synthetically and used esp. against cocci.

penile of or relating to the penis.

penis the male organ of copulation, composed of erectile tissue and containing the urethra.

penitis inflammation of the penis.

pentobarbital a barbiturate used as an antispasmodic, sedative, and hypnotic.

Pentothal Sodium a trademark for the barbiturate thiopental sodium.

peptic of, relating to, or affecting the stomach or digestion.

peptic ulcer an ulcerous lesion in the mucous membrane lining the stomach or duodenum.

percussion the technique of tapping the surface of the body to diagnose from the resultant sound the condition of the parts beneath. —**percuss** *vb.*

perforation a hole in an organ produced by disease or injury. —**perforate** *vb.*

peri- *prefix* all around; about.

perianal located around the area of the anus; surrounding the anus.

pericarditis inflammation of the pericardium.

pericardium *pl.* **pericardia** the membranous sac surrounding the heart. —**pericardial** *adj.*

pericranium *pl.* **pericrania** the thick, fibrous membrane covering the surface of the bones of the skull; the periosteum of the skull.

perineum *pl.* **perinea** the region of the pelvic floor between the anus and the anterior portion of the external genitalia. —**perineal** *adj.*

periodontics the dental practice specializing in diseases of the gum and their treatment. —**periodontist** *n.* —**periodontal** *adj.*

peripheral nervous system the system of nerves and their associated organs and tissues outside of the brain and spinal column.

peristalsis the involuntary muscular waves of the intestine that move the contents onward. —**peristaltic** *adj.* —**peristaltically** *adv.*

peritoneum *pl.* **peritoneums** *or* **peritonea** the transparent membrane that lines the abdominal cavity. —**peritoneal** *adj.*

peritonitis inflammation of the peritoneum.

permanent tooth any one of the 32 teeth normally developed after childhood.

pernicious highly destructive or injurious; deadly: *pernicious anemia.*

peroral occurring through or taken by way of the mouth. —**perorally** *adv.*

peroxide hydrogen peroxide.

pertussis whooping cough.

perversion an aberrant sexual practice.

pes *pl.* **pedes** foot.

pessary *pl.* **pessaries** 1. a device placed in the vagina to support the uterus or prevent conception. 2. a vaginal suppository.

pestilence an epidemic disease.

petit mal a mild form of epilepsy.

peyote mescaline or the cactus from which it is derived.

phagocyte a white blood corpuscle that typically consumes and destroys debris and foreign bodies.

phalanx *pl.* **phalanxes** *or* **phalanges** one of the digital bones of the hand or foot.

phallus *pl.* **phalluses** *or* **phalli** 1. the penis. 2. anything resembling or suggestive of a penis. —**phallic** *adj.*

phantom limb the sensation sometimes experienced after amputation of a limb that the limb is still there.

pharmaceutical 1. of or relating to pharmacy or to pharmacists. 2. of or relating to a drug or drugs. 3. a medicinal drug. —**pharmaceutically** *adv.*

pharmaco- *prefix* medicine; drug.

pharmacology the science dealing with medicinal drugs

and their action on the body. —**pharmacological** *adj.* —**pharmacologist** *n.*

pharmacopoeia an official book describing drugs, medicinal preparations, and chemicals.

pharmacy *pl.* **pharmacies** 1. the practice of preparing, compounding, and dispensing drugs. 2. a place where drugs and medicines are compounded and dispensed. —**pharmacist** *n.*

pharyngeal of or relating to the pharynx.

pharyngitis inflammation of the pharynx.

pharynx the part of the alimentary canal between the mouth and the esophagus; the lower back part of the throat.

phenacetin a painkilling drug.

phenobarbital an anticonvulsant barbiturate also used as a sedative and hypnotic.

phenolphthalein a laxative drug.

phimosis severe contraction of the foreskin usually requiring circumcision.

phlebectomy *pl.* **phlebectomies** excision of a vein.

phlebitis inflammation of a vein.

phlebotomy *pl.* **phlebotomies** the bleeding of a patient by the opening of a vein, as in the treatment of polycythemia.

phlegm a thick mucus produced in abnormal quantities by the respiratory passages.

phosphoprotein any of various proteins combined with a compound containing phosphorus.

photophobia abnormal sensitivity of the eyes to light.

phrenic 1. of or relating to the diaphragm. 2. relating to the mind.

phthisis an older name for tuberculosis of the lungs.

physical examination a medical examination to determine the subject's state of health.

physical therapy physiotherapy.

physician a medical doctor.

physiology a branch of biology dealing with the structure and function of living organisms. —**physiological** *adj.* —**physiologist** *n.*

physiotherapy therapy involving the use of heat, massage and exercise rather than medication. —**physiotherapist** *n.*

piles the informal name for hemorrhoids.

pilomotor reflex goose pimples or bumps; horripilation.

pimple a small, inflamed, pus-filled elevation of the skin; pustule. —**pimpled** *adj.* —**pimply** *adj.*

pink eye infectious conjunctivitis.

pituitary gland an endocrine gland at the base of the brain producing various essential hormones.

placebo a chemically inactive agent given to reassure a patient or used in the double-blind or single-blind evaluation of active drugs, where one group of patients receives the test drug and another the inactive agent.

placenta the vascular organ surrounding the fetus within the uterus. —**placental** *adj.*

plague an acute, infectious bacterial disease transmitted to man by rat fleas.

plantar relating to, affecting, or occurring on the sole of the foot: *plantar wart.*

plaque *or* **dental plaque** a film on the teeth susceptible to bacterial infection and subsequent periodontal disease.

plasma the liquid portion of the blood, in which the corpuscles are suspended.

Plasmodium the genus of several species of protozoa that cause different types of malaria.

plastic surgery surgical repair or restoration of damaged or deformed tissue. —**plastic surgeon.**

platelet a disk-shaped blood cell containing no hemoglobin.

pledget a small, flat gauze compress.

pleura *pl.* **pleurae** *or* **pleuras** a thin membrane lining the lungs and the inner surface of the chest cavity.

pleurisy inflammation of the pleura.

plexus a network of interlacing nerves or blood vessels.

pneumoconiosis fibrosis of the lungs from prolonged inhalation of irritant dust particles.

pneumonia a disease marked by severe inflammation of the lungs.

pneumonic plague an often fatal form of bubonic plague with bronchopneumonia.

pneumonitis inflammation of one or both lungs.

pockmark a cavity of the skin caused by a pustule, as from smallpox or acne.

podiatrist a physician specializing in the care and treatment of the feet. —**podiatry** *n.*

poliomyelitis a viral disease marked by inflammation of the nerve cells of the spinal cord, deformity, and paralysis. Also called *infantile paralysis, polio.*

polycythemia an abnormal increase in the total number of circulating red blood cells.

polyp a small projecting tumor, esp. in a body cavity or passage.

polyuria excretion of abnormally large amounts of urine from any cause.

pons the bridge of tissue at the base of the brain that connects the medulla oblongata with the cerebral hemispheres and the cerebellum. Also called *pons Varolii.*

postmenopausal occurring after the menopause.

post mortem necropsy; autopsy.

postnasal drip a persistent dripping of nasal mucus into the pharynx.

postpartum following parturition.

postprandial following meals: *postprandial medication.*

poultice a moist bandage applied over a wound.

prednisone a steroid hormone used as an anti-inflammatory drug.

pregnancy the condition of a woman from conception till the delivery of an infant from her womb, usually about nine months. —**pregnant,** *adj.*

premature characterizing an infant born before the full term of pregnancy of the mother.

prenatal before birth, in reference either to a pregnant woman or to an unborn infant.

prepuce foreskin.

presbyopia farsightedness associated with advancing age.

prescribe to write a prescription.

prescription an order for a drug written by a qualified medical practitioner to a pharmacist, often including dosage instructions.

prescription drug a drug that is legally obtainable only by prescription.

pressure acupuncture a system of treatment similar to acupuncture in which, instead of inserting needles, pressure is applied to certain points of the body with the fingers. Also called **acupressure.**

pressure point a point at which pressure may be applied to check hemorrhage.

preventive characterized by a policy, treatment, or practice directed at avoiding disease by maintaining good health.

prickly heat inflammation around the sweat ducts causing redness and itching.

primipara a woman who has borne only one child.

probe a slender instrument for exploring wounds.

process a natural growth.

proctology a branch of medicine dealing chiefly with the structure and diseases of the lower bowel. **—protological** *adj.* **—proctologist** *n.*

proctoscope an instrument for examining the interior of the rectum.

progesterone a hormone, produced by the corpus luteum, that prepares the uterus for gestation.

prognosis an estimate, usually by a qualified medical person, of the course of a disease or condition.

prolapsed fallen; dislocated: *a prolapsed uterus.*

prophylaxis prevention of or protection from disease. **—prophylactic,** *adj.*, *n.*

proprietary drug a drug manufactured and sold for profit and protected by patent, trademark, or copyright.

proprioception the detection of sensation from within the body. **—proprioceptor,** *n.*

prostaglandin a natural fatty acid, resembling a hormone, synthesized as a drug with a variety of uses.

prostatectomy *pl.* **prostatectomies** surgical removal of the prostate gland.

prostate gland a muscular gland at the base of the male urethra that secretes the viscid fluid that is a major constituent of semen. **—prostatic** *adj.*

prostatitis inflammation of the prostate gland.

prosthesis replacement of an absent organ or limb with an artificial one. **—prosthetics** *n.*

protein a natural compound of several amino acids that is essential for building bodily tissue.

proteinuria the presence of abnormal amounts of protein in the urine.

proximal situated nearer to the trunk of the body.

pruritis an itching of the skin.

psilocybin a hallucinogenic drug extracted from a variety of Mexican mushroom.

psittacosis a viral disease of birds, as parrots, transmittable to man.

psoriasis a skin disease marked by the formation of red scaly patches.

psychiatrist a physician who specializes in psychiatry.

psychiatry a branch of medicine that deals with mental, emotional, or behavioral disorders. —**psychiatric** *adj.* —**psychiatrically** *adv.*

psychoanalysis a method of treating emotional disorders in which the patient talks freely about himself and esp. about his dreams and childhood to an analyst. —**psychoanalytic** *adj.*

psychogenic originating in the mind; imaginary or psychosomatic.

psychology the science concerned with the mind and human behavior. —**psychological** *adj.* —**psychologist** *n.*

psychopath a mentally deranged person. —**psychopathic** *adj.*

psychosis severe, disabling mental derangement marked esp. by a loss of contact with reality. —**psychotic** *n. & adj.*

psychosomatic relating to or involving both psychological and physical factors: *psychosomatic illness.*

psychotherapy any system of psychological treatment for psychopathic, neurotic, or other mental and emotional disorders.

ptosis abnormal drooping of the upper eyelid.

puberty the age at which a person becomes capable of reproducing sexually and during which the genitals mature and the secondary sex characteristics appear; generally between the ages of 12 and 14.

pubes 1. the hair that appears just above the external genital organs at puberty. 2. the two bones forming the front of the pelvis. —**pubic** *adj.*

pudendum, *n., pl.* **pudenda** the external genitals, esp. of women. **—pudendal,** *adj.*

puerperal fever a condition following childbirth and associated with infection, usually as a result of unhygienic conditions.

pulmonary of or relating to the lungs or to the respiratory organs.

pulse the rhythmical beating, detected in superficial arteries, that corresponds to the beating of the heart.

pupil the round, contractive area in the center of the eye.

purgative a medicine for inducing evacuation of the bowels.

purulent characterized by the presence of pus.

pus a thick, opaque whitish fluid containing cellular debris and being a product of inflammation or infection.

pustule a small elevation of the skin containing pus. **—pustular** *adj.*

pyelitis inflammation of the pelvis of the kidney.

pylorus *pl.* **pylori** the valve-like opening of the stomach into the duodenum. **—pyloric** *adj.*

pyogenic producing pus.

pyorrhea an inflammation of the gums that produces pus.

Q

q.d. *abbr.* quaque die: every day.

q.i.d. *abbr.* quater in die: four times daily.

Quaalude a tradename for a drug, methaqualone, used as a sedative and hypnotic.

quack a pretender to medical skills. —**quackery** *n.*

quadrate having four sides that are equal; square.

quadriceps a muscle having four heads, such as a muscle of the thigh (*musculus quadriceps femoris*) or the calf (*musculus quadriceps surae*).

quadricepsplasty a surgical procedure to repair the quadriceps muscle of the thigh.

quadricuspid having four cusps. Also called *tetracuspid.*

quadridigitate having four digits.

quadriplegia paralysis of both legs and arms.

quadriplegic 1. relating to quadriplegia. 2. one with paralysis of all four limbs.

quadrisect to divide or separate into four parts. —**quadrisection** *n.*

quadruplet one of four children born at one birth.

quantum *pl.* **quanta** 1. a unit of radiant energy. 2. a definite amount.

quarantine a restraint upon the activities or movements of anyone with a communicable disease in order to inhibit its spread; detention and isolation from others for a given period of anyone with a contagious disease.

quartan recurring every fourth day.

quater in die (in prescription writing) four times daily.

quaternary 1. (of a chemical compound) containing four elements. 2. coming fourth in a series.

quick 1. pregnant with a child whose movement can be felt within the uterus. 2. any sensitive part that is particularly painful to touch. 3. the part of a finger or toe to which the nail is attached.

quickening the first indications of movement of the fetus within the uterus, usually noted within the first 16 to 20 weeks of pregnancy.

quicksilver mercury.

quin- *or* **quino-** *prefix* relating to or containing quinoline or quinine.

quinine a white, crystalline alkaloid derived from cinchona bark and used as an analgesic, antipyretic and antimalarial agent.

quinoline a substance derived from coal tar and used medically as an analgesic, antipyretic and in the treatment of amoebic dysentery and related infections.

quinsy inflammation of the throat with swelling and fever.

quintan recurring every fifth day.

quinti- *prefix* fifth.

quintipara a woman who has given birth five times.

quintuplet one of five children born at one birth.

quotidian occurring each day; recurring daily.

quotidian fever a malarial fever that flares up every day during the illness.

R

rabbit fever tularemia.

rabiate suffering from rabies.

rabic relating to or concerning rabies.

rabicidal destructive to the virus that causes rabies.

rabid affected with rabies.

rabies an acute and inevitably fatal viral disease transmitted by the bite of a rabid animal.

racemose (esp. of a gland) resembling a bunch of grapes.

rachi- *or* **rachio-** *prefix* relating to or indicating the spinal column.

rachialgia pain in the spine. Also called *rachiodynia.*

rachianalgesia spinal anesthesia.

rachidian relating to the spinal column.

rachiodynia pain in the spine. Also called *rachialgia.*

rachis *pl.* **rachises** *also* **rachides** spinal column.

rachitic relating to or affected with rickets; rickety.

radectomy surgical removal of all or part of the root of a tooth.

radiad in the direction of a radius or the radial side of a structure or part.

radiation sickness an abnormal condition resulting from exposure to radioactive materials. Headache and gastric problems are symptomatic of moderate exposure; sterility, carcinomas, cataracts, and death may result from longer exposure.

radical 1. (in chemistry) a group of atoms that act as a single unit, capable of passing unchanged from one chemical compound to another. 2. relating to or being anything that attacks or reaches an origin or root of something else.

radical mastectomy surgical excision of the breast and its associated muscles and tissues as treatment of cancer of the breast.

radiobiology a branch of biology dealing with the effects on living organisms of radioactive materials or ionizing radiation. —**radiobiological** *adj.* —**radiobiologist** *n.*

radiograph a picture of internal structures of the body using X-rays or gamma rays on a sensitive photographic surface. —**radiographic** *adj.* —**radiography** *n.*

radiology the use of radiant energy, as X-rays, in the diagnosis and treatment of disease. —**radiological** *adj.* —**radiologist** *n.*

radiosensitive sensitive to the effects of radiant energy.

radiotherapy the treatment of disease by the use of radioactive substances or X-rays. —**radiotherapist** *n.*

radium a radioactive and fluorescent metallic element, used in the treatment of various tumors esp. by implantation or insertion into the tissues.

radium therapy the therapeutic use of radium, esp. in controlling the spread of tumors.

radius *pl.* **radii** *or* **radiuses** the outer and shorter bone of the forearm.

radix the root of anything, such as the root portion of a spinal or cranial nerve.

rale an abnormal respiratory sound.

ramus *pl.* **rami** a secondary branch of a bodily structure, as a nerve or vessel.

ranula a cyst formed in a mucous membrane, as that under the tongue. —**ranular** *adj.*

rape sexual intercourse with a female without her consent or when she is legally under age or mentally incapable of making moral decisions.

raphe a ridge, crease or fibrous junction uniting two parts of an organ or part.

rash a usually minor eruption on the skin.

rat-bite fever a febrile, bacterial disease transmitted by the bite of an infected rat.

reaction a bodily response to a stimulus. —**reactive** *adj.*

Read method a system of preparation for natural childbirth developed by Dr. Grantly Dick-Read.

recalcitrant resistant to treatment: *a recalcitrant disease.*

receptor an organ that receives stimuli.

recessive tending to recede or be of minor importance.

recipient one who receives.

recombinant DNA a molecule of DNA in which the arrangement of the genes has been artificially altered.

recrudescence a recurrence of symptoms after an abatement. —**recrudesce** *vb.* —**recrudescent** *adj.*

rectal relating to, being near, or involving the rectum.

rectum *pl.* **rectums** *or* **recta** the part of the intestine from the sigmoid flexure to the anus.

rectus *pl.* **recti** a straight muscle, as one sustaining the abdomen.

recumbent lying down.

recuperate to recover health; become well. —**recuperative** *adj.* —**recuperation** *n.*

recurrent 1. turning back in an opposite direction. 2. repeated; returning after an intermission: *a recurrent head cold.*

red blood cell any of the hemoglobin-containing cells that carry oxygen to the tissues and give redness to the blood; erythrocyte.

reduction the correction of a hernia, fracture, or luxation.

referred pain pain felt in a part of the body different from the site of an injury or disease.

reflex an automatic response to a stimulus that involves a nerve impulse passing to a nerve center and outward again, producing an automatic reaction. Also called *reflex act, reflex action.*

refractory resistant to cure or treatment: *a refractory wound.*

regeneration renewal or restoration of a structure or part of the body, esp. after injury. —**regenerate** *vb.*

regimen a strict plan of diet, medication, or exercise for the purpose of maintaining or restoring health.

regression 1. the decline of a symptom of a disease. 2. gradual loss of function of a body part, esp. as the result of the process of aging.

regurgitation 1. the casting up of incompletely digested food. 2. the backward flow of blood from a defective heart valve. —**regurgitate** *vb.*

Reiter's syndrome *or* **Reiter's disease** arthritis, conjunctivitis, and urethritis occurring simultaneously and of unknown cause.

rejection an immune reaction against grafted tissue or a transplanted organ.

relapse the recurrence of the symptoms of a disease after a period of recovery. —**relapse** *vb.*

relapsing fever any of various acute infectious diseases marked by recurrent high fever for periods of about a week and caused by various spirochetes.

remission a condition or period during which the symptoms of a disease subside.

renal relating to, affecting, or located in the area of the kidneys; nephritic.

resection the surgical excision of part of an organ or structure. —**resect** *vb.* —**resectable** *adj.*

reserpine a drug used to reduce hypertension.

resolution the diminution of inflammation.

resonance the sound produced by percussion of the chest.

respiration the intake of oxygen and expulsion of carbon dioxide from the lungs; breathing. —**respiratory** *adj.*

respirator 1. a device covering the mouth and nose for protecting the respiratory tract. 2. a device for aiding in artificial respiration.

respiratory system the system or organs, as the lungs, their circulatory and nervous supply, and their connecting channels, by which air is conducted to and from the body.

restless legs syndrome a sensation, of undetermined cause, of discomfort and itching within the leg muscles, sometimes accompanied by pain.

resuscitation the action of reviving a person from apparent death or from unconsciousness. —**resuscitate** *vb.*

retardation a less than normal degree of intellectual development. —**retard** *vb.* —**retardant** *adj & n.*

retch to strain in an effort to vomit. —**retch** *n.*

retention abnormal holding in of a secretion or fluid of the body.

reticular of or resembling a net or network: *reticular tissues.*

retina *pl.* **retinas** *or* **retinae** a sensory membrane that lines the interior of the eye, contains the light-sensitive receptors. receives the optical image formed by the lens, and is connected by the optic nerve to the brain. —**retinal** *adj.*

retinitis inflammation of the retina.

retinol vitamin A.

retinopathy any noninflammatory disorder of the retina.

retinoscopy the projection of a beam of light into the eye to observe abnormalities of the retina.

retractor 1. an instrument used in surgery to hold back the edges of a wound. 2. a muscle that draws back or in an organ or part.

retro- *prefix* back; behind.

retroflexion *or* **retroflection** the turning back of a bodily organ upon itself.

retroperitoneal located behind the peritoneum.

retroversion a bending backward of the cervix and uterus.

rheum a watery discharge from the eyes. —**rheumy** *adj.*

rheumatic relating to, affected with, or associated with rheumatism.

rheumatic fever an acute febrile disease marked chiefly by pain and inflammation of the joints and inflammation of the heart valves and the endocardium.

rheumatism inflammation or pain in joints, fibrous tissues, or muscles.

rheumatoid arthritis a progressive disease marked by inflammation, swelling, and sometimes deformation of the joints.

Rh factor a substance present in the red blood cells capable of producing antigenic reactions.

rhinal of, relating to, or affecting the nose; nasal.

rhinitis inflammation of the mucous membranes of the nose.

rhinopharyngitis inflammation of the nose and pharynx.

rhinoplasty plastic surgery to the nose.

rhinoscope a speculum for examining the nasal passages.

rhinoscopy examination of the nasal passages.

rhodopsin a red photosensitive pigment in the rods of the retina of the eye.

rhonchus *pl.* **rhonchi** a hoarse whistling sound heard upon ausculation of the chest and caused by obstruction of the air passages.

rib any one of the twelve pairs of curved bones that enclose the lungs and protect the viscera of the chest.

riboflavin vitamin B.

ribonuclease an enzyme active in catalyzing the hydrolysis of RNA.

ribonucleic acid RNA.

ribosome any of the cytoplasmic granules that are rich in RNA and are central to protein synthesis. **—ribosomal** *adj.*

rickets a disease of childhood caused by insufficient assimilation of calcium and phosphorus from inadequate vitamin D and sunlight and marked by softening and deformation of the bones.

rickettsia *pl.* **rickettsias** *or* **rickettsiae** any of a family of microorganisms, intermediate in size between bacteria and viruses, that cause various diseases, as typhus and Rocky Mountain spotted fever. **—rickettsial** *adj.*

right-handedness dextrality; the condition of being right-handed.

rigor mortis stiffening of the muscles in a dead body.

ringworm any of several diseases of the skin or scalp caused by fungi and marked by ring-shaped, scaly, pigmented patches.

risus sardonicus a fixed, grinning expression caused by spasm of the facial muscles and associated chiefly with tetanus.

RNA ribonucleic acid; any of various nucleic acids found mainly in the nucleolus and mitochondria of cells and being important to the control of cellular chemical action, as protein synthesis.

Rocky Mountain spotted fever an infectious disease caused by a *Rickettsia* organism and transmitted by a tick.

rod any of the rod-shaped, photosensitive receptors in the retina of the eye.

roentgen 1. of or relating to X-rays. 2. the international unit of X-radiation or gamma radiation.

roentgenology a branch of radiology using X-rays for the diagnosis and treatment of disease. **—roentgenologic** *or* **roentgenological** *adj.* **—roentgenologist** *n.*

roentgenoscope fluoroscope. **—roentgenoscopic** *adj.* **—roentgenoscopy** *n.*

roentgen ray X-ray.

root 1. the basal, enlarged part of a hair within the skin. 2. the part of a tooth within the socket. 3. either of the two bundles of nerve fibers that emerge from the spinal cord, joining to form a single spinal nerve.

rose fever an allergic reaction to airborne pollen, not the pollen of roses, which is dispersed by insects, not the wind.

roseola a rose-colored rash, as that occurring as a symptom of German measles.

roughage food containing dietary fiber that is not readily digestible and therefore stimulates peristalsis and is considered essential to maintain the health of the intestinal tract.

rubefacient a substance that causes the skin to redden. **—rubefacient** *adj.*

rubella an infectious viral disease that is less severe than measles but is harmful to the fetus during pregnancy. Also called *German measles.*

ruga *pl.* **rugae** an anatomical wrinkle or fold, as one of the many folds of mucous membrane that lines the stomach.

rugose full of wrinkles; wrinkled.

rupture hernia.

S

Sabin vaccine an orally administered vaccine for protection against poliomyelitis, containing attenuated strains of live polio virus.

sabulous gritty or sandy; resembling coarse sand.

sac a small, internal, usually fluid-containing pouch. —**sacular** *adj.* —**saculated** *adj.*

saccharin a white crystalline compound that is much sweeter than cane sugar and is used in food and liquid as a calorie-free sweetener.

saccharine relating to sugar or sweetness; sweet.

saccharo- *or* **sacchar-** *or* **sacchari-** *prefix* relating to sugar.

saccus *pl.* **sacci** a sac.

sacrad in the direction of or toward the sacrum.

sacralgia pain in the region of the sacrum. Also called *sacrodynia.*

sacro- *or* **sacr-** *prefix* relating to the sacrum.

sacrococcygeal relating to both the sacrum and the coccyx.

sacrodynia pain in the region of the sacrum. Also called *sacralgia.*

sacroiliac 1. relating to both the sacrum and the ilium. 2. (informal) the lower part of the back, including the base of the spine.

sacrolumbar relating to both the sacrum and the lumbar region. Also called *lumbosacral.*

sacrum *pl.* **sacra** the lower part of the vertebral column that connects with and forms part of the pelvis. —**sacral** *adj.*

sadism sexual pleasure derived from inflicting physical or mental pain on others; delight in cruelty. —**sadist** *adj. & n.* —**sadistic** *adj.* —**sadistically** *adv.*

sadomasochism sexual pleasure derived from both inflicting pain and cruelty on others and being the recipient of cruelty or physical pain.

sagittal relating to or located in the median plane of the body. —**sagittally** *adv.*

Saint Vitus's dance chorea.

sal *pl.* **sales** salt.

salify to convert or change into a salt.

saline consisting of or containing salt: *a saline solution.*

saliva the clear, alkaline, somewhat viscid liquid secretion of the salivary glands.

salivary of or relating to saliva or the salivary glands.

salivary gland any of the glands of the oral cavity that secrete saliva.

salivate to produce marked quantities of saliva.

salivation the production of saliva.

Salk vaccine a vaccine that contains three types of polio viruses that have been inactivated for inoculation against poliomyelitis.

salmonella *pl.* **salmonellae** *or* **salmonellas** any of a genus of microorganisms causing food poisoning, diseases of the genital tract, and inflammation of the gastrointestinal tract.

salmonellosis infection with salmonellae.

salpingectomy surgical removal of a fallopian tube.

salpingemphraxis obstruction of a eustachian or a fallopian tube.

salpingian relating to the eustachian or the fallopian tube.

salpingioma any tumor or growth developing in a fallopian tube.

salpingitis inflammation of a eustachian tube or a fallopian tube. —**salpingitic** *adj.*

salpingo- *or* **salping-** *prefix* relating to or denoting a tube, usually a fallopian or eustachian tube.

salpingocele hernia involving a fallopian tube.

salpingolysis the surgical or manual freeing from adhesions of a fallopian tube.

salpingo-oophor- *or* **salpingo-oophoro-** *prefix* relating to a fallopian tube and ovary.

salpingo-oophorectomy surgical removal of a fallopian tube and ovary.

salpingo-oophoritis inflammation of both a fallopian tube and ovary.

salpingoplasty plastic surgery involving the fallopian tubes.

salpingorrhagia bleeding from a fallopian tube.

salpingorrhaphy the procedure of suturing a fallopian tube.

salpinx *pl.* **salpinges** a eustachian or fallopian tube.

saltpeter potassium nitrate.

salubrious favoring health or healthy conditions; healthful. —**salubrity** *n.*

saluresis the excretion in the urine of sodium.

saluretic enhancing or favoring the excretion of sodium by the kidneys.

salutarium sanitarium.

salutary wholesome or healthful.

salve an adhesive, unctuous ointment for soothing wounds or sores.

sanative healing or curative.

sanatorium *pl.* **sanatoriums** *or* **sanatoria** an institution for the convalescent or for the chronically ill.

sandfly fever a febrile, viral disease transmitted by any of various biting, two-winged flies. Also called *phlebotomus fever.*

sanguine of, relating to, or filled with blood. **—sanguinary** *adj.* **—sanguineous** *adj.*

sanitarium *pl.* **sanitariums** *or* **sanitaria** sanatorium.

sanitary of or relating to health or cleanliness. **—sanitation** *n.*

sanitary napkin a soft, disposable, absorbent pad worn to absorb blood flow during the menstrual period.

sanitize to make sanitary.

sanity soundness of mind; rationality. **—sane** *adj.*

saphenous relating to or being either of the two chief superficial veins of the leg.

sapo- *or* **sapon-** *prefix* relating to soap.

saponaceous relating to or resembling soap; soapy.

saponify to convert into soap.

sapphic lesbian. **—sapphism** *n.*

sarapus one who has flatfoot.

sarcoid 1. relating to or resembling flesh; fleshy. 2. a tumor resembling a sarcoma.

sarcoidosis a chronic, progressive disease of unknown origin that is marked chiefly by the appearance of nodules on various bodily organs or tissues or on parts of the body.

sarcolemma a thin membrane enclosing a striated muscle fiber.

sarcoma *pl.* **sarcomas** *or* **sarcomata** an often malignant tumor of connective tissue, striated muscle, bone, or cartilage. **—sarcomatous** *adj.*

sarcomatosis *pl.* **sarcomatoses** a disease marked by the development and spreading of sarcomas.

sartorius a long muscle that crosses the front of the thigh.

sawbones *Slang.* physician; surgeon.

scab a crust over a wound formed of hardened blood, pus, and serum. —**scabby** *adj.*

scabies a contagious skin disease caused by mites and marked by intense itching. —**scabietic** *adj.*

scald a burn caused by hot liquid or steam. —**scald** *vb.*

scale a thin, dry aggregation of cells shed from the skin in some skin diseases. —**scale** *vb.*

scalp the skin covering the top of the head, normally covered with hair.

scapula *pl.* **scapulae** *or* **scapulas** either of the flat triangular bones forming the back of the shoulder; shoulder blade.

scar a mark on the skin remaining after the healing of a wound.

scarification the making of small incisions in the skin, as for a vaccination. —**scarify** *vb.*

scarlatina scarlet fever. —**scarlatinal** *adj.*

scarlet fever an acute, contagious disease marked by fever, extensive skin rash, tonsillitis, and generalized toxemia.

Schick test a test for susceptibility to diphtheria by skin injection of a dilution of diphtheria toxin.

schistosomiasis *pl.* **schistosomiases** a parasitic disease caused by infestation with blood flukes and marked by loss of blood and damage to tissues caused mainly by the deposition in the vessels and tissues of the worms' eggs. Also called *bilharzia.*

schizophrenia a psychotic condition marked chiefly by withdrawal from reality, hallucinations, delusions, and bizarre behavior. Also called (informal) *split personality.* —**schizophrenic** *adj. & n.*

sciatica pain radiating from the lower back to the buttocks and the lower extremities. —**sciatic** *adj.*

sciatic nerve either of a pair of large nerves of the posterior limb and pelvic region passing down the back of the thigh.

scissura 1. a fissure; cleft. 2. a splitting.

sclera the hard white outer coating of the eyeball excluding the cornea. —**scleral** *adj.*

scleradenitis inflammation and hardening of a gland.

sclerema a hardening of subcutaneous fat.

sclero- *or* **scler-** *prefix* 1. hard. 2. relating to the sclera.

scleroderma a skin disease marked by the hardening and thickening of the skin. —**sclerodermatous** *adj.*

sclerosis hardening of tissue. —**sclerotic** *adj.*

scolecoiditis appendicitis.

scolex *pl.* **scolices** the head of a tapeworm.

scoliosis *pl.* **scolioses** lateral curvature of the spine. —**scoliotic** *adj.*

scopolamine an alkaloid derived from the roots of plants of the nightshade family and used as a sedative and as a so-called truth serum.

scorbutic relating to or suffering from scurvy.

scorbutus scurvy.

scotoma *pl.* **scotomas** *or* **scotomata** a blind spot in the field of vision. —**scotomatous** *adj.*

scotophobia an abnormal fear of the dark.

scrofula an obsolete term for primary tuberculosis in which abscesses are present.

scrotum *pl.* **scrotums** *or* **scrota** the external pouch that holds the testes. —**scrotal** *adj.*

scurf dry thin scales shed from the epidermis esp. in some skin diseases. —**scurfy** *adj.*

scurvy a disease caused by deficiency of ascorbic acid and marked chiefly by sponginess of the gums and loosening of the teeth.

sebaceous relating to, resembling, or secreting fatty material; fatty: *sebaceous glands.*

seborrhea abnormally profuse production and discharge of sebum. —**seborrheic** *adj.*

sebum a lubricant, fatty substance secreted by the sebaceous glands of the skin.

secobarbital a drug used as a sedative and hypnotic.

Seconal a tradename for secobarbital.

secondary sex characteristic a physical characteristic, as the appearance of facial hair in boys, that appears at the time of puberty but is not directly related to reproduction.

secondary syphilis the second stage of syphilis that appears from 2 to 6 months after the primary stage and is marked by lesions in the skin, organs, and tissues and has a duration of 3 to 12 weeks.

section 1. a surgical division of a structure or part; cut. 2. a cut surface. 3. an extremely thin slice of tissue taken for microscopic examination.

secundigravida a woman who is pregnant for the second time.

sedative 1. tending to calm or neutralize nervousness or excitement. 2. an agent or drug that has a sedative effect. —**sedate** *vb.* —**sedation** *n.*

segmentum *pl.* **segmenta** 1. a section or part of a structure. 2. the part or region of an organ that has an independent function, separate nerve or vascular supply, etc.

semen a whitish, viscid fluid produced by the male reproductory tract that serves as the vehicle for spermatozoa.

semicircular canal a loop-shaped canal of the inner ear associated with maintenance of the sense of equilibrium.

seminal of, relating to, or consisting of semen.

senescence the condition or process of aging.

senile dementia deteriorated mental ability in the aged, caused by atrophy of the brain that is not associated with disease. Also **senile psychosis.**

senility the loss of mental faculties owing to old age. **—senile** *adj.*

senna pods or leaflets of the plant *Cassia augustifolia* or *C. acutifolia,* used as a cathartic drug.

sensation a mental process, as seeing or smelling, that is a direct response to bodily stimulation.

sense organ a structure of the body, as an eye or ear, that receives stimuli and transmits the excitation to nerve fibers continuous with the central nervous system where the stimuli are interpreted as sensations.

sensitive highly susceptible; hypersensitive: *sensitive to ragweed pollen.*

sensitization the condition of being sensitive or hypersensitive to an antigen or drug. **—sensitize** *vb.*

sensory carrying nerve impulses from the sense organs to the nerve centers; afferent. **—sensorial** *adj.*

sepsis *pl.* **sepses** a toxic condition resulting from the spread of bacteria or the products of bacteria from an infection. **—septic** *adj.*

septicemia circulation of virulent microorganisms in the bloodstream. Also called *blood poisoning.*

septum *pl.* **septa** a dividing wall or membrane between two bodily cavities.

sequela, *pl.* **sequelae** the event or condition following upon and the result of a disease, injury, etc.

sequestrum *pl.* **sequestrums** *or* **sequestra** a fragment of dead bone; bony necrosis.

serology the study of blood serum.

serosa a serous membrane. **—serosal** *adj.*

serotonin a vasoconstrictor and neurotransmitter that occurs naturally in the brain and intestine.

serous relating to or resembling serum; watery and thin.

Serpasil a tradename for reserpine.

serum *pl.* **serums** *or* **sera** the watery part of a fluid, as blood, remaining after coagulation or removal of the other parts.

serum sickness an allergic reaction following an injection of foreign serum and marked by skin rash, pain in the joints, swelling, fever, and prostration.

sesamoid of or relating to a mass of cartilage or bone at a joint or bony prominence. —**sesamoid** *n.*

sessile attached to a base; not free to move: *sessile polyps.*

sex 1. either of two divisions of living organisms distinguished as male or female respectively. 2. the functional, structural, and behavioral characteristics of the male or female sex. 3. sexual activity. 4. (informal) sexual intercourse.

sex chromosome a chromosome inherited differently in the two sexes and concerned with the determination of sex.

sex-linked characterizing any disease or disorder resulting from an abnormality in sex chromosome.

sexual 1. relating to or associated with sex or the sexes. 2. erotic in nature or character. —**sexually** *adv.*

sexual intercourse sexual connection esp. between human beings; penetration of the vagina by the penis, usually leading to orgasm; coitus.

sexuality sexual feelings and interests.

shell shock a former name for combat fatigue.

shield a material used to block radiation, as lucite or aluminum, which block beta radiation, and lead, which blocks gamma radiation.

shigellosis infection of the bowel caused by the *Shigella* bacterium, transmitted by contact with the feces of an infected carrier.

shinbone tibia.

shingles an acute viral inflammation of the spinal and cranial nerves marked by neuralgic pains and vesicular eruptions; herpes zoster.

shin splints a painful disorder of the lower leg caused by strain of the muscles of the toes, commonly resulting from strenuous activity, as running.

shock severe circulatory disturbance with markedly reduced blood pressure and volume caused typically by a severe injury, burn, or the like.

show (informal) a discharge of bloodstained mucus from the vagina occurring chiefly at the beginning of labor.

sialogogue any substance or other stimulus that increases the flow of saliva.

Siamese twins twins from the same ovum that are physically joined at birth.

sibling one of two or more individuals having the same parent.

sick bay an infirmary on a naval ship or at a naval station.

sick call a military formation at which individuals can report if in need of medical attention.

sickle to form into a crescent.

sickle-cell anemia an inherited anemia occurring chiefly among people of Negro ancestry and in which a large proportion or the majority of the red blood cells tend to sickle.

sigmoid curved like the letter *S*.

sigmoid flexure the contracted and crooked part of the colon just above the rectum.

silicon a nonmetallic element that is the most abundant element (25 per cent) next to oxygen in the earth's crust.

silicone an organic compound in which the carbon has been replaced by silicon.

silicosis a disease of the lungs marked by shortness of breath and caused by prolonged inhalation of silica dust.

simethicone a drug used to reduce stomach gas.

simple fracture a bone fracture having no secondary complications.

simple mastectomy surgical excision of the breast in which the associated muscles and tissues are left intact.

sinciput the upper and fore part of the cranium. —**sinciputal** *adj.*

sinew a tendon connecting a muscle to a bone. —**sinewy** *adj.*

singultus a hiccup.

sinistral relating to or situated on the left side.

sinoatrial of, relating to, or involving a cluster of cells in the right wall of the atrium of the heart.

sinus 1. a passage leading from an abscess to an external opening of the body. 2. a dilated channel for venous blood. 3. an air-filled passage communicating from the bones of the skull to the nostrils.

sinusitis inflammation of a sinus of the skull.

sinusoid 1. resembling a sinus. 2. a blood channel in certain organs. —**sinusoidal** *adj.* —**sinusoidally** *adv.*

siriasis sunstroke.

skeleton the rigid, supportive bony framework of the body. —**skeletal** *adj.* —**skeletally** *adv.*

skin the outer integument of the body.

skin graft skin transferred surgically from one part of a person's body to another part that has been injured, burned, or surgically removed because of disease.

skull the bony skeleton of the head protecting the brain and the major sense organs.

sleeping pill any drug taken to induce sleep.

sleeping sickness an acute infectious protozoal disease

chiefly of Africa that is marked by fever, tremors, intense lethargy and is transmitted by tsetse flies.

slipped disk the rupture of one of the disks of cartilage that lies between the vertebrae; herniated intervertebral disk.

slough dead tissue cast off from the body or a bodily part.

small intestine the portion of the digestive tract between the stomach and the opening into the large intestine, approximately 23 feet long.

smallpox a highly infectious viral disease marked by fever and scarring skin eruptions with pustules.

smear a thin film of tissue put on a glass slide for use as a specimen for microscopic examination.

smegma a cheesy sebaceous substance collecting between the glans penis and the foreskin or around the labia minora and clitoris.

smooth muscle involuntary muscle composed of long cells, esp. that of the stomach and intestines.

snare a surgical instrument consisting of a wire loop contracted by a mechanism in the handle and used for removing masses of tissue, such as the tonsils.

snow blindness inflammation and photophobia of the eyes resulting from exposure to ultraviolet light reflected from snow or ice. —**snow-blind** *adj.*

sociopath a psychopath.

sodium bicarbonate a drug used chiefly as an antacid; baking soda.

sodium chloride common table salt.

sodium pentobarbital a sodium salt of pentobarbital used esp. as a sedative and as an adjunct to other anesthesia.

soft palate the palate at the upper rear part of the mouth, between the hard palate and the pharynx.

solar plexus a nerve plexus in the abdomen.

soleus a muscle in the calf of the leg.

solvent a liquid capable of dissolving a substance.

somatic of, relating to, or affecting the body, esp. as distinct from the psyche.

somnambulism the habit of walking while asleep. **—somnambular** *adj.* **—somnambulist** *n.* **—somnambulistic** *adj.*

soporific an agent that tends to induce sleep; hypnotic. **—soporific** *adj.*

sore throat inflammation of the lining of the throat, esp. caused by a bacterial infection.

spasm an involuntary, abnormal muscular contraction. **—spasmodic** *adj.* **—spasmodically** *adv.*

spasmolytic capable of relieving spasms.

spastic 1. relating to or characterized by spasms. 2. marked by spastic paralysis. **—spastic** *n.*

spectroscope an instrument for forming and examining optical spectra. **—spectroscopy** *n.*

speculum *pl.* **specula** *or* **speculums** an instrument for insertion into a body passage for inspection or applying medication.

speech center the part of the brain controlling speech.

sperm 1. semen. 2. a spermatozoon; male sex cell.

spermatic cord a cord that suspends the testis within the scrotum and contains the vas deferens.

spermatozoon *pl.* **spermatozoa** a motile male gamete having a flagellum for propulsion and being the means for fertilizing the human egg.

spermicide *also* **spermatocide** a substance that destroys spermatozoa.

sphenoid bone a bone at the base of the skull.

sphincter an annular muscle for contracting a body opening.

sphygmomanometer an instrument for measuring blood pressure. **—sphygmomanometry** *n.*

spina bifida a birth defect in which the spine is partly open.

spinal anesthetic an anesthetic injected into the base of the spinal column, used to avoid giving a general anesthetic in surgery.

spinal column the backbone; vertebral column; spine.

spinal cord the cord of nerve tissue extending from the brain through the spinal column.

spine the backbone; spinal column; vertebral column.

spirochete *also* **spirochaete** any slender, spirally undulating bacterium.

splanchnic of, relating to, or involving the organs of the stomach; visceral.

spleen a vascular organ involved with destruction of blood cells, storage of blood, and production of lymphocytes. —**splenic** *adj.*

splenectomy *pl.* **splenectomies** surgical removal of the spleen.

splenomegaly abnormal enlargement of the spleen.

splint a rigid or flexible device for immobilizing or limiting movement of a part of the body.

spondylitis inflammation of a vertebra.

spontaneous abortion naturally occurring abortion before the 20th week of pregnancy, resulting from abnormality of the fetus or the mother.

spotted fever any of various eruptive fevers, as typhus.

sprain a wrench of a joint with stretching or tearing of the ligaments.

sprue a chronic disease with chronic diarrhea, soreness of the tongue and mouth, and anemia.

sputum *pl.* **sputa** expectorated matter composed chiefly of mucus but sometimes also of discharge from the respiratory passages.

squamous scaly.

stapes *pl.* **stapes** *or* **stapedes** the innermost of the three conducting bones of the middle ear; stirrup.

staph staphylococcus.

staphylococcus *pl.* **staphylococci** any of various round (coccal) bacteria that include parasites of the skin and mucous membranes. —**staphylococcal** *adj.*

stasis *pl.* **stases** a slowing or stopping of the normal flow of body fluids.

steat- *or* **steato-** *prefix* fat.

steatopygia an abnormal development of fat on the buttocks. —**steatopygic** *or* **steatopygous** *adj.*

stenosis the abnormal narrowing of an opening or duct in an organ.

sterile unable to produce offspring. —**sterility** *n.*

sterilization deprivation of the ability to produce offspring, esp. by removal of the ovaries or by vasectomy. —**sterilize** *vb.*

sternum *pl.* **sternums** *or* **sterna** the breastbone.

stertor rasping, wheezing respiration during deep sleep; a snore. —**stertorous** *adj.*

stethoscope an instrument for listening to and diagnosing sounds produced within the body, esp. those of the heart and lungs.

stillborn dead at birth. —**stillborn** *n.*

stimulant a substance that produces alertness and a temporary increase in functional activity. —**stimulant** *adj.* —**stimulate** *vb.* —**stimulation** *n.*

St. Louis encephalitis a brain infection carried from birds to man by the bite of an infected mosquito.

stoma, *pl.* **stomas** *or* **stomata** any natural or artificial opening, as in the surface of the skin, between two organs, etc.

stomach an expansion of the alimentary canal, extending

from the esophagus to the duodenum, in which food is first digested before entering the small intestine.

stomachic an agent that stimulates the digestion of food in the stomach.

stomach pump a device for emptying the contents of the stomach through a tube inserted through the nose or throat.

stomatitis inflammation of the mouth.

stone calculus.

stool a discharge of fecal matter.

strabismus an inability of one eye to focus in conjunction with the other through muscle weakness.

strangulated constricted so as to be cut off from a supply of blood: *strangulated hernia.*

strep throat sore throat and associated symptoms caused by a streptococcus.

streptococcus any of a genus of parasitic bacteria that includes many important pathogens. **—streptococcal** *adj.*

streptomycin sulfate an antibiotic drug.

striated muscle voluntary muscle composed of thin parallel fibers.

stroke cardiovascular accident, often causing sensory or motor impairment.

sty *or* **stye** an inflamed swelling at the margin of an eyelid.

styptic tending to arrest bleeding.

subcutaneous beneath the skin.

sudden infant death syndrome the sudden, unexpected death from unknown causes of an apparently healthy, normal infant between two weeks and one year of age.

sudorific inducing sweat.

sulcus, *pl.* **sulci** a groove on the surface of an organ.

sulfadiazine an antibacterial drug.

sulfonamide a group of antibacterial drugs.

sunstroke heat exhaustion.

suppository a medication in the form of a small capsule, etc., that melts at body temperatures and is administered esp. by means of the rectum or vagina.

suppuration the formation or discharge of pus. —**suppurate** *vb.* —**suppurative** *adj.*

surgery 1. the branch of medical science concerned with diseases and conditions requiring operations. 2. a specially equipped room where surgical operations are performed.

surgical of, relating to, or used in surgery. —**surgically** *adv.*

suspensory *pl.* **suspensories** a fabric supporter for the testicles.

suture a fiber or strand used to sew parts of the body that are wounded or have undergone surgery. —**suture** *vb.*

swab a wad of absorbent material, as cotton, used alone or wrapped around the end of a small stick to cleanse a wound or remove material from an area. —**swab** *vb.*

sweat to exude moisture through the skin, esp. profusely; perspire. —**sweat** *n.*

sycosis inflammation of the hair follicles esp. of the beard.

sympathetic nervous system autonomic nervous system.

symphysis *pl.* **symphyses** an articulation of various bones joined together by fibrous cartilage.

symptom a bodily change experienced by a patient that is indicative of a disease or disorder. —**symptomatic** *adj.*

syncope temporary loss of consciousness; faint.

syndrome the aggregate of signs and symptoms characteristic of a particular disease.

synovia a transparent fluid secreted by a membrane of a joint or bursa. —**synovial** *adj.*

synovitis inflammation of the synovial membrane of a joint.

syphilis a chronic disease usually transmitted during sexual intercourse with an infected partner, caused by a spirochete and characteristically marked by three sequential degenerative stages occurring over the course of many years. —**syphilitic** *n. & adj.*

syringe 1. an instrument for injecting a drug or medication and consisting of a hollow barrel with a plunger to hold the substance and a hollow needle. 2. an instrument with a nozzle and compressible bulb used for irrigation of a cavity.

systemic of, relating to, or involving the entire body, rather than a part.

systole the contraction of the heart by which the blood is forced through the circulatory system.

T

tabella *pl.* **tabellae** a medicated mass of compressed material such as a tablet or lozenge.

tabes *pl.* **tabes** wasting of the body associated with a chronic disease, as syphilis. —**tabetic** *adj.*

tabescence the state or condition of wasting away.

tablespoon (as a unit of measure) one-half fluid ounce; 15 milliliters.

tache a small area of discoloration on the skin or a mucous membrane, such as a freckle or macule. —**tachetic** *adj.*

tachycardia increased heart beat.

tachypnea abnormally rapid breathing.

tactile relating to the sense of touch.

tactus the sense of touch; touch.

taenia *also* **tenia** 1. any bandlike structure or part. 2. a tapeworm.

Taenia saginata the beef tapeworm, acquired by humans as the result of eating inadequately cooked infected beef and causing the condition known as teniasis.

taeniasis teniasis.

Taenia solium the pork tapeworm, acquired by humans as the result of eating inadequately cooked infected pork and causing the condition known as cysticercosis.

talipes club foot.

tapeworm any of a variety of taenia that infest the digestive tract.

tarsus 1. the seven bones that together constitute the articulation between the foot and leg; ankle. 2. the cartilaginous connective tissue supporting the eyelids. —**tarsal** *adj.*

tartar a calcium deposit forming on the teeth in combination with saliva and food particles.

taste bud an end organ lying chiefly on the surface of the tongue and conveying the sense of taste.

Tay-Sachs disease an inherited disorder, occurring chiefly among people of eastern European Jewish origin and usually fatal by the age of four.

tear a drop of saline fluid secreted by the lacrimal glands. —**tear** *vb.* —**teary** *adj.*

teeth *pl. of* tooth.

tegument the skin; integument.

temperature degree of heat.

temple the flattened area on each side of the forehead. —**temporal** *adj.*

tendinitis inflammation of a tendon.

tendon a tough band or cord of dense connective tissue that joins a muscle with some other part. —**tendinous** *adj.*

tenesmus ineffectual, painful straining to evacuate the bowel or bladder.

teniasis *also* **taeniasis** the presence of tapeworms in the body; infestation with tapeworms.

tennis elbow epicondylitis.

tenorrhaphy suture of the cut ends of a tendon. Also called *tenosuture.*

tenosynovitis inflammation of both a tendon and its enclosing sheath. Also called *tendosynovitis.*

tenotomy surgical incision of a tendon, as in the treatment of a deformity caused by abnormal shortening of a muscle.

teratogenic tending to cause malformation of a fetus. —**teratogen** *n.* —**teratogenesis** *n.*

ter in die (in prescription writing) three times daily. Abbr. *t.i.d.*

terpin hydrate and codeine elixir a liquid medicine given for a cold, sore throat, etc.

Terramycin a tradename for an antibiotic.

tertiary syphilis the third degenerative and usually fatal stage of syphilis.

testicle testis.

testis *pl.* **testes** either of two male reproductive glands suspended in the scrotum.

testosterone a male hormone produced in the testes or synthetically and responsible for male secondary sex characteristics.

tetanus an acute infectious disease characterized by spasms of the muscles esp. of the jaw and caused by a bacillic toxin introduced through a wound.

tetany muscular spasms caused by mineral deficiency.

tetracycline a broad-spectrum antibiotic.

thalamus a mass of nerve cells at the base of the brain that is the main receptor for sensory impulses, which it transmits to the cerebral cortex.

thalassemia a form of hemolytic anemia occurring chiefly among people of Mediterranean origin.

thalidomide a hypnotic, sedative drug no longer in use because it was found to produce malformation of the fetus when taken during pregnancy.

theca *pl.* **thecae** an enveloping sheath of a bodily part. **—thecal** *adj.*

therapeutics a branch of medical science dealing with methods of treating disease. **—therapeutic** *adj.*

thermography a technique for measuring the heat in various parts of the body and transforming the signals received into a diagnostic photographic record. **—thermograph** *n.* **—thermographic** *adj.*

thermometer an instrument, typically a liquid-filled glass tube with a numbered scale, used for recording variations in temperature. —**thermometric** *adj.*

thiamine *also* **thiamin** a B vitamin essential to metabolism and nerve function.

thigh the part of the leg between the pelvis and the knee.

thighbone femur.

thiopental sodium a barbiturate used as a general anesthetic for procedures lasting less than 15 minutes.

thoracic relating to, involving, or located within the thorax.

thorax *pl.* **thoraxes** *or* **thoraces** the part of the body between the neck and the abdomen including the heart and lungs contained within it; chest.

thromb- *or* **thrombo-** *prefix* blood clot; relating to a blood clot or to clotting.

thromboembolism the blocking of a blood vessel by an embolus.

thrombophlebitis inflammation of a vein with thrombosis.

thrombosis *pl.* **thromboses** the formation of a clot within a blood vessel. —**thrombotic** *adj.*

thrombus *pl.* **thrombi** a blood clot formed within a blood vessel and remaining attached to its point of origin. Compare *embolus.*

thrush a fungus disease marked by the formation of white patches in the mucous membranes esp. of the mouth.

thymus a glandular structure of uncertain function that is present in the upper chest or base of the neck of the young and tends to atrophy with age.

thyroid 1. a large endocrine gland at the base of the neck producing the hormone thyroxine. Also called *thyroid gland.* 2. of or relating to the thyroid gland.

thyroidectomy *pl.* **thyroidectomies** surgical removal of tissue of the thyroid gland.

thyroiditis inflammation of the thyroid gland.

tibia the larger of the two bones of the lower leg extending from the knee to the ankle; shin bone.

tic spasmodic, habitual twitching of a muscle, esp. of the face.

tic douloureux trigeminal neuralgia.

t.i.d. *abbr.* ter in die: three times daily.

tincture a medicinal substance diluted with alcohol. **—tincture** *vb.*

tinea any of various fungal skin diseases. Also called *ringworm.*

tinnitus a sensation of noise, as roaring or ringing, in the ears.

tissue an aggregate of cells of a particular kind together with its intercellular substance forming part of the body's structural material.

tissue culture the method of causing tissue to grow in a medium outside of the parent source.

tolerance 1. the ability to endure the effects of a drug, food, or other agent without adverse reaction. 2. the development of a decreased effect of a particular drug at a given dose, requiring that the dose be increased in order to achieve the original effect. **—tolerable** *adj.* **—tolerant** *adj.* **—tolerate** *vb.* **—toleration** *n.*

tomography a technique for producing a detailed x-ray radiograph at a specific depth.

tone the condition of the body or any of its parts in relation to a standard of vigorous health.

tongue the muscular organ on the floor of the mouth equipped with the end organs providing the sense of taste and functioning as an organ of speech.

tongue-tie shortening of the frenum of the tongue resulting in restricted mobility. —**tongue-tied** *adj.*

tonic 1. any remedy that is considered to be invigorating. 2. relating to or characterized by tonus.

tonsil either of two masses of lymphoid tissue that lie one on each side of the throat.

tonsillectomy surgical removal of the tonsils.

tonsillitis inflammation of the tonsils.

tonus a condition of mild contraction characteristic of normal muscle.

tooth *pl.* **teeth** one of the hard bony appendages lining the jaws and used in mastication.

tophus *pl.* **tophi** deposits of urate or crystals of uric acid in tissue characteristic of advanced or chronic gout, typically seen in the fleshy folds of the external ear.

topical intended for external application to a local area: *a topical anesthetic.*

torpor extreme sluggishness; lethargy.

torsion the act of twisting or the state of being twisted.

torso *pl.* **torsoes** *or* **torsi** the trunk of the body.

torticollis contraction of the neck muscles resulting in a twisted, unnatural carriage of the head. Also called *wryneck.*

tourniquet an instrument or device, as a bandage twisted and held fast with a stick, formerly recommended to check the flow of arterial bleeding.

toxemia the presence of a toxic substance in the blood. —**toxemic** *adj.*

toxic of, relating to, or caused by poison.

toxic- *or* **toxico-** *prefix* poison.

toxicant a toxic agent. —**toxicant** *adj.*

toxicology a branch of science dealing with poisons and their effects. —**toxicological** *or* **toxicologic** *adj.*

toxicosis *pl.* **toxicoses** a disease caused by poisoning.

toxic shock syndrome an acute staphylococcal infection, most common in menstruating women who use highly absorbent tampons.

toxigenic producing toxin. —**toxigenicity** *n.*

toxin a poisonous substance of bacterial or other origin that is capable of causing antibody formation.

toxoid a toxin that has had its toxicity neutralized so as to be functional as an antitoxin for injection.

toxoplasma any of a genus of parasitic protozoal microorganisms that are pathogens of vertebrate organisms. —**toxoplasmic** *adj.*

toxoplasmosis *pl.* **toxoplasmoses** a disease caused by infection with toxoplasmas and marked by severe damaging effects on the central nervous system.

trabecula *pl.* **trabeculae** *or* **trabeculas** a strand of connective tissue in the structure of a bodily part or organ.

trachea *pl.* **tracheae** *or* **tracheas** the main trunk of the air passages from the larynx to the bronchi. —**tracheal** *adj.*

tracheitis inflammation of the trachea.

tracheostomy the insertion of a tube into the trachea directly through an incision in the neck to allow a patient with an obstructed pharynx to breathe.

tracheotomy *pl.* **tracheotomies** surgical incision of the trachea through the muscles and skin of the neck.

trachoma a chronic, contagious form of conjunctivitis.

traction a constant pulling force exerted on a skeletal part as a means of achieving proper alignment of bones.

tragus *pl.* **tragi** the cartilaginous prominence central to the opening of the outer ear.

trance an abnormal, profound state of sleep.

tranquilizer *also* **tranquillizer** a drug used to reduce or modify tension or anxiety. —**tranquilize** *also* **tranquillize** *vb.*

transfusion the transference of a fluid, as blood, into a vein.

transplant an organ or tissue used for transplantation. —**transplant** *vb.*

transplantation the transfer of an organ or tissue from one part of the body to another or from one individual to another.

transsexual one having a psychological urge to be a member of the opposite sex and often seeking surgical and hormonal remedy to alter gender. —**transsexualism** *n.*

transudation the passage of a fluid from a tissue or through a membrane. —**transude** *vb.*

transvestism the adoption of the attire and often the behavior of the opposite sex. —**transvestite** *n.*

trapezium *pl.* **trapeziums** *or* **trapezia** a wrist bone at the base of the thumb.

trapezius a large triangular muscle at each side of the back.

trauma *pl.* **traumas** *or* **traumata** physical or psychological injury. —**traumatic** *adj.* —**traumatically** *adv.*

treatment any of various means of curing or alleviating the signs and symptoms of a disease or disorder.

tremor a physical trembling caused typically by neurological disease, debility, or emotional stress. —**tremulous** *adj.*

trench mouth Vincent's angina.

trephine 1. a circular incision, as one made surgically on the skull or a cornea. 2. a surgical instrument for performing a trephine. —**trephination** *n.*

triage the classification of ill and injured according to their need for treatment.

triceps a muscle arising from three heads, esp. the large muscle of the back of the upper arm.

trichinosis a serious disease, sometimes fatal, resulting from eating undercooked or raw pork.

trichomoniasis an infection of the vagina or (in males) the urethra caused by a protozoan.

tricuspid valve a valve of three flaps preventing the return of blood from the right ventricle to the right auricle of the heart.

trigeminal nerve either of two major nerves supplying motor and sensory fibers chiefly to the face.

trigeminal neuralgia intense paroxysmal pain of the trigeminal nerves. Also called: *tic douloureux.*

trimester a three-month period; one of the three divisions of the term of pregnancy.

triplet any of three children born at one birth.

trismus a spasm of the muscles of the jaw; lockjaw.

trocar *also* **trochar** a sharp-pointed instrument used with a cannula for drawing off body fluids.

trochlear of, relating to, or affecting a trochlear nerve.

trochlear nerve a cranial nerve supplying motor fibers to the eye muscles.

trophic of, relating to, or involving nourishment. **—trophically** *adv.*

trunk the part of the body exclusive of the head or limbs; torso.

truss a device worn to retain a hernia by external pressure. **—truss** *vb.*

trypanosome any of a genus of parasitic protozoans that infest the blood, are usually transmitted by the bite of an insect, and cause serious disease, as sleeping sickness.

trypanosomiasis *pl.* **trypanosomiases** disease caused by trypanosomes.

tsetse fly a two-winged fly of Africa, south of the Sahara, that is a vector of trypanosomes. Also called *tsetse.*

tubal of or involving a tube, esp. a fallopian tube.

tubercle a small knobby excrescence or prominence; nodule.

tubercle bacillus a bacterium causing tuberculosis.

tubercul- *or* **tuberculo-** *prefix* tubercle; tubercle bacillus.

tubercular relating to or affected by tuberculosis.

tuberculin a sterile liquid extracted from the tubercle bacillus and used in the diagnosis of tuberculosis.

tuberculin test a test for hypersensitivity to tuberculin.

tuberculosis *pl.* **tuberculoses** a communicable disease caused by infection with the tubercle bacillus and characterized by toxic symptoms partly affecting the lungs. **—tuberculous** *adj.*

tubule a small, slender, anatomical channel.

tularemia an infectious plague-like disease transmitted by the bite of blood-sucking insects.

tumefaction the process or action of becoming swollen. **—tumefactive** *adj.*

tumescence the condition or process of becoming swollen. **—tumesce** *vb.* **—tumescent** *adj.*

tumor an abnormal growth or mass of tissue that is not inflammatory and may be either benign or malignant; neoplasm. **—tumorous** *adj.*

turgid marked by a state of swollenness; distended. **—turgidity** *n.* **—turgor** *n.*

tussive of, relating to, or involved in coughing.

twin either of two children born at one birth.

Tylenol a tradename for the drug acetaminophen.

tympanic membrane a membrane that separates the external ear and the middle ear and serves in the reception and transmission of sound waves; eardrum.

tympanites distension of the abdomen caused by retention of abdominal gas.

tympanum *pl.* **tympana** *or* **tympanums** tympanic membrane; eardrum.

typhoid typhoid fever. —**typhoid** *adj.*

typhoid fever an acute, infectious bacterial disease marked by fever, headache, diarrhea and prostration.

typhus a severe febrile rickettsial disease marked by stupor and delirium in alternation, body rash, and violent headache and transmitted by body lice.

THE THYROID GLAND

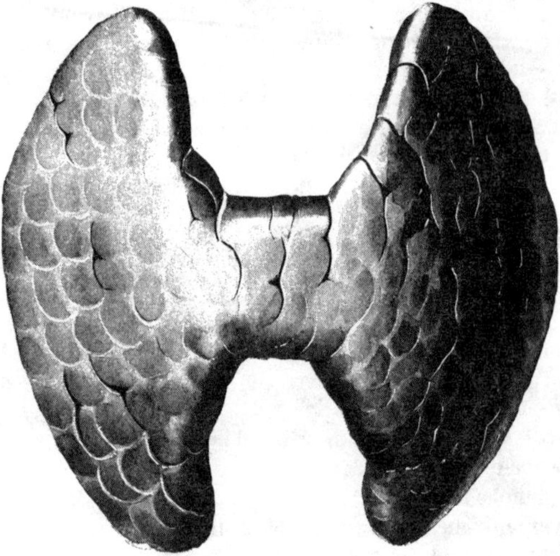

The thyroid is a large reddish, endocrine (ductless) gland located in front of, and on either side of, the trachea. It consists of two lateral lobes and a connecting isthmus.

U

ulcer a break in mucous membrane or skin resulting in the development of an open sore. **—ulcerate** *vb.* **—ulceration** *n.* **—ulcerative** *adj.*

ulcerous relating to or marked by an ulcer.

ulcus *pl.* **ulcera** ulcer.

ulcus hypostaticum a bedsore; decubitus ulcer.

ulectomy surgical removal of scar tissue.

uletic relating to a scar; scarred.

uletomy surgical incision of a scar to relieve tension.

ulna the inner of two bones of the forearm between the elbow and the wrist. **—ulnar** *adj.*

ulnad toward the ulna.

ulo- *or* **ule-** *prefix* relating to or denoting a scar or scarring.

ulosis scar formation; cicatrization.

ultrafiltration filtration of a colloidal substance through a semipermeable membrane or other filter to separate it from its dispersion medium and crystalloids.

ultramicroscope a device using scattered light to make visible those particles too small for viewing by an ordinary microscope.

ultramicroscopic smaller than can be perceived with an ordinary microscope.

ultrasonics the diagnostic or therapeutic use of extremely high-frequency sound waves. **—ultrasonic** *adj.*

ultrasonogram a record obtained from the use of ultrasonography.

ultrasonography the diagnostic use of ultrasonic waves to locate, delineate or measure deep structures of the body by measuring their relative ability to reflect or transmit these extreme high-frequency sound waves.

ultraviolet ray a light ray beyond the visible spectrum at its violet end but having a wavelength longer than that of an X-ray.

umbilical of, relating to, or situated at the navel.

umbilical cord a cord from the navel of a fetus that connects with the mother's placenta.

umbilicus *pl.* **umbilici** *or* **umbilicuses** a small depression (or sometimes a slight elevation) in the center of the abdomen marking the original connective point of the umbilical cord.

uncinariasis infection with hookworms.

uncinate shaped like or resembling a hook; hook-shaped.

unconscious 1. not conscious; unable to perceive or respond to external stimuli. 2. (in psychoanalytic theory) the part of the mind that influences impulses, thoughts, desires, etc., but of which the individual is not aware.

undulant fever an acute, infectious, febrile disease marked by recurring attacks of fever and weakness; brucellosis.

unguent a healing or soothing ointment or salve.

unicellular consisting of a single cell: *unicellular microorganism.*

uniparous having borne only one child.

upper respiratory tract the nose and associated structures, larynx, and trachea.

ur- *or* **uro-** *prefix* urine; urinary.

urea a white, crystalline substance found in urine, constituting the chief nitrogenous waste product of metabolism.

uremia a severe toxic condition caused by retention in the blood of high levels of the waste product urea, which is normally eliminated in the urine. —**uremic** *adj.*

ureter the long, narrow tube that carries the urine from the kidney to the bladder. —**ureteral** *adj.*

urethr- *or* **urethro-** *prefix* urethra: *urethritis.*

urethra *pl.* **urethras** *or* **urethrae** the canal that carries the urine from the bladder for excretion and in the male also serves as the conduit for semen. —**urethral** *adj.*

urethritis inflammation of the urethra.

urethroscope an instrument for viewing the interior of the urethra.

uric acid a waste product normally present in small quantities in urine, but which in larger amounts can form crystals of urate in the joints and give rise to the painful symptoms of gout or gouty arthritis.

urinalysis *pl.* **urinalyses** a chemical analysis of the constituents of urine.

urinary relating to or involving urine or the urinary bladder.

urinary bladder a membranous sac for retaining urine.

urination the act of excreting urine. —**urinate** *vb.*

urine fluid waste material secreted by the kidneys, temporarily stored in the urinary bladder, and eventually discharged from the body through the urethra.

urinometer a small hydrometer for determining the specific gravity of urine. —**urinometric** *adj.*

urogenital of, relating to, or involving the urinary and genital organs. —**urogenitally** *adv.*

urography X-ray examination of the urinary tract. —**urographologist** *n.*

urolith a calculus in the urinary tract.

urologist a specialist in urology.

urology a branch of medicine concerned with diseases or

problems of the urinary or urogenital tracts. **—urologic** *or* **urological** *adj.*

urticaria an allergic reaction marked by an eruptive skin rash; nettle rash; hives.

uterus *pl.* **uteri** *or* **uteruses** an organ of the female for containing and nourishing the developing fetus; womb. **—uterine** *adj.*

uvea the posterior, pigmented layer of the iris of the eye.

uveitis inflammation of the uvea.

uvula *pl.* **uvulas** *or* **uvulae** a pendant lobe at the back of the soft palate. **—uvular** *adj.*

uvulectomy *pl.* **uvulectomies** surgical removal of the uvula.

uvulitis inflammation of the uvula.

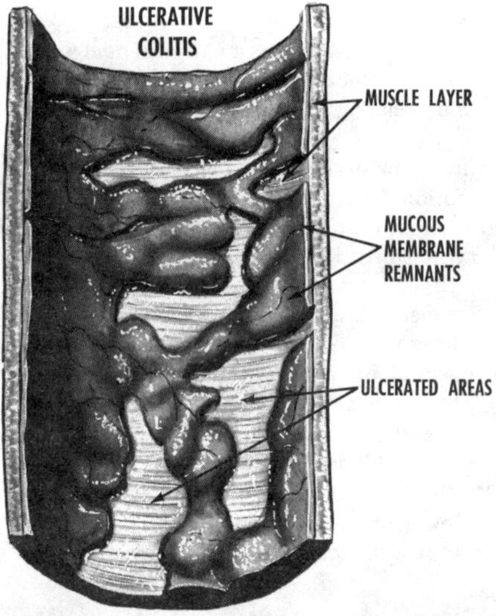

V

vaccination 1. the inoculation with a vaccine to prevent smallpox. 2. inoculation with any bacterial vaccine. 3. the scar left by a vaccination. —**vaccinate** *vb.*

vaccine a suspension made from killed or attenuated organisms for inoculation to establish resistance to an infectious disease.

vaccinia cowpox.

vacciniform resembling cowpox (vaccinia).

vagal of or relating to the vagus nerve.

vagina a canal leading in the female from the external genital orifice to the uterus. —**vaginal** *adj.*

vaginectomy surgical removal of all or part of the vagina.

vaginismus painful contraction of the vaginal muscles, often associated with a psychological aversion to sexual intercourse and preventing insertion or withdrawal of the penis.

vaginitis inflammation of the vagina.

vaginopathy any disease or disorder of the vagina.

vaginoplasty plastic surgery involving the vagina.

vagus *pl.* **vagi** either one of the tenth pair of cranial nerves which supply chiefly the viscera with sensory and motor fibers.

valgus an abnormal outward turning or twisting of a joint.

Valium a trademark for a tranquilizing drug, diazepam.

valva *pl.* **valvae** valve. —**valval** *adj.* —**valvar** *adj.*

valve a fold of membranous tissue in a passage or channel that permits the flow of a fluid in just one direction. —**valvular** *adj.*

valvula *pl.* **valvulae** a small fold or valve.

valvulitis inflammation of the valves of the heart.

varicella chickenpox.

varicocele varicose enlargement of the veins of the spermatic cord.

varicose *also* **varicosed** abnormally swollen or dilated: *varicose veins.* —**varicosity** *n.*

variola smallpox. —**variolous** *adj.*

varioloid 1. resembling smallpox. 2. a mild form of smallpox occurring chiefly in persons who have previously had smallpox or who have been vaccinated.

varix *pl.* **varices** an abnormally dilated vein, artery or lymphatic vessel.

varus an abnormal condition of inward turning of a joint.

vas *pl.* **vasa** an anatomical duct.

vas- *or* **vaso-** *prefix* 1. vessel; blood vessel. 2. vas deferens.

vascular relating to or being a channel for the conveyance of a body fluid. —**vascularity** *n.*

vas deferens the excretory duct of the testis, through which semen is conveyed during ejaculation.

vasectomy *pl.* **vasectomies** surgical incision of the vas deferens chiefly as a permanent method of male contraception.

vasoconstriction narrowing of the diameter of blood vessels.

vasodilatation widening of the diameter of blood vessels.

vasomotor relating to or being nerves controlling the inner diameter of blood vessels.

vasoparalysis paralysis or lack of tone of blood vessels.

vasoparesis a slight degree of vasoparalysis.

vasopressin a hormone secreted by the posterior lobe of the pituitary gland that acts to elevate blood pressure and inhibit the excretion of urine.

vasospasm spasmodic contraction of a blood vessel. **—vasospastic** *adj.*

vastus one of three large muscles of the thigh.

vector an organism, as an insect, that transmits disease. **—vectorial** *adj.*

vegan a strict vegetarian who not only excludes meat but all animal products from the diet.

vegetation an abnormal concretion or outgrowth upon part of the body, as the valves of the heart.

vein any of the tubular vessels that branch throughout the body and carry oxygen-depleted blood to the heart (except the pulmonary veins, which convey oxygen-rich blood from the lungs to the heart).

vena cava *pl.* **venae cavae** either one of the two large veins (inferior and superior venae cavae) that carry the blood to the right atrium of the heart.

venepuncture venipuncture.

venereal 1. contracted or transmitted during sexual intercourse: *venereal disease.* 2. relating to or resulting from sexual intercourse.

venereal disease an infectious disease, esp. gonorrhea or syphilis, contracted through sexual intercourse or other sexual contact with an infected partner.

venereology *or* **venerology** a branch of medicine dealing with venereal diseases. **—venereological** *or* **venerological** *adj.* **—venereologist** *or* **venerologist** *n.*

venesection the opening of a vein for the letting of blood, as in the treatment of polycythemia.

venipuncture *also* **venepuncture** puncture of a vein, esp. for the withdrawal of a sample of blood for laboratory analysis.

venography X-ray examination of a vein after injection with a radiopaque substance.

venous relating to or affecting the veins.

ventral of or relating to the belly; abdominal. —**ventrally** *adv.*

ventricle 1. a chamber of the heart from which blood is forced into the arteries. 2. any one of the cavities of the brain that contain cerebrospinal fluid. —**ventricular** *adj.*

ventriculus *pl.* **ventriculi** a digestive cavity; stomach. —**ventricular** *adj.*

venule a small vein.

vermicide an agent for destroying intestinal worms. —**vermicidal** *adj.*

vermiform appendix appendix (def. 2).

vermifuge causing worms to be expelled or destroyed. —**vermifuge** *n.*

verminosis *pl.* **verminoses** infestation with parasitic worms.

verruca *pl.* **verrucae** a wart.

version manual alteration in the uterine position of a fetus to achieve normal delivery.

vertebra *pl.* **vertebrae** *or* **vertebras** any of the thirty-three bony and cartilaginous segments that make up the spinal column. —**vertebral** *adj.*

vertex *pl.* **vertexes** *or* **vertices** the crown of the skull; top of the head.

vertigo *pl.* **vertigoes** *or* **vertigos** a state of disorientation in which an individual or his surroundings seem to be whirling; giddiness; dizziness. —**vertiginous** *adj.*

vesical of or relating to the urinary bladder.

vesicant an agent, as a gas, that induces blistering. —**vesicant** *adj.*

vesicate to blister.

vesicle a small, often painful elevation on the skin filled with watery fluid; blister. —**vesicular** *adj.*

vesiculate 1. covered with or containing vesicles. 2. to form or become covered with vesicles.

vestibule 1. the bony cavity of the labyrinth of the inner ear. 2. the opening between the labia minora of the vulva. —**vestibular** *adj.*

vestige the remnant of a bodily structure formerly having a functional purpose. —**vestigial** *adj.*

viable born in a fully normal and developed condition; fit for life: *viable fetus.* —**viability** *n.*

vibrio *pl.* **vibrios** any of a genus of bacteria in the form of an *S* or a comma, one of which causes cholera.

villus *pl.* **villi** a small, protruding, cellular process found on the surface of certain membranes. —**villous** *adj.*

Vincent's angina a mildly contagious bacterial disease marked chiefly by ulceration of the mucous membrane of the mouth and adjacent parts.

viremia the presence of viruses in the blood. —**viremic** *adj.*

viricide *or* **virucide** an agent that inactivates or destroys viruses. —**viricidal** *or* **virucidal** *adj.*

virilism 1. the development in a female of male secondary sex characteristics. 2. early development of secondary sex characteristics in a male.

virology a branch of science concerned with the study of viruses and the diagnosis and treatment of diseases they cause. —**virologic** *or* **virological** *adj.* —**virologically** *adv.* —**virologist** *n.*

virulence the ability of microorganisms to produce a disease with a rapid, severe, and malignant course. —**virulent** *adj.*

virus any of a large group of infective, submicroscopic

agents that are capable of growing only in living cells and are the cause of many significant diseases.

viscera *pl. of* viscus.

viscid sticky in quality; adhesive; glutinous: *a viscid fluid.*

viscous viscid.

viscus *pl.* **viscera** an internal bodily organ.

vision the act or state of perceiving with the eyes.

visual of or relating to vision.

vital relating to life; essential to maintaining life: *the vital organs are the heart, lungs, brain, kidneys and liver.*

vital signs the body temperature, pulse and respiratory rates, and blood pressure, the existence of which indicates a person is alive.

vitamin any of various organic substances that are essential in the diet in very small quantities to maintain health; they act as metabolic regulators and are present chiefly in natural foodstuffs.

vitamin A any of various fat-soluble vitamins found typically in the oils of fish liver, in egg yolk, and in milk, deficiency of which results in impaired vision.

vitamin B_1 thiamine.

vitamin B_2 riboflavin; a vitamin of the B complex concerned with oxidative processes and found in kidney, liver, milk, grass, eggs, and other sources.

vitamin B_6 pyridoxide; a vitamin of the B complex that is necessary for protein metabolism.

vitamin B_{12} a complex compound containing cobalt, found in liver, and essential to blood formation, growth, and the functioning of the nervous system.

vitamin B complex a group of water-soluble vitamins that include niacin, riboflavin, thiamine, and niacinamide.

vitamin C a vitamin found esp. in fruits and leafy vegetables and used in the prevention and treatment of scurvy and as a nutritional additive.

vitamin D a vitamin essential to the development of bones and teeth and found chiefly in milk, egg yolk, and the oil of fish liver.

vitamin E any of various vitamins important to the development of muscle and to fertility.

vitamin G riboflavin; vitamin B_2.

vitamin H biotin.

vitaminize to supplement with vitamins. —**vitaminization** *n.*

vitamin K either of two vitamins (vitamins K_1 and K_2) essential to the ability of the blood to clot.

vitiligo a skin condition marked by white, depigmented spots or patches on the body.

vitreous relating to or constituting the vitreous humor of the eye.

vitreous humor the transparent, clear, colorless substance between the lens and the retina of the eye.

vivisection surgery performed on living animals chiefly for purposes of research. —**vivisect** *vb.* —**vivisectionist** *n.*

vocal cords either of two pairs of folds of mucous membranes extending into the cavity of the larynx, which when vibrated by the passage of air act in the production of the voice.

voluntary functioning under conscious control: *voluntary muscles.*

volvulus a twisting of the intestine upon itself causing obstruction.

vomer a bone forming part of the septum of the nose.

vomit 1. to disgorge (the contents of the stomach) through the mouth. 2. the matter disgorged by vomiting.

vomiturition repeated, ineffectual attempts to vomit.

vomitus matter ejected by vomiting.

vulva *pl.* **vulvae** the external parts of the female genital organs; pudendum. —**vulval** *or* **vulvar** *adj.*

vulvectomy surgical excision of all or part of the vulvar tissues.

vulvitis inflammation of the vulva.

vulvovaginitis inflammation of the vulva and vagina.

PEPTIC ULCER

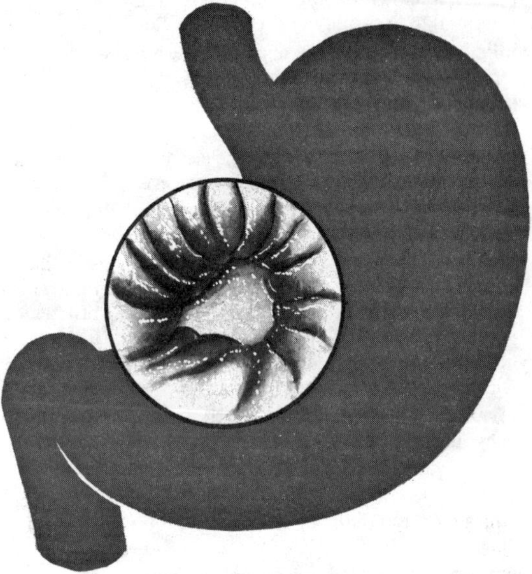

W

wadding surgical dressing of carded cotton or sheets of wool.

waddle a swaying or side-to-side walk seen in some forms of muscular dystrophy or nervous disorders.

wale a linear weal, as one produced by the sharp blow of a stick or whip.

walk 1. the manner in which one moves; gait. 2. to move about on foot.

ward a room or area in a hospital equipped with beds for patients: *surgical ward.*

warfarin sodium a drug used as an anticoagulant.

wart an epithelial tumor occurring typically as a horny projection on the skin of the extremities and caused by a virus. Also called *verruca.* —**warty** *adj.*

wash a lotion.

Wassermann reaction a test for the detection of syphilis. Also called *Wassermann, Wassermann test.*

waste 1. to lose tissue bulk; grow thin; emaciate. 2. excrement.

wasting emaciation.

waterborne carried by water: *waterborne infections.*

water brash a burning sensation in the stomach and esophagus with acid regurgitation; heartburn.

waters (colloquial) amniotic fluid.

Watson-Crick helix the double-stranded helical structure of deoxyribonucleic acid (DNA).

watt the unit of electrical power.

weal a lump or ridge raised on the skin, usually by a blow; welt.

wean to accustom (a child) to take nourishment other than by nursing. —**weaning** *n.*

webbing a congenital condition marked by the abnormal existence of a sheet or band of tissues joining two adjacent structures or parts.

welt a weal.

wen a cyst formed by obstruction of a sebaceous gland; a sebaceous cyst.

wheal a slightly elevated, reddened, itching patch on the skin typically associated with an insect bite or urticaria.

wheatgerm oil an oil rich in vitamin E, obtained from the germs of wheat seeds.

wheeze a high-pitched whining sound, heard during inhalation and exhalation, caused by a temporary or permanent obstruction or stenosis.

whiplash injury injury to the vertebrae and soft tissues of the neck produced by a sudden and violent jerking backward or forward of the head, as can occur to passengers involved in a rear-end collision of a motor vehicle.

whipworm a parasitic worm of the human intestine.

white blood cell leucocyte.

whitlow an abscess or purulent infection of the bed of a nail or the distal end of a finger. Also called *felon.*

whooping cough an infectious disease typically of children marked by paroxysms of violent coughing followed by a shrill, whooping drawing in of the breath. Also called *pertussis.*

Wilson's disease a rare hereditary disease marked by toxic deposits of copper in tissues, organs and the central nervous system and characterized esp. by symptoms of severe mental disorder.

windburn irritation and redness of the face caused by prolonged exposure to strong wind.

windpipe trachea.

wink 1. to open and close the eyelids very quickly, either as a conscious action or (usually) as an involuntary response. 2. the act or movement of opening and closing the eyelids quickly.

winter itch itching associated with exposure to cold, dry weather, thought to be caused by the drying of skin that is deficient in natural oils.

wisdom tooth the rearmost molar tooth in each half of each jaw, typically being the final teeth to erupt (as late as age 25 or so).

withdrawal 1. a pathological retreat from objective reality. 2. the complex of symptoms attending an addict following abstention from addictive drugs.

wolfram tungsten.

womb uterus.

wood alcohol an alcohol obtained from the distillation of wood, being poisonous and capable of causing blindness if ingested.

wood tick a species of tick occurring in North America and responsible for transmitting the micoorganisms that cause tularemia and Rocky Mountain spotted fever.

wool fat a fatty substance obtained from the wool of sheep, used as a base in the preparation of various ointments.

woolsorter's disease pulmonary anthrax caused by handling wool contaminated with the infecting microorganism *Bacillus anthrax.*

wound 1. an injury to the body involving piercing or laceration of the skin. 2. a surgical incision. 3. to injure; inflict a wound or wounds (on or upon).

W.r. *abbr.* Wassermann reaction.

wrinkle any crease or fold in the skin.

wrist the joint between the hand and the forearm; carpus.

writer's cramp muscular spasm of the hand induced by prolonged writing.

wryneck torticollis; stiff neck.

wuchereriasis infestation with threadlike worms of the genus *Wuchereria.* Also called *filariasis.*

X

xanthic 1. yellow or yellowish. 2. relating to xanthine.

xanthine a precursor of uric acid sometimes forming renal or urinary calculi.

xanthinuria the excretion of abnormally large quantities of xanthine in the urine.

xantho- *or* **xanth-** *prefix* yellow or yellowish.

xanthochromatic yellow-colored.

xanthochromia a condition characterized by the abnormal formation of yellow patches in the skin. Also called *xanthopathy.*

xanthochroous having a light or fair complexion; blond.

xanthocyanopsia a type of color blindness in which red and green are not distinguished but yellow and blue are; red-green blindness.

xanthoderma any yellowish discoloration of the skin. Also called *xanthoplasty.*

xanthodont a person with a yellowish discoloration of the teeth.

xanthoma a yellowish nodule or plaque in the skin caused by the deposition of certain lipids. **—xanthomatous** *adj.*

xanthomatosis a condition characterized by the multiple occurrence of xanthomas, esp. on the knees and elbows.

xanthone an agent that kills moth eggs.

xanthopathy xanthochromia.

xanthoplasty xanthoderma.

xanthopsia a visual defect in which all objects appear to be colored yellow.

xanthopsydracia a skin eruption characterized by the formation of small yellowish pustules.

xanthosis a yellowish discoloration seen in some malignant tumors and degenerating tissues.

xanthous yellow.

xanthylic relating to xanthine.

X chromosome a sex chromosome occurring paired in each female cell and zygote and singly in each male cell and zygote.

xenophobia an abnormal fear of meeting strangers.

xenophthalmia inflammation of the eye caused by the presence of a foreign particle.

Xenopsylla a genus of fleas, including the rat flea (*Xenopsylla cheopis*) which transmits the bacteria that cause the plague.

xenopus test a test for pregnancy in which the patient's urine is injected into the dorsal lymph sac of a toad.

xer- *or* **xero-** *prefix* dry.

xeransis a loss of moisture in the tissues.

xerantic causing dryness.

xerasia a condition characterized by abnormally dry and brittle hair.

xerochilia dryness of the lips.

xeroderma a dry, rough condition of the skin.

xeroma xeroph thalmia.

xeromycteria a condition characterized by abnormal dryness of the mucous membranes of the nose.

xeronosus xerosis.

xerophagia subsisting on a diet that is dry or lacking in moisture.

xerophthalmia a dry, thickened condition of the eyeball resulting from a deficiency of vitamin A.

xerosis severe dryness of the skin, mouth, or eye.

xerostomia excessive dryness of the mouth.

xerotes dryness.

xiphisternum *pl.* **xiphisterna** the posterior segment of the sternum.

xiphoid of, relating to or being the xiphisternum.

X-linked associated with or transmitted by X chromosomes, hence occuring predominantly in males, as hemophilia.

x-ray to photograph, examine, or treat with X rays.

X ray a photon having a frequency distribution that is higher than the ultraviolet range of the electromagnetic spectrum and has the ability of penetrating various thicknesses of all solids.

X-ray therapy treatment of a disease, as cancer, with the use of X rays.

Y

yaws an infectious tropical disease with symptoms resembling syphilis and caused by a spirochete. Also called *frambesia.*

Y chromosome a sex chromosome that is characteristic of male cells.

yeast any of various true fungi that are active fermenters of carbohydrates.

yellow fever an acute viral disease transmitted by a mosquito and marked by fever, prostration, jaundice, and occasionally bleeding. Also called *yellow jack.*

yerba a herb.

Y-linked associated with or transmitted by Y chromosomes.

yolk the stored nutrient portion of an ovum.

yperite a type of mustard gas.

ytterbium a metallic element of the rare earth group.

yttrium a metallic element.

Z

zein a protein present in corn (maize).

zelotypia pathologically excessive zeal in the support or advocacy of a cause.

zero gravity *also* **zerogravity** the phenomenon or state of weightlessness resulting from the absence of the pull of gravity as occurs during flights into outer space.

zestocausis cautery achieved by the use of hot steam.

zinc a metallic element.

zincoid resembling or relating to zinc.

zinc oxide an ointment used in the treatment of many skin irritations.

zingiber ginger.

zoanthropy a mental delusion of being a lower animal, such as a dog or cat.

zoetic relating to life.

zona *pl.* **zonae** an encircling area, as in shingles. —**zonal** *adj.*

zonula any small zone. —**zonular** *adj.*

zonula ciliaris suspensory ligament of the lens of the eye.

zoo- *prefix* relating to or denoting animal life or an animal.

zooblast any animal cell.

zooerastia human sexual gratification involving a lower animal.

zoograft a tissue graft obtained from a lower animal.

zoology the branch of science concerned with the study of animal life and its classifications. —**zoological** *adj.* —**zoologist** *n.*

zoomania an abnormal or exaggerated fondness or love of animals.

zoopathology the branch of pathology concerned with lower animals; veterinary pathology.

zoophagous eating the flesh of animals; carnivorous.

zoophobia an abnormal fear of animals.

zoster herpes zoster; shingles.

zygoma *pl.* **zygomata** *also* **zygomas** zygomatic arch.

zygomatic relating to or situated near the zygomatic arch.

zygomatic arch an arch of bone of the side of the face below the eyes; cheekbone. Also called *zygomatic bone.*

zygote a cell developing from the union of two gametes.

'Amber, I am *talking* to you. Look, I'm already late for work—'

'So go. I'm not stopping you.'

'All right, I will go.' But she stands at the door. 'Amber. You're worrying me so. I thought you'd get up today. I thought it was just school getting you down. Is it? Or is it something else? If you'll only say.'

She waits. I wait for her to get fed up.

And Amber's mum, Jay, does get fed up and slams out of the door. Amber is so frightened she is going to grow up to be like Jay that she rejects everything and takes to her bed.

'Amber's escape from the responsibility of Jay and her growth into true maturity are well developed. The characters are as convincing and the storyline as strong as one expects from Jacqueline Wilson.' *Punch*

Also available in Lions

Face at the Edge of World *Eve Bunting*
If This Is Love, I'll Take Spaghetti *Ellen Conford*
Granny Was a Buffer Girl *Berlie Doherty*
There Will Be a Next Time *Tony Drake*
Sixteen *Donald R. Gallo (ed.)*
The Green Behind the Glass *Adèle Geras*
Hey, Dollface *Deborah Hautzig*
Isaac Campion *Janni Howker*
Badger on the Barge *Janni Howker*
A Formal Feeling *Zibby Oneal*
More to Life Than Mr Right *Rosemary Stones (ed.)*
Breaking Training *Sandy Welch*
The Other Side *Jacqueline Wilson*
Waiting for the Sky to Fall *Jacqueline Wilson*
Nobody's Perfect *Jacqueline Wilson*
Hollywood Dream Machine *Bonnie Zindel*

Jacqueline Wilson

Amber

Lions

First published in Great Britain 1986
by Oxford University Press
First published in Lions 1988
8 Grafton Street, London W1X 3LA

Lions is an imprint of
the Children's Division, part of
the Collins Publishing Group

Printed in Great Britain by
William Collins Sons & Co. Ltd, Glasgow

Chapter 1

THE alarm is ringing. I'm almost asleep, my eyes aren't open yet, but I remember. Oh God. What am I going to do? No. I'm not going to think about it. The alarm is still ringing. I huddle away from it under my covers. Why should I always be the one to switch it off? It's Jay's clock, isn't it? A huge orange enamel affair patterned with purple and lime green swirls in a style that used to be called psychedelic. Time stands still in our room.

Is it going to go on ringing for ever? A cry of alarm, signifying danger. Stop it. It stops too. At last. Jay mumbles something but doesn't otherwise stir. I'm not going to either. I shut my eyes so tightly I can feel the blood beating in my lids. I watch my own private purple swirls. My thoughts swirl too so I listen for the clock and count each tick and tock until all the words in my mind stop spinning and stirring and march to a regimented beat. I will not get up. I will not get up. I will not get up. The minutes tut. They increase and multiply and Jay still does not go forth. She's going to be very late. And so am I. But I will not get up.

'Oh my God!' Jay sits up and grabs the clock. 'Amber. Get up. We've slept in.'

I will not get up.

'Do wake up, you great lump.'

I twitch, hating her. I can feel my body expanding, rising like dough. Just because she's so thin. She scratches her sparse hair. It's getting thinner and thinner. It's all that backcombing when she was my age in those stupid swinging sixties. She'll be bald by the time she's forty.

Justin told me a story of a cat of his that started to moult in middle age. The vet prescribed hormone treatment. I think the cat's fur grew again but she started to get very fat, so fat she could only waddle. Justin's mother put her on a strict diet and the poor cat didn't like this one bit and wailed and complained and Justin felt so sorry for her that he stole a cold chicken from the fridge and fed it all to her, legs, breast, the lot. She was tremendously grateful and ate it all up with enthusiasm but an hour later she had a stroke and died.

Poor Justin. How could I . . . ? No. I will not get up. I will not think of yesterday. I will not start today. Or tomorrow or tomorrow or tomorrow. Fit tomorrow to the ticks. To-mor Row-to Mor-ow To . . . .

'Amber! What's up with you this morning? Can't you even get the kettle on?' Jay grumbles, sitting up on her mattress and doing a silent-movie version of her Yoga exercises. Her screwed up face and whizzing limbs do not convey Inner Peace and Harmony. Her bones crack and creak. She's much too old to sleep on a mattress on the floor. I used to have no alternative, but I saved up for a proper bed this summer. Not a new bed, of course, but there are often second-hand divans advertised in the local newspaper. Mine cost thirty pounds. I could have got one even cheaper but I didn't want any old bug-ridden cast-off. My divan came from a spotlessly clean three-storey town house near the park. The woman was very kind and invited me into her Elizabeth Ann kitchen and gave me coffee in a Habitat mug and a big slice of Marks and Spencer blackcurrant cheesecake. Justin calls me the Namer of Parts. Show me a brand and I can name it.

I made a lot of money at the craft market so I treated myself to new bedclothes too, two new pairs of single sheets with matching pillowcases, hyacinth blue. I embroidered little pink and blue hyacinths at the edge of the pillowcases to make them even prettier. Jay scoffed of course. If beds are bourgeois then embroidered bed-linen is the ultimate banality.

'Amber, it is twenty-five past eight,' she hisses, rising unsteadily from her mattress and running round the room. She puts the kettle on, wriggles into her knickers and pokes her head through her rainbow sweater. She still doesn't wear a bra. I've been waiting for her to droop down to her waist like an old native woman but there's not enough of her.

'Amber!' She tugs at my pillow and tugs some of my hair too.

'You're hurting.' I burrow away from her.

'Well, get *up*.'

I burrow deeper. The sheets are over my head so I can't see her.

'What's got into you?'

I think about the words and start shaking. I'm trying not to laugh. No, I'm trying not to cry.

'Amber?' She sounds disconcerted. Her hands scrabble at my sheets, uncovering my face. She touches my forehead. 'Don't you feel well?'

I duck away.

'O.K., be like that. Stay in bed. I don't care.'

Jay rushes round, still in her knickers. She brews herself a mug of herbal tea and sips it, stepping into her jeans. She's been wearing them all week so there are little knobbles where her knees go. The zip's broken too but she sticks in a safety-pin carelessly. If my arm or leg had fallen off when I was little, Jay would have fastened me up with a couple of safety-pins and counted me as good as new. She searches the airer for her socks and it collapses under her assault, spilling underwear. She swears and leaves everything lying on the dusty floor.

'I can't find my stripy socks,' she wails helplessly.

Every morning I bet millions of mothers help their children find their socks. In our room the roles are reversed. I always help Jay. I wake her up and roll her off her mattress and make her muesli and kit her out in her crumpled clothes.

But I'm not going to do it now. I'm not going to get up

because then today will start and I'll have to think about yesterday. I gabble it under my breath. It sounds like one of Jay's idiotic mantras. Today and yesterday become meaningless if you repeat them often enough. I am going to lurk in this no man's land between the two.

Jay munches her breakfast, moans at me, and sticks her unsocked feet into her cowboy boots. They were shiny scarlet hand-stitched leather back in the seventies but now they're like old crumbling bricks.

'I'm off,' she announces, approaching my bed. 'You look O.K. to me, you know. Have you got a pain? Amber! You make me so mad when you won't tell me what's wrong.'

'You're going to be late,' I say in the calm flat tone that infuriates her.

'I know that, thank you very much. *You* are going to be late too. Very, very late. Or aren't you going to school at all today?'

I close my eyes.

'Look, I thought this stupid school meant so much to you. That's why we're stuck in this dump, isn't it. Why I'm stuck in this boring boring boring nine to five routine.'

'It's going to be quarter past nine to five today.'

'Oh to hell with you. I'm going.'

She pulls her splitting jacket from the peg on the door but she still hovers uneasily.

'Look, if you really feel bad you can always ring me at the shop. Or go round the corner for Wendy.'

Another pause.

'Aren't you even going to say goodbye?'

No. I watch her walk out of the room. She swaggers in those shabby old boots. She's fluffed out her hair at the front but she hasn't managed the back. It hangs in little limp straggles and the mouse shows through the henna. I call out goodbye after all but she's already shut the door on me so she won't have heard.

I burrow back under my clean sheets. I change them once a week, sometimes even twice. I can't afford the launderette so I wash them myself. Wendy's said I can shove them in with her washing in her automatic but I don't want my sheets winding themselves round Gordon's grubby boxer shorts and Naomi's nappies etc. I wash my sheets separately in the sink, helping myself to Wendy's Lux flakes when she isn't looking. I breathe the fresh soapy smell of my sheets now, but I can smell my own warm body too. It sickens me. It makes me remember. I want to scour all the smell away but that means getting up. I'm not getting up, not yet, not today, not ever. So I bury my face in the pillow and lie still.

I listen to the thump and bustle in the house underneath me. They are not much better at getting up and out than Jay. Gordon has jogged off long ago, of course, but I can hear Leonora and Polly yelling at each other and Naomi wailing. Wendy stays serene, as sweet as the honey on her wholemeal toast.

The door bangs. Leonora clatters off down the path. Then Polly. And eventually I hear Naomi fussing as Wendy slots her into her snowsuit and straps her into her push-chair. Naomi is off to the nursery, Wendy to Alladin's Cave. I am on my own.

I think about it. I don't think I have ever been alone in this house before. It is extraordinary. I think of all the homes I've ever had, the communes and caravans, the seaside chalets and the squats. I run through them like a litany. I exaggerate the shambles and the squalor. My eyes prick with self-pity. But I'm not going to cry. I cried enough last night when Jay was asleep. I thump my head on my pillow to stun my thoughts. I stretch out my arms and cling to the sides of my beautiful bed. I imagine the girl who used to sleep in it. I saw her bedroom. She has Laura Ashley wallpaper and curtains, David Hamilton ballet posters on the walls, a white portable television set, perfume bottles on her dressing-table (Charlie for every day, Paris for parties) and a huge snow-white Snoopy dog snoozing on her new Slumberland.

If I shut my eyes I can pretend I am in her new bed, not her old one. I am not Amber any more, I am . . . . Elizabeth Ann, like the kitchen. Yes, I'm Elizabeth Ann sharing my bed with Snoopy and my mother's cheerfully calling me to get up because my bacon and eggs are getting cold. Would it be a fried breakfast? No, that's on Sundays. This is a weekday, so it's cornflakes and I can sprinkle on as much sugar as I fancy, *white* sugar. Everything is wonderfully white in this house, the sugar, the bread, the scented soap, the school blouses, the underwear, the cooker, the bath-tub, the lavatory bowl, our gleaming teeth when we smile. Yes, she smiles at me and I smile at her, and she asks me if I've done my homework and hands me my laundered games kit and my packed lunch. Let's see, egg mayonnaise sandwiches, a sausage roll, a tomato, salt and vinegar crisps, a KitKat, a Peach Melba yoghurt, a can of coke and a Granny Smith, *yes*. She kisses me goodbye at the door. No she doesn't, she's got her own car, just a second-hand mini but it's neat and nippy and it gets me to school on time every day. Not my school, no fear, now I'm Elizabeth Ann I go to Parkside, the one that used to be the grammar school, only now you need to be rich as well as clever to go there. Well I'm rich now and I'm clever too, not a boring swot but I'm in the top stream and I'm going to be taking heaps of O levels and I bet I'll pass them all . . . .

I'm taking two. I'm in the lowest stream. I'm stupid. I didn't even learn to read for ages. Well, it wasn't really my fault, how could I learn when I didn't go to school? And anyway I'm not me, I'm Elizabeth Ann. I'm sure her mother used to read to her when she was little, Topsy and Tim and Mrs Tiggywinkle and Miffy, all those lovely baby books I finger in Smiths; and so if I'm her I can read bits already when I go to school at five years old. I whizz through all my Jane and Peters with no bother at all and I get to read aloud to the class, I even stand up on the stage in Assembly and read to the whole school . . . .

Elizabeth Ann and I must have dozed off. I peer at the alarm. It's twenty past eleven. I'm obviously not going to school today. I'm not going to get up at all. I'll pull the sheets back over my head. Sleep.

Go on. Think of Elizabeth Ann. Is she fifteen too? Yes, I'm Elizabeth Ann and I'm fifteen and I have a fitted wardrobe and different clothes for every day of the week. My father gives me a monthly allowance, *yes*, how much? Oh it doesn't matter, it's very generous, and I go to Chelsea Girl and Miss Selfridge and Top Shop with my friends on Saturdays and I choose . . . I can't decide. Nothing looks right on me anyway. No, I'm not Amber, I'm not blonde and bulging, I'm Elizabeth Ann and I think I'm little and dark and cute. Not like Leonora, I'm not a bit weird or way out. I'm as everyday as cornflakes. What wouldn't I give for a big bowl of cornflakes with sugar and top of the milk. I always eat cornflakes at Justin's. I used to eat cornflakes at Justin's. Stop it. It's like picking at a huge hangnail. It hurts so much but I can't seem to help doing it.

I'm not Elizabeth Ann, I'm Amber, and I can't sleep any more and I hate myself and I'm starving hungry and I badly need to pee. I can't lie here all day long with an empty stomach and a bladder full to bursting. I'll have to get up or I'll wet the bed, so I patter downstairs to the bathroom.

It's in a disgusting state as usual. Jay and I share it with Leonora and Polly. Well, Jay doesn't do much sharing. She is neither cleanly nor godly. Polly is both but she whispers in and out like a wraith and never disturbs anything. But Leonora . . . . She's been dyeing her hair again for a start. There are magenta daubs all over the wash-hand basin and she's spattered the wallpaper too. Her green woolly leg warmers are draped over the towels like giant caterpillars. I snatch my towel away. Pale green smudges smear the sugar pink. I bought that towel myself. I throw it down in a rage, hating Leonora. I'd like to hurl her to the floor too. But I won't. I won't even whine about the towel. I don't shout and scream. I don't let it all hang out, Jay's hateful expression. I keep everything tightly sewn inside.

Years ago in the Black Mountains I climbed Hay Bluff with Davie and then he took my hand and we ran all the way down it together. My feet ran of their own accord, hurtling me forwards, and I screamed in dread and delight while Davie hung on to my hand and I went on screaming for the sheer thrill of it, screaming all the way to the valley below.

I flush the lavatory and switch on the shower as hard as it will go. Leonora's multicoloured hair makes a paisley pattern on the tiled floor so I fish that out first, shuddering, and then I pull off my nightie and get under the storm of the shower and open my mouth and I scream.

It doesn't work. I feel silly and I'm swallowing water and someone might hear. What if Wendy slips back from her shop as she sometimes does? If she catches me she'll think I've gone crazy. Well she thinks I'm crazy already, they all do.

I soap myself savagely. I scrub the soft places until they sting. They deserve punishment. The water is unbearably hot, nearly boiling, but I stand under it for a full five minutes.

I am still scarlet when I'm dry and in my night-dress. My head throbs and I feel sick. I creep shakily back to my room and poke about for food. I'm so fed up with muesli. Leonora once said it was like dried sick and I've never been able to forget it. I find an elderly banana instead. It is dark and mushy inside and I give it up half-way. I go back to bed chewing a mouthful of withered prunes. And this is supposed to be *health* food? Sometimes I don't think I'm the crazy one at all. They are. Lots of people would agree with me too. Elizabeth Ann and her family for a start. And all the people on their estate and all the pupils at Parkside school. All the pupils at my own school, come to that. All the pupils at all the hundreds of schools I've attended. They called me a hippy and a gypsy and a tinker and a druggie and a flower child and a squatter and a lot of other uglier things. Only I'm not, *I'm* not. As soon as I'm sixteen and can legally live on my own then I'll be off. Jay's going to get a surprise one day when she wakes up and finds me gone. Only it shouldn't be that much of a surprise. That's what she did to her mother.

I suck prune stones and think about Jay's mother. My

grandmother. I haven't seen her for ages. I don't expect she knows where we're living now. But I know where she lives.

I get out of bed and search my school-bag for scrap paper. I am going to write my grandmother a letter.

Chapter 2

I DON'T know what to say. I don't know what she's like. I've met her of course. Several times. I stayed with her for a fortnight when I was little. Jay was in hospital. I'm not sure why. They told me she had a bad pain and she had to go to hospital so the doctors could make her better. It could have been a respectable emergency like a burst appendix. It could have been a drug overdose or even a suicide attempt. I didn't suspect anything like that at the time, naturally. I was simply scared. Jay had been spirited away in the night and I didn't know if I'd ever see her again.

I cried when I was dumped at Grandma's and she did her best to comfort me. I think she even picked me up and cuddled me, which was noble of her because I was very dirty in those days.

'Don't cry, dear, Mummy will be all right,' she said, but I wasn't crying because of Jay, I was crying because I'd left my bit of blanket behind and I couldn't get to sleep without it. That's mostly what I can remember: lying wide awake night after night in Grandma's spare room, trying to nuzzle my nose against her cold stiff sheets. And then one day, when she was cooking in her shining kitchen or having her afternoon nap on the rose velvet sofa in the living-room or whatever, I crept into her bedroom and peeped inside her wardrobe.

It was the most fantastic discovery for me. Nobody I knew had a proper wardrobe for a start. At best clothes were hung up behind an old curtain; more usually they stayed crumpled in a case. My grandmother would need trunk after trunk for her clothes. I hadn't realised one person could possibly own so many. They were so strange too, sombre and plain. I knew at once that these were real clothes and that Jay's beaded batik patchworks were bogus.

Grandma's dresses and suits and skirts were all immaculately turned out on their padded hangers, like a line of soldiers on parade. Her shoes stood to attention too, pair after pair, all polished to perfection. I tried on the black patent high heels, hobbling across the bedroom carpet. Then I stumbled and got scared Grandma might hear, so I tried the other shoes on my hands, making them perform little tap-dances in thin air. There were shelves on the right-hand side of the wardrobe and these were treasure chests too: soft sweaters that smelt of talcum; suede gloves clasping empty fingers; silk scarves folded into smooth squares. I stroked one as if it were a little animal, but my bitten nails snagged the fine material and I hid it quickly at the bottom of the pile, my heart thudding. I searched hopefully for Grandma's underwear but she obviously kept it elsewhere.

I crawled right inside the wardrobe and felt around at the back, behind the shoes. I found a bumpy little box that didn't feel particularly promising, but when I held it out into the light I started trembling. It was a little jewelled casket, exactly the same size and design as Miranda's secret casket from India.

Miranda was staying in the commune that summer recovering from the death of her boy-friend, who had been someone big in the music world. She mourned him by taking a moonlight walk every evening and crooning his name aloud, but she didn't seem particularly down-hearted otherwise. I never saw her cry. She didn't laugh either. Her face was a china doll mask, big glassy blue eyes and tiny pursed mouth. I suppose she was permanently dazed with drugs but this didn't occur to me then. I worshipped Miranda. I loved the buttercups and daisies she threaded through her golden plaits. I loved her

Afghanistan dresses so stiffly embroidered they could stand up by themselves. I loved her jewellery, the diamond winking unexpectedly above her nostril, the tinkling silver bangles that manacled her tiny ankles. I loved her secret casket most of all. The boy-friend had taken her on a trip to India to meet the Maharishi and she'd come back bearing a little jewelled casket on a purple velvet cushion, stepping right out of a fairy-tale. She wouldn't tell anyone what was inside. She shook her head mysteriously when people asked her about it. I thought about the casket constantly and longed to know its secret, but I was shocked when Leonora suggested we take a look for ourselves. Polly and I didn't dare so Leonora went by herself and peeped in the casket when Miranda was off on her moonlight amble.

'I looked right inside,' she boasted.

'What did you see, what did you see?' we begged.

Leonora was too clever to tell us straight away. She kept us in suspense for days while we bribed her with stolen hair ribbons and chocolate and coloured pencils (like all the commune children we were accomplished thieves). Then one day she tied the bright ribbon we had brought round her forehead, like a Red Indian, rearranged her coloured pencils in their little cardboard packet and munched her way through a Mars and a Milky Way and a Fry's Turkish Delight without offering us a single bite. Then she told us what was in Miranda's secret casket.

'Nothing,' said Leonora. Her dark eyes glittered as she waited for our reaction. 'Nothing at all,' she spluttered. Her mouth opened wide as she laughed, showing her chocolatey teeth. 'That's the secret.'

I was sure she was lying. How could such a fabulous casket contain nothing at all? I'd imagined the contents so often I was almost positive the casket contained an emerald as big as an egg or a golden butterfly with moving wings or a silver pot of perfume with scent so strange it could cast spells.

'Nothing!' Leonora cackled.

Perhaps she was too coarse or cruel to see the secret for

herself. I remembered all the tales that Davie told us. That was it. Leonora simply wasn't worthy.

I decided that I'd have to peep into the secret casket for myself, but then Jay disappeared and the police came and I was whisked away to Grandma's. It was as if someone had really cast a spell and scattered us in seconds. And now it looked as if I was still enchanted because here was Miranda's secret casket at the back of my grandmother's wardrobe.

I could discover the secret for myself.

I squatted at the edge of the wardrobe with Grandma's gaberdine suits brushing my head and her pointed shoes pecking my bottom. I slowly opened the casket, my hands shaking, and then I jumped and very nearly screamed. There was a full set of false teeth inside, huge great choppers set in salmon pink gums. I stared at them in horror. Could they possibly belong to Grandma? But she had her own teeth, I'd seen them when she smiled dutifully at me. Then Grandpa? He was a shadowy figure who stayed at his office almost all the time. He didn't smile, but I'd watched him chewing his roast beef on Sunday. He had teeth too. Perhaps these were a spare set.

Miranda must have false teeth now. I was told she tried to fly out of the commune window one night. I can just see her, flower-strewn hair a golden cloud, embroidered dress billowing, legs kicking in her silver bangles, flying for one, two, three magical seconds—and then plummeting downwards and landing with a shriek and splatter on the pavement. She didn't die. Perhaps the Afghanistan dress acted as a parachute. She was lucky not to break her neck, but she broke everything else, arms, legs, ribs, nose and teeth. Leonora said she wasn't recognisable even when she came out of hospital months later. She tried going back to the commune but she had changed inside as well as out. She let her long hair grow lank, her dresses stiffened with dirt as well as embroidery, even her bangles tarnished. Her parents came and collected her one day and put her in a private Nursing Home.

'A loony-bin,' said Leonora.

I wondered if she'd taken her secret casket with her. I found jewels in Grandma's casket once I'd dared edge the false teeth to one side. Pearls and a brooch of pink and yellow china roses, and necklaces that made an exciting shivery noise when I ran them through my fingers. They must have belonged to Grandma although I never saw her wearing any jewellery at all apart from the three rings on her left hand, diamond engagement ring, gold wedding-ring, and diamond eternity ring. Jay had lots of rings but she'd never had a ring symbolising eternity or a wedding vow or even an engagement.

I didn't realise what that made me. It was Grandma who hissed the word the next time I went to see her. I was eleven or twelve. Jay was with me too. We'd gone to see Grandma because we'd bumped into some old neighbour in an Oxfam shop and she'd sympathised with Jay about the loss of her father.

It turned out Grandpa had died three months ago.

'Why didn't you *tell* me?' Jay demanded. 'You knew where to get hold of me. For God's sake, you could at least have asked me to his funeral.'

We were living in the caravan then and so we had a permanent address.

Grandma didn't seem to hear. She sat staring straight in front of her. She wasn't wearing black, but her navy frock and navy cardigan and navy silk scarf were as melancholy as mourning. Her hair was tightly permed but her face sagged underneath. She blinked her swollen eyelids and focused on Jay.

'Why didn't I tell you?' she whispered, but there was a snap to her voice that made Jay's head jerk. 'I didn't tell you, Joyce, because I didn't want you to come anywhere near your poor father. I didn't want you or your little bastard.'

It was a second or two before I realised she meant me.

'You killed him,' said Grandma, her voice rising. She leant forward in her armchair, rage flooding her ghostly face. 'You killed him!' she shrieked, spit spilling in little runnels at the edges of her lips.

I didn't understand. I thought Grandma meant Jay had murdered Grandpa. I stared at her, thinking she had gone quite mad.

'The angina started the day you left home, Joyce. Daddy read your note, went as white as a sheet and clutched his chest. I was sure he was having a heart attack. It might have been more merciful if he'd died there and then. But no, he had to live on with the knowledge that his little girl was flaunting every decent convention, behaving like a slut, grubbing in the gutter. That knowledge was more deadly than poison. It killed him.'

'You're talking nonsense,' said Jay calmly, but she was shaking.

Grandma was shaking too, her whole body vibrating as if she were on a bus.

'You killed him,' Grandma repeated emphatically. 'You broke his heart. That's why I didn't want you at his funeral. I'd have *spat* at you if you'd dared put in an appearance.'

Jay flinched. She looked as if she might start crying but she smiled instead.

'Still worried what the neighbours will think, is that it?' she said, smirking defiantly.

Grandma sucked in her lips.

'Trust you to be flippant about it, you filthy little slut. Look at you. Look at your child. Tarred with the same brush, I dare say.' Grandma was looking and we were making her shudder.

I looked too although I didn't want to. It was as if I were seeing us with Grandma's eyes. Jay had bleached her hair so it hung to her shoulders like half-eaten candy-floss. She renewed the black smudges round her eyes every morning. The black under her long nails happened naturally. We didn't have a proper water supply and it was hard to keep clean. The ballooning sleeves of her smock were grey with grime, her long skirt was patterned with stains and her bare feet were filthy. I was filthy too. I ran my fingers through the greasy straggles of my hair and looked down at my own tattered T-shirt and my bald blue velvet jeans splitting at every seam.

No wonder Grandma didn't want us. I started crying. Grandma and Jay glared at me. I went on crying like a baby even though I was much too old for such howling.

Careful. I'll start now, four years later.

Concentrate on the letter.

Dear Grandma.

What else? What can I say to her? I haven't seen her since the day she called me a bastard. If my own grandmother can call me that then why write to her anyway? The last thing she wants is a letter from me. I haven't even got any proper writing-paper. I can't see Grandma accepting a scrap torn from an old exercise book, all lines and ragged edges. My writing's hopeless too. I hate the way it scratches and slopes. Grandma will sneer at my illiterate scrawl. I was never taught how to do proper joined-up writing. I didn't even learn to print for ages because I couldn't read. I pretended I could, but the schools always found out in the end. They thought I was stupid. I was even sent to a special unit for the Educationally Subnormal. They showed me pretty pictures and asked me to name them. I didn't recognise a lot of them, things like pyjamas, tooth-brush, a birthday cake and candles, an iron, a rocking-horse, monkeys and giraffes and lions in a zoo. I'd never set eyes on any of them so I couldn't name them. I didn't go back to the E.S.N. Unit. Perhaps they thought me too thick even for that.

Davie was staying with us then and he found me crying over a Ladybird first reader I'd stolen from one of the schools. I'd stared at the big black print until it blurred but I couldn't get it to make any sense. The pictures weren't much help either, although I loved looking at them. Jane and Peter lived a life so clean, so cheerful and so cosy that it seemed more fantastic than Fairyland. I fingered the pictures, patting the paper dog, playing with Jane's paper doll, pinching a paper cake from a plate, and I made up a long story: Jane died and her mother and father adopted me instead so I had all Jane's pretty dresses and dolls and I played with Peter and Pat the dog and my new mother cooked me tasty teas and my new father tucked me up in my own clean comfortable bed at night. I could say my story for hours but I couldn't write it down and the only words I could read were Jane and Peter and Pat the dog and Mother and Father.

'I can't read any other words, I'm too thick,' I sobbed.

'Rubbish,' said Davie, pulling me on to his lap.

I curled up and snuffled his warm woolly smell. He hitched me over to one side and found an old biro in his pocket. He smoothed out a brown-paper bag and drew a picture of a little fat tear-stained girl saying 'I can't read any other words, I'm too thick,' and a picture of a man with curly hair and a patchwork jacket saying, 'Rubbish.' He read me what I was saying and then he made me guess what he was saying, and even I could manage that. Then he drew a pretty little girl with crazy witch hair and a long trailing dress—'Leonora!'—and he made her say all sorts of short rude words, most of which I recognised already. Then he drew Polly and he did her hair all sad little wisps the way it went after Leonora made her play hairdressers. Poor Polly was saying, 'I don't like Leonora.' He covered the paper bag with drawings of all the children from the commune. He even drew the baby and made it say 'Mum Mum Mum' and then 'Yum Yum Yum' after it had been fed. I stopped crying and started laughing and read every word on the paper bag.

Davie wrote me some stories the next day.

'Amber has a pretty pink dress from a posh shop. Amber has a pretty pink ice cream in a fancy café. Get Amber! Amber licks up her pretty pink ice cream. Oh dear. It spills all down her pretty pink dress. But nobody sees. It does not even show because the ice cream is pink and the dress is pink. And

Amber's tongue is pink as it goes lick lick lick. Amber's lips are pink as she smiles. So let's give her a kiss.'

And he did. I read all Davie's stories until I knew them by heart and when I went back to my stolen Jane and Peter book I found I could read that too. I read the next Jane and Peter and the next. I wasn't so stupid after all. I could read.

I can't imagine not being able to read now. It's what I like doing most, next to needlework. Only I still have so much catching up to do. I have forty-three books of my own but they are all a little odd and old. I got them from the 10p shelves of the Cinema Bookshop at Hay. I paid 10p for every single one. I don't steal any more.

I lean out of bed and look at my books, touching the covers, brown and red and blue. Forty-four. There's a paperback that isn't mine, it's Justin's. He's been lending me all his old favourites: *Just William* and *Treehorn* and *The Hobbit* and *Wind in the Willows* and now I'm on *Winnie-the-Pooh*. He knows them nearly off by heart so he has no difficulty reading them. He reads Pooh to me sometimes, doing different voices for all the animals. He makes Kanga sound like Edna Everage and it always makes me laugh.

I'm not laughing, I'm crying. Oh Justin, I'm sorry. I didn't mean to—

Yes I did. I did. It's no use. I'm just like Jay. I've tried and tried not to be, I've stopped stealing and I wash all over every day and I keep my clothes neat and I study as hard as I can at school and I work too and I've bought my bed and I've made so many plans but *it's no use*.

Tarred with the same brush. That's what Grandma said.

Dear Grandma,

I know you will be surprised to get a letter from me. I am sorry I haven't got any proper writing-paper. I am sorry that my writing's so bad. I am sorry that I was so dirty and untidy the last time I came to see you. I know you don't like me very much but I badly want to change and be different and behave properly. I don't like my mother any more and I don't like the way we live. I don't want to be this sort of person but I can't seem to help it here. So please couldn't I come and live with you? I am very quiet and very clean now and I'll do all sorts of errands for you and I can sew and I already work part time and I can get a full-time job the minute I'm sixteen if you want. Please say yes.

Yours faithfully
Your loving granddaughter

Amber.

Chapter 3

'WHAT are you up to then, Amber?'

I jump and knock the biscuit tin flying.

'Clumsy,' says Leonora, shaking her head at me.

I kneel on the cold kitchen floor and try to scoop the shattered biscuits back into the tin. They're not my biscuits, that's the awful thing. They're Leonora's. I got so hungry and there's nothing anywhere near edible in our room (if I eat any more prunes I'll be groaning in the lavatory all tomorrow) so I came creeping downstairs to raid Wendy's larder. I couldn't stop thinking about her home-made chocolate chip cookies.

But now Leonora's caught me. She lolls against the fridge, laughing.

'They're all broken,' I mumble. 'And these bits have got fluff on them.'

'Throw them away,' says Leonora carelessly, opening the fridge and helping herself to some milk. She drinks it straight from the bottle in great greedy gulps, and then bites into a slab of Double Gloucester, leaving milky teeth-marks.

'Leonora!'

'Want some?' She breaks me off a chunk.

I shake my head but my hand reaches out and I gobble it down and then I eat all the fluffy bits of cookie too. Leonora starts on a big red apple from the bowl. I want one too but I haven't quite got the nerve to help myself.

'What are you doing hanging around at home?' Leonora asks. She peers at my night-dress. 'Are you ill?'

I shake my head. 'I just didn't feel like school today, that's all.'

Leonora raises her eyebrows. She's plucked them out of existence and pencilled new ones in purple, but Leonora stays pretty with or without eyebrows. She's wearing hideous chocolate brown uniform but she even gives that a certain style. She's resewn the skirt so that it's much shorter and tighter than it should be, and she's wearing a white boy's shirt with a high hard collar that looks incongruously prim. Her tie draggles decoratively, the knot bouncing on her chest. She's got a ladder running right up her dark tights but somehow even that looks sexy.

'What are you home for anyway?' I ask irritably.

Leonora shrugs. 'Oh, I've got boring old Latin this afternoon and I just couldn't face it. I mean, what is the point of it all? It's just a dry dead old language, utterly obsolete.'

I cram another cookie in my mouth, hating her. It's so unfair. Leonora's clever, much cleverer than me. She doesn't even have to try. She missed out on school like me but the moment she started she shone. I bet she looked at the Jane and Peter book and read it just like that. By the time she started junior school Gordon had decided alternative living was losing its appeal and went back into advertising. He was soon rich enough to send Leonora and Polly to posh private schools. Leonora's in the top stream in the fifth year at her public day-school now, studying for ten O levels. I bet she passes them all, even Latin, though she doesn't do a stroke of work.

I am in the bottom stream at my school. I'm taking two O levels, English Language and Needlework. I can't even do C.S.E.s in French or Maths or Science or anything, I'm hopeless at all of them. I don't know one single word of Latin and Leonora knows it.

'What shall we do then? Shall we get dolled up and go into town?' Leonora suggests, although we've never once been out together before.

'No thanks. I'm going back to bed.'

'Oh don't be so boring, Amber,' says Leonora, following me out of the kitchen and up the stairs. 'Come on, I'll lend you something to wear.'

She knows all her things are much too small for me. And they wouldn't look right on me even if they fitted.

'I'm going to bed,' I repeat, but Leonora follows me right up to my room.

I wish it was my room. It is our room, and Jay's things are everywhere.

'It is weird you living with us,' Leonora says tactlessly. 'I keep expecting all our table-tennis things to be here. I used to like playing the old ping-pong.'

She picks up a dirty plate, pretending it's a table-tennis bat and swots a stripy sock in the air. The plate has honey on it and the sock sticks comically to the ceiling. We both stare up at it in surprise, and then Leonora shrieks with laughter. I join in too.

'Jay was looking for that sock this morning.'

'Well, she knows where to find it now.'

'How am I going to get it down?' I say, standing on a rickety chair. I am tall, but my arm waves uselessly well below the ceiling.

'Oh no, you must leave it there. It looks very avant-garde,' says Leonora. 'Come on, Am. Let's go into town. I've got money, I'll treat you. I'll buy you a big squidgy cream cake in Patisserie Valerie, how about that?'

'No thanks,' I say. Though I can't help coveting the cream cake. I've never eaten in Patisserie Valerie, I've never even seen it, but it's one of Leonora's favourite haunts and she often describes their cakes in taunting detail.

Leonora stares at me appraisingly. I wish I was dressed. I know the white winceyette of my night-dress is utterly opaque but Leonora looks as if she can see every tip and tendril.

'Why are you looking so furtive?' she asks. 'I know! You're going to see that weird boy-friend of yours. He's coming over this afternoon, isn't he?'

'No he's not. And he's not weird. Look, I'm going back to bed.' I get in but Leonora comes and sits on the end of my bed, grinning at me.

'Going to bed, eh?' she says, eyes sparkling. 'Really, Amber! And I thought you were such a goody-goody. So you and your weirdo go to bed, right?'

'No. Shut up. And stop calling him weirdo,' I snap, my face burning.

'You're blushing. Look at you, like a lobster! Oh, Amber, come on, you can tell me, for God's sake. What's it like with weirdo? Sorry, *Justin*. He doesn't keep that silly puppet on his hand while he's doing it, does he?'

'No he doesn't! Oh do shut *up* about it.'

'So he does do it?'

'No! Just because you and everyone else in this house are obsessed with sex don't assume other people rut like rabbits all the time.'

'Do rabbits rut? I thought that was deer. Remember that time we went for a picnic in Richmond Park? Were you living with us then? Anyway, it was in the Autumn and all the deer were at it, and this stag, honestly, the noise he was making, I've never heard anything like it, utterly *gross*.' Leonora snorts enthusiastically in imitation. Then she pauses, looking thoughtful. 'Although there was one man I met on holiday and when he—'

'Leonora, I do not want to know. I just want to go to sleep. Alone. Please.'

Leonora sighs impatiently. 'O.K., O.K. I'll go into town by myself. I shall eat cream cakes and meet lots of lovely new men and get asked to all sorts of exciting new clubs and have a Moby Dick of a time and when I get back I'll wake you up and tell you all about it and won't you be jealous.'

'Desperately,' I say, attempting sarcasm—although perhaps she's right.

I lie down and close my eyes and hear Leonora sauntering out of the room. Then I remember.

'Leonora!' I call, sitting up again. 'Will you be going past a post-box?'

I fumble under my pillow for my letter. I've put it inside an old brown envelope of Jay's. She hadn't even opened it. She never opens any envelope that's brown because she says it will be Bad News. She is so stupid. The bills have all got to be paid eventually. But Jay just waits and pretends not to worry and when she's about to be thrown into jail she generally gets some other mug to pay. I suppose it will be Gordon now. I can't bear to think about it, even though he's so rich I don't suppose he'll ever miss the money.

Leonora glances at my letter. 'Writing to the weirdo?'

'Oh forget it,' I say, sighing, pretending to put the letter back.

She takes it from me as I know she will.

'Have you got a stamp?' I ask, trying to sound casual. Leonora has several *books* of stamps in her Victorian mahogany writing-slope. I'd give anything to own that beautiful box. Leonora doesn't even look after it, she's scratched her name on it.

'Sure,' says Leonora, peering at the address on the envelope. 'Your writing, Amber!'

It's so unfair. I cannot believe in graphology. Leonora's own handwriting is very neat, very tidy, very controlled. She's never practised it in her life. She just picked up a pen and it came out that way right from the start.

'I'll give you the 17p.'

'It's O.K.,' says Leonora, as I know she will. I am as bad as Jay in many ways. In all ways.

'Who's Mrs Elephant then?' asks Leonora.

'What? Mrs *Elliston*. My grandmother.'

'It looks like Elephant to me. Why are you writing to your granny? I didn't think you and Jay had anything to do with your family.'

'I just wanted to write to her, that's all,' I say, lying down again. 'You will remember to post it, won't you?'

'Sure. Oh well. See you.'

I hear her pottering around beneath me in her bedroom and then she clatters down the stairs and swears as she trips in her Oxfam stilettos. Gordon gives her a monthly allowance and she's got her own bank account but she buys half her things from Oxfam shops by choice.

The house is silent again. Polly will get home from school about half-past four but she's even shyer than I am and certainly won't come up here. Wendy gets back with Naomi about quarter-past five. Jay comes home around six. Gordon probably won't be back till nine at the earliest. Does he really work all that time or is he playing around? Wendy doesn't seem to mind if he is. But then Wendy's used to not minding. I think Jay and Gordon used to sleep together back in the commune days. That's why Gordon offered Jay and me this room rent-free.

I was scared at first that there might be more to it than that. I kept looking at Gordon. He is a square man, going soft at the stomach for all his jogging and gym sessions. His trendy hair is pale yellow, the eyes behind his aviator glasses are blue. It was not hard to imagine a slight resemblance. It was driving me so mad I had to ask Jay outright.

'Is Gordon my father?'

She burst out laughing. 'Of course he's not. If he was, do you think we'd be scrimping and scraping like this? And I told you who your father was. I don't lie to you, do I?'

I don't suppose she does. Maybe I wish she did. I think I'd even prefer Gordon to my real father. He is dead, if Jay is to be trusted. He died a month before I was born.

Some crazy fans still mourn on February 13th, the anniversary of the day Olim Boyd was killed in a car crash. Olim Boyd the pop star. He was very big in the sixties. From London, not Liverpool, but his group The Sparklers had six records in the top twenty, and one went right to number two in the charts. It was called 'Be Boppy'. Honestly. Jay told me all this rubbish as if I'd actually be impressed. She played me 'Be

Boppy', listening with a reverent expression as if all that Boppy baby-talk was Beethoven with knobs on. It wasn't as if Daddy was Olim Boyd himself. He wasn't even a member of The Sparklers. He was the Roadie. The bloke who drove Olim Boyd and the Sparklers from gig to gig. He was driving Olim Boyd's Jensen on February 13th. Olim was giggling in the back, smashed out of his mind. He was smashed out of his body too because my daddy failed to notice a roundabout and drove right through it.

His name was in the newspapers. 'Olim Boyd's Road Manager, Norman Titmarsh, was also killed outright.' Norman Titmarsh. I'd never have known his name otherwise. Jay and my daddy had a fifteen minute acquaintanceship. I still can't quite believe it. Jay was only my age too. No wonder Grandma spat at her.

What did your mother do when she left school? Oh, she took up a career very common in the sixties. Common being the operative word. She was a groupie. She hung around all the pop stars and tried to sleep with as many as she could. She wasn't even particularly successful. She never got near John Lennon or Mick Jagger or anyone with style. She made it with Olim Boyd's Roadie, and she didn't even manage that very well because she got herself pregnant.

She managed it last year too, when the doctor said she had to come off the pill. Even Jay wasn't crazy enough to see Pete the Potter and her and me and a new baby all playing Happy Families together. She told Pete she was going to a week-end women's conference and went to hospital and had an abortion instead. She wouldn't talk about it to me. She seemed all right at first but weeks later she started bursting into tears for no reason and it irritated Pete and they had a row and Jay told him what she'd done. I think she wanted him to be sensitive and sorry for her but Pete the Potter was a pig. He decided Jay had had the abortion because she was worried the baby wasn't his. That shows his mentality, because the three of us were living in a damp shack at the top of a wet Welsh mountain and

Pete was the only man Jay ever saw week in, week out. But he got all worked up and started shouting and swearing and then he started hitting. He hit Jay so hard he knocked her to the ground and then he kicked her and when I screamed and tried to get her away he kicked me too. I thought he was going to kill us both. Perhaps Jay did too, because when he eventually stormed off we packed our bags in a hurry and slithered down the mountain and hitched a lift half-way to London.

And that evening we were drinking tepid tea in an all-night transport café and I was still crying and Jay was just sitting there like a zombie with her eyes shut, not even trying to think what we were going to do next, when a whole fleet of Range Rovers and fancy vans pulled into the car-park and a film crew piled into the café after filming a couple in a meadow at sunset for some breath freshener advertisement. This pretentious twit in a leather waistcoat and faded jeans and daffodil yellow boots suddenly peered through his aviator glasses and pounced on us.

Gordon took us home with him. And here we've stayed. At first I shared with Leonora and Jay shared with Polly (they both have twin beds in their rooms) but when it was obvious we'd become semi-permanent members of the household Gordon offered us the attic room for ourselves.

I hated the idea. 'We can't sponge off them for ever. They don't want us here. We'll have to go, Jay.'

'O.K. Tell me where.'

'I don't know. Can't you go to the council again?'

We'd tried that several times in the past but it hadn't been a success. They'd put us in a derelict flat in a multi-storey and a gang of skinheads had kicked their way through the front door in the middle of the night. They didn't actually do anything except call us names but it scared us so badly we moved out the next day. Then we were put in bed and breakfast accommodation, but the bed had bugs and the breakfast was one slice of stale bread and a tea-bag in water, and we had to share a room with three other women, one of whom was a drunk and kept wetting her bed so the whole room stank.

Maybe it wasn't such a bright idea going to the council. We didn't seem to have any alternative so we stayed where we were.

'But I'm going to pay my way from now on,' said Jay. 'I'll get a job. And we'll get you into the local school and you can do some exams. Well, that's what you've been nagging me about, isn't it. Maybe it's time we settled down a bit.'

I think the Pete episode had worried her a lot. She didn't sleep properly for a while and she got very thin. I started to worry too, but then she got the job in the health food shop and started eating all their left-overs and soon looked a bit better. I worked all summer at the craft market and had money for the first time ever, and in September I started in the fifth year at Mallford comprehensive. In 5e.

'With the odds and the sods and the clods,' as Justin puts it.

Oh Justin. You're the only real friend I've ever had. Why did I spoil everything? Just like Jay. Tarred with the same brush. Black and dirty. Who am I kidding? I can't wash it away.

Chapter 4

'AMBER. *Amber*. AMBER!' Jay pulls my arm so hard my night-dress splits at the seam.

'Look. You've torn it now.'

'Well, answer me. Sit up. Come on. You are going to *talk* to me.'

Jay's cold hands scrabble at my shoulders until I sit up. I blink at her resentfully through my tangled hair. It smells. I smell too. I didn't wash yesterday. Or the day before.

'Amber. This has gone on long enough. Are you getting up today?'

I shake my head.

'It's Saturday. Aren't you going to go to the craft market?'

'No.'

'*Why?*'

'I don't feel like it.' It's true. I don't feel like anything any more. I've become so sodden with sleep that I can't even think properly when I'm awake.

'You've been in bed three days. This is getting farcical. You're going to get up right this minute and start acting normally again,' says Jay, poking me with her fingers, literally trying to prod me into action. I brush her fingers away but she catches hold of me. 'What's your big game, eh? Are you trying to scare me silly, is that it? Well, congratulations, you've succeeded. Amber, look at me. I'm worried about you.'

I know she is. She's had a little pow-wow and dispatched first Leonora, then Wendy, even *Gordon*, to have a little chat with me. They chat. I lie and try not to listen, waiting for them to go away. Then I go back to sleep. I don't know why I found it so difficult the first day. I'm getting really good at it now. The nights are still a nuisance but I've got the days under control. I'm almost new-born baby standard, sleeping three hours out of every four. I wish I could feed like a baby too. I wouldn't mind a meal every four hours. The only part of my body still one hundred per cent awake is my stomach. I'm so *starving*. Jay thought she'd outwit me yesterday. She didn't leave anything at all for me to eat, she even took the muesli packet to work with her, and when she got home she didn't bring me any supper. She abandoned her vegetarian principles and fried bacon on our little gas ring and made beautiful buttery bacon rolls. Just for herself.

'You can have some too, Amber,' she called. 'Only get yourself up and dressed first.'

I didn't get up, I didn't get dressed, and so I didn't eat. The smell of the bacon stayed in the room for hours. I can still smell it faintly now.

'Can I have some breakfast?'

'Yes, when you get up and—'

'O.K., forget it.'

'Look, you're not going all anorexic like Polly, are you? Is that what all this is about?'

I shake my head.

'You just can't be bothered to get up and get it yourself, is that it? Well, you needn't think I'm going to run round in circles after you.'

'I'd have to be mad to expect you to do that.'

'Oh God, are you going to start all that poor-little-you rubbish? All right, I haven't been the best mother in the whole world, you haven't always had conventional three course lunches and clean white socks—'

'Sometimes I didn't have any sort of lunch. Or socks, come to think of it.'

'Oh yes, I know, you think you've been so deprived. If I'd

had the freedom and variety and wealth of experience that you've had in *my* childhood I'd have counted myself bloody lucky. You think I lived in some kind of privileged paradise, don't you? You want to try living that kind of life.'

I do, I do. Only Grandma hasn't written back. She can't want anything to do with me. She'd write back straight away if she did. And surely she'd use a first class stamp? Did Leonora? Did Leonora forget to post the letter?

'Amber, I am *talking* to you. Look, I'm already late for work—'

'So go. I'm not stopping you.'

'All right, I will go.' But she stands at the door. 'Amber. You're worrying me so. I thought you'd get up today. I thought it was just school getting you down. Is it? Or is it something else? If you'll only *say*.'

She waits. I wait for her to get fed up.

'Look, this has gone on long enough. You must be ill. I'm going to get a doctor. Do you hear? I'm going to phone for a doctor right this minute.'

'There's no surgery on Saturdays.'

'Oh shut up. You're enjoying yourself, aren't you? All right, carry on this stupid game. Turn into sodding Sleeping Beauty.' She slams out of the door.

I give a huge sigh of relief, hoping she hears, and then snuggle down under the covers. I wait. Only it doesn't work this time. I still feel a bit het up from talking to Jay. She won't really get a doctor, will she? And my hair is driving me mad. It smells like a vile little animal. I shove it back behind my ears but stray strands worm round my shoulders. I've always hated my hair. It probably looked fine when I was a baby and blonde wisps were appropriate. The trouble is that my hair hasn't grown up with the rest of me. It's so fine that it needs washing once a day. I know it might thicken up if I had it cut but I can't stand the thought of short hair. I once had to have my hair chopped right off. I had some sort of disgusting infestation. We were camping in tents at that time and the only water was from a sullen stream that was obviously polluted. I had diarrhoea all that summer too. Presumably these little health hiccups are part of my Wealth of Experience. Jay talks such wicked rubbish. I hate her. I really hate her. She hasn't left me any food again. Honestly, how can my own mother deliberately starve me? Did she leave any bacon from last night? Or a roll?

I crawl out of bed and examine the cupboard. Nothing. Nothing at all. The bitch. I dive back into bed and pull the covers right up over my horrible hair and lie twitching in the dark. My stomach growls. I put my hands on it. It's empty and yet it's still as plump as a pumpkin. Any one would think I was shut up shut up shut up. You'll have to get up anyway, you need a pee, and that bang below, I think it was the post.

I go flying downstairs, scared of bumping into any of the Smallwoods, but thank God the only one around is Naomi. She is sitting at the bottom of the stairs in her night-dress, with her anorak on inside out and her bare feet stuck in Leonora's stilettos. She is clutching a large loaf of brown bread, breaking off little bits and scattering them wildly all over the hall carpet.

'Me feeding the ducks,' she announces.

'Mm, that's nice,' I mumble, searching through the pile on the mat. I examine them expertly. Bills for Gordon, three letters for Leonora (one from Prague, one from India, and one from Islington written in gold on black paper, typical) some bumph in big buff envelopes for Wendy (news of antique and collectors' fairs, National Association of Gifted Children news-letter and holiday cottages in Cornwall) and a self-addressed foolscap envelope for Polly, obviously a new diet sheet. Nothing for me. Perhaps I should have put in a stamped addressed envelope. No, you surely don't have to do that with your own grandmother?

She isn't going to write back. She can't even be bothered to scribble 'I don't want to see you' on a post card. Maybe Jay was right about her all along.

One of Naomi's chunks of bread lands on my foot. I bend

down, mutter 'quack,' and eat the bread in one gulp. Naomi chuckles. The bread is wonderful. I usually hate wholemeal on principle, but now that I'm so hungry it tastes so good, strong and sustaining. I quack some more hopefully. Naomi stares at me in surprise because I don't usually play games with her but when she decides I am serious she throws me another piece of bread. And another and another. But I'm getting a bit fed up with this. I feel ridiculous crouching in this draughty hall in my grubby night-dress. I shall die if Leonora discovers me. And Naomi isn't breaking off big enough pieces. My mouth is literally watering.

'Duckie's growing big now,' I say, getting up and towering over her. 'Duckie's turned into a great big swan. A great big naughty swan who might peck you hard with his beak. You'd better give him all the bread just to keep him quiet.'

I edge it out of Naomi's hands. She blinks at me worriedly, not sure whether to cry or not. She opens her mouth and I quickly pop a chunk of bread inside.

'That's it, you're the duckie now, and this is your tea, and now you can go for a long swim up and down the river,' I say, pointing to the carpet.

Naomi toddles obediently up the hall, mumbling 'quack quack quack' through her mouthful of bread.

I run back to bed with my stolen loaf. I ought to eke it out throughout the day but I'm too greedy. I gnaw at it eagerly, washing it down with a mug of water. In five minutes it's gone, every last crumb. I wonder if Naomi will tell on me. She can't really talk enough to explain properly. And anyway, it isn't as if the Smallwoods will actually miss it. I've seen Wendy scatter whole loaves to the birds before now. Well, half loaves anyway. If Jay continues my starvation regime I suppose I could always creep into the garden every day and forage from the bird-table.

I wish I'd helped myself to a few papers while I was downstairs. I'd give anything for something to read. This is nonsense. I've got heaps of books up here. I can't read the

Pooh book without hearing Justin's voice and then I start crying, but I have forty-three books of my own. I lean out of bed and peer at the pile. I love them, they're my most precious possessions, and yet somehow I don't really fancy reading any of them just at the moment. I've read most of them two or three times. All right, there's some I haven't actually started yet because they look a bit difficult but I'll read them all some day, I know I will. I was a bit limited in my choice. They had some very odd books on the tenpenny shelf outside the Cinema Bookshop in Hay-on-Wye. Books like *The Ladies' New Medical Guide* by Doctor Pancoast. It's lost its covers, but it's still got a title page and most of its contents. It's not surprising it's falling to bits because it's almost a hundred years old. It's got the weirdest illustrations inside and I hoped it might help me with Human Biology at school but bodies seem to have changed considerably. I chose a *Child's Own Geography* book but countries have changed too, and *Notable Women Authors* isn't much help with Literature because when I mentioned Mrs Lynn Linton and Florence Marryat and Rosa Nouchette Carey to the English teacher at school he hadn't heard of any of them. I suppose History stays the same because it's already happened and finished with, but the only History book I could find in the tenpennies was *Scenes and Characters of the Middle Ages*.

I pick it up now. It's by the Rev. Edward L. Cutts. I try to read the first page. I don't understand much of it. It doesn't explain what the Middle Ages are. When were the Beginning and Ending Ages? I flick through the pages, looking for pictures. It seems to be about monks and friars and knights. Weren't there any ordinary people in the Middle Ages? Any women? Oh, there's a chapter on nuns. Jay was sent to a convent when she was a little girl and she says she still gets nightmares about those nuns even now. They used to prod her with a ruler when she talked in class and when she was really naughty they rapped her hard over the knuckles. Good for those nuns.

What's this chapter on anchoresses? What an odd name. As in anchor? Did sailors tie a woman to a rope and throw her overboard? I look for an illustration. No, an anchoress is only a female recluse. That's me!

I'd have been in good company in the Middle Ages. Only of course, that's exactly what they don't have. It says here they go into their little cell and a bishop puts his seal upon the door and then it mustn't ever be opened again except in time of sickness or approach to death. Which must occur pretty soon if you're locked up without any food or drink—no, wait a minute, you get that, you have a little window and someone brings it to you each day. It says you live upon the alms of pious and charitable people. You have an alms-box hanging up outside. I'd like that. Maybe I'll stick my own special alms-box outside the door. Whenever Wendy is feeling pious and charitable she'll put in a plate of her magical macaroni cheese. Gordon could leave me some *petits fours* from his business lunches: he often brings home a handful of Turkish Delight or candied grapes for Naomi. Leonora can contribute a Patisserie Valerie cake. Polly can slip in a carton of plain yoghurt and a lettuce leaf or two. Naomi might manage to donate the odd tube of Smarties. No use hoping for alms from Jay. She's never felt pious and charitable in her life.

It says you are restricted as to the times you can eat flesh-meat. Well, there's no flesh-meat in macaroni cheese or sweets or cakes or yoghurt or lettuce so I'm all right there. But what am I meant to do all day long? Pray, I suppose. I know the Lord's Prayer in my battered Bible from the Cinema Bookshop. 'Give us this day our daily bread.' I'll pray that all right. And it's worked today. I feel full for the first time since I took to my bed. 'And lead us not into temptation.' I'll certainly pray that. Again and again. There's the bit about forgiveness too, isn't there? Only I don't deserve to be forgiven. When I think about no don't, don't think.

Read this odd old book instead. These anchoresses indulged in frequent devotions. What does that mean? How can they behave devotedly when they're on their own? I imagine one kissing the wall passionately, another stroking the floor, a third scooping up the hem of her skirt and cradling it in her arms—no, it can't mean that. Wait, I've got half a dictionary from the tenpenny shelves; as long as a word comes before 'M' I can track it down. How boring, here's devotions and it just means prayers. So I've got to say the Lord's Prayer over and over again if I want to be an anchoress and that's going to get very tedious indeed. Aha! No, they *don't* just pray and eat up their alms. 'They occupied themselves, beside their frequent devotions, in reading, writing, illuminating, and needlework; and though the recluses attached to some monasteries seem to have been under an obligation of silence, yet in the usual case the recluse held a perpetual levee at the open window, and gossiping and scandal appear to have been among her besetting sins.'

Oh well, Leonora can come and tell me all the gossip and scandal, she'll be very good at that. Only I don't want to sin any more so I won't open my window very often. I'd like doing all the other things though. Reading. Well, I'm doing that now. And writing's all right, so long as I can take my time. What's illuminating? Dictionary. 'To throw light in or into'? Like a human torch? No, idiot, read on. 'To decorate (a letter, page etc) by the application of colours, gold or silver.' I'd like to do that, I'm quite good at art. And I could get one of those gold pens. If Leonora's friend has got one then she's bound to have one too.

I'm not sure I want to illuminate holy pictures though. One Christmas when I was little, a teacher told me to draw a beautiful picture of Mary and Joseph and the new-born baby Jesus. This teacher read us the nativity story and then handed out sugar paper and tins of wax crayons. The other kids made sure I had the torn piece of paper and the tin with all the broken crayons because I was the new queer dirty hippy girl. For once I didn't mind. I was too keen to get on with my drawing because at last I felt I knew what I was doing. Magda, one of the women at the commune, had given birth to a baby only a fortnight before and we had all welcomed the baby minutes after he was born. I felt sick as soon as I stumbled into that reeking room but everyone else seemed in raptures. They said it was beautiful. I didn't think Magda beautiful with her hair all stringy with sweat and blood all over her legs, and the red and wrinkled baby seemed perfectly hideous, but I obediently agreed that it was beautiful. So now at school I coloured a picture of a beautiful nativity. My Joseph and the infant Jesus were unremarkable. It was my Mary that attracted attention. I'd drawn her just like Magda, with her nightie hitched up under her armpits and her legs still wide apart. The children sitting near me nudged each other and bit their lips, their faces red with suppressed giggles, but I was used to that. I didn't realise there was anything unusual about my picture until the teacher saw it and gasped. She tore it into tiny shreds and shouted that it was just the sort of disgusting behaviour she expected from a child like me.

Oh, stop feeling so sorry for yourself, you fool. You should have known better. Leonora never made mistakes like that. Or if she did then it was deliberate, to shock or impress. I've shocked lots of people but I don't think I've ever impressed. No, that's not absolutely true. Needlework. I'm good at that. Better than all the other girls in my class. I've always sewn, ever since I could hold a needle and thread. I sewed up the holes in my clothes and patched them and turned the patches into pictures. I converted Jay's long skirts into dresses for me and when they got too short and tight I made them into smocks and then lots of little dresses for my dolls. I made *them* too, I had lots of little families like the Jane and Peter people. Their clothes were as neat and conventional as I could make them, and they all had spotless pale pink bodies and very neat short wool hair. I threw them away the moment they started to look scruffy. They kept me amused all the time so Jay didn't mind too much, although she was embarrassed that a girl of hers could enjoy anything as sexually stereotyped as sewing.

I didn't realise my sewing could ever earn me money until I went round the craft market last summer and saw the junky old tat on the stalls: dresses with crooked seams and uneven hems, dolls with vacant stares and lumpy limbs, tapestry bags already losing their handles. I knew I could do much better so I got Wendy to talk to Jeff, the man who runs the market (Aladdin's Cave is just around the corner) and I had my own stall there every Saturday.

Not this Saturday though. I've missed it and if you start mucking Jeff about then he soon gives your pitch to someone else. I've got five rag dolls and five teddies and a carpet-bag and two shoulder-bags and three little smocked dresses all neatly folded in a big black plastic bag by my bed. It's a wonder I haven't worn out Wendy's sewing machine. On a good day I can sometimes sell half my stock. There's only been one day when I didn't sell anything. I wanted to save up for a proper winter coat and a bookshelf for my forty-three books—oh what does it matter? The books can stay where they are and if I stay where I am too I won't need a winter coat, will I?

Maybe I'll be an anchoress and stay here in this room for ever. What do they wear? It says here a black habit and veil. I don't think I've got anything black. Jay's got black underwear but that won't do, of course. Wait a minute, she's got a black shawl. It would make a perfect veil. And I wonder if Leonora's still got any black dye left from the time she turned her whole bedroom black? Then this night-dress would do as a habit.

I flick on through the anchoress chapter, still playing with the idea, until I come to an account of a woman called Thaysis. She was locked up by an abbot as a penance for her sinful life—'and now and then throughout the subsequent ages the self-hatred of an earnest, impassioned nature, suddenly roused to a feeling of exceeding sinfulness, might urge women to such self-revenges, to such penances, as these.'

Chapter 5

JUSTIN. Remember that first day in 5e. He stood out from all the other boys. He couldn't help standing out, he's over six foot two in his socks. You can tell he's not used to being so tall because he walks awkwardly, as if he's on stilts. He was small until he was fourteen and then he grew six inches in six months and hasn't stopped since. His naturally anguished expression makes him look as if he's been stretched on the rack. He is not good-looking. He wouldn't be even if his hair didn't wave wildly out of control, even if he didn't need his much-mended spectacles. And there is also his voice.

It's the most amazingly unfortunate upper-class voice. It sounds petulant and pedantic at the best of times: when Justin gets excited it increases in pitch, petulance and pedantry to a positively unbearable level. Justin talked a great deal that first day and at first I couldn't understand why the other fifth years didn't punch him in the teeth. They often laughed when Justin said something, but it was with him, not at him. Then I realised why. It wasn't Justin who talked like that. It was Sleeve. Justin tucked his long bony wrist inside the sleeve of his grey pullover and kept his hand bunched inside. He'd inked a face on the stretched sleeve and every time Justin talked he moved his thumb and forefinger so that it looked as if Sleeve were saying it instead. In some lessons Justin did this openly, resting on his elbow and making Sleeve bob up and down. Paul Stokes, the English teacher, took this in his stride and addressed Sleeve personally; he and Justin developed quite a little comedy routine. Most of the teachers tried to ignore Sleeve, although he was obviously a distraction. Justin didn't chance his Sleeve arm with stiff old Mr Chapman, the History teacher. He was the sort who might have a cane down his trouser leg. Justin confined Sleeve to the cover of his desk in History lessons but whenever Mr Chapman chalked something on the board Sleeve peeped out and did a defiant dance while everyone grinned.

Justin wasn't exactly popular. He didn't have any real friends among the boys and the girls treated him as a joke. But nobody picked on him and threw his things around or mimicked his incredible voice. He was often called a nut-case or a twit or a weirdo, but it was affectionate abuse.

I thought Justin very clever to capitalise on his eccentricities. At first I was sure he was conventionally clever too: Sleeve answered and argued so articulately. But when I got used to those professorial tones I realised he didn't always make sense. And when it came to written work Justin couldn't use the Sleeve subterfuge. The long flowing stream of his words dried to a muddy puddle. He botched and blotted, his spelling faltered and punctuation disappeared, he missed out words or whole sentences, he could not add the simplest sum without making a mistake, he could not even copy correctly.

'You don't think, Justin Popper, that's your trouble. You're a clever enough lad, but you don't think. Think, boy, *think*', Mr Chapman commanded that first day of term.

'I do think,' Justin told me when I got to know him. 'That's the trouble. I've got too many thoughts in my head. They're all buzzing away and I can't get them to shut up so I can concentrate.'

He'd been to a lot of other schools before Mallford. They'd tried coaxing Justin, coaching him, caning him. Eventually his parents ran out of posh private schools and Justin ended up at the comprehensive. In 5e.

It was a come-down for Justin, but Mallford was a step up

for me. A new start. I had my own money from the craft market so I could start the way I wanted too. I went to Boots and bought blusher and eye-shadow and mascara. (Jay doesn't wear any make-up. Does she think she doesn't need it?) I bought a big bottle of Head and Shoulders (I hate that herbal muck Jay brings home from the shop). I bought a stick of Mum Rollette (Jay thinks deodorants interfere with the body's natural chemical balance). And I bought clothes.

I'd been making my own for years but they made me conspicuous. So I went to Miss Selfridge and bought new clothes, a grey dress with a navy check, a grey skirt, a navy sweater.

Jay was appalled when she saw me. 'They make you look so ordinary.'

She couldn't have paid me a greater compliment.

I tried hard to act ordinary at school. I kept quiet and copied the other girls. After the first few days they lost interest in me, although they didn't seem to mind when I tagged along with them. None of the boys bothered me. The teachers decided I was as colourless as my clothes and took no notice of me. I knew this wasn't such a good idea. I wanted to start learning. I wanted to be entered for exams. I tried very hard in lessons but they seemed to be talking in another language and I even found English puzzling. I was so looking forward to English. I had read my Hay bumper edition of the novels of Jane Austen until the pages fell out. A lot were already missing when I bought it but *Emma* and *Pride and Prejudice* and most of *Mansfield Park* were still intact so it was good value for 10p. Leonora had read *Pride and Prejudice* at her posh school and I'd flipped through her English Literature exercise book to see what work she'd done on it. It didn't look too difficult. I could have a go at writing a character study of two of the Bennet sisters. I could compare and contrast two proposals. I read Leonora's efforts and I thought I could do as well. Better.

But we didn't study *Pride and Prejudice* in 5e. We read *The Loneliness of the Long-Distance Runner* and *The L-Shaped Room* and *The Liverpool Poets*. The English teacher thought they were modern.

The only lesson I liked was Needlework. We were given the simplest of night-dresses to make, one of those special easy-to-sew patterns, and yet a lot of the girls couldn't even manage that. It was a good way of getting them to like me a little. I did a lot of stitching for them at break or in the lunch hour. Then we were taught basic embroidery stitches and told to decorate our long white shrouds. Most of the girls sewed a few half-hearted lazy daisies on the yoke and round the hem. I decided to do the same, but it was very boring sewing an entire field of lazy daisies right round my nightie and back again. So at home I added bluebells and poppies and then I got a bit bolder and chain-stitched creepers and bushes and trees, and I feather-stitched a flock of birds and added a monkey hanging from a branch and a tiger stalking through my jungle and then I couldn't stop. I embroidered an emerald Tree of Knowledge with a grinning serpent winding round it and a little pink Adam and Eve and a bearded God in his own white night-gown sitting up in a cloud. I was scared to take it back to school because I thought the other girls would laugh and think me weird, but they all seemed impressed and the teacher pinned my night-dress up on the wall for Open Day. I didn't tell Jay. I didn't want her coming to the school. She probably wouldn't have bothered anyway.

The girls kept fingering my nightie and passing remarks and one said it would cost a fortune in the shops. I wondered whether to tell them about my Saturday stall at the craft market but then they drifted off and I lost the opportunity.

That was how I got friendly with Justin: we met at the craft market. I was sitting stitching away when a familiar voice said, 'I say! Fancy finding you here, young lady. What attractive little doll personages. Might I say how do you do?' It was Sleeve slithering about on the end of Justin's arm.

I laughed uneasily, hoping no one was watching.

'Did you make all these beauteous artefacts?' Sleeve

enquired, and when I didn't reply he tapped me on the nose. 'I say, do you suffer from some kind of hearing impediment? I asked if—'

'Do shut up, Justin, people will think you're mad,' I mumbled.

'It's not me, it's Sleeve. I find his exuberance equally exhausting,' said Justin in his own watered-down voice, while Sleeve went on scrabbling through my display.

'Please don't,' I begged, grabbing two shoulder-bags that Sleeve sent flying.

'I'm sorry, but he's totally out of my control. I've tried sitting on him but he just bites my bottom. He's got a savage bite, you know, even though he hasn't a tooth in his woolly old gums. I wouldn't get too stroppy with him if I were you, or he'll go for you too. He's a very vicious nose-tweaker, you know. Sleeve. No, Sleeve. Down, boy, down!' Sleeve was tweaking my nose for all he was worth. We were attracting a little crowd and I couldn't bear it.

'Stop it, Justin, please!'

'I wish I could stop him, but—Sleeve, sir, it'll be the cold wash-tub treatment for you if you don't desist. Sleeve! No, not the lady's ear, it's tender—'

'You're *hurting*. And it's not funny. Please, can't you leave me alone, I'm trying to *sell* things. Justin, why don't you simply take off your jumper?'

'And expose me in all my fleshly pink nakedness! What an outrageous idea. Justin, this young lady's positively depraved,' Sleeve protested.

'Do you go on like this all the time?' I asked weakly.

'You must try to make allowances for Justin,' said Sleeve. 'Poor boy. He's too old for these attention seeking devices. Imagine what it's like for me. It's positive purgatory being permanently attached to such an uncouth yobbo.'

Sleeve sighed histrionically. I tried to ignore him. I looked at Justin instead. His mouth hardly moved when Sleeve talked. It was almost as if they were two separate entities.

'You're not paying attention, young lady,' said Sleeve, digging me sharply in the ribs.

I picked up one of my large paper bags and put it over his head.

'Help! Let me out! What a monstrous outrage!' Sleeve shouted, his voice actually sounding muffled.

'He'd better not talk. He'll use up all the oxygen,' I said. 'And he mustn't scrabble like that, he'll tear my paper bag and I haven't got many left. Justin. *Please*.'

'All right, I agree. I could do with a break from him too,' said Justin. He smiled at me sheepishly. 'These are really good,' he said, picking up a bag with his un-Sleeve hand. 'Who taught you? Your mother?'

'No! No one. I've always been able to do it. Who taught you ventriloquism? Your father?'

'No! Oh. Point taken.' He looked at me, fidgeting. 'You're not a bit like the other girls at school, Amber.'

'Thanks,' I said, bitterly.

'No, I'm *glad* you're not.'

There was another silence. Justin glanced longingly at Sleeve.

'Your things are really good,' he repeated. 'And I loved that night-dress thing of yours, with the Garden of Eden.'

'Thank you.'

'Oh well. I suppose I'd better be off. Will you unleash Sleeve or shall I? I'd better shove him in my pocket quick.'

As he did so he spilled several old sepia photographs.

'Look, you've dropped something. What are they?' I glimpsed an Edwardian gent in a natty bowler hat. 'Is that your great grandad?'

'No, I've only just bought them. From a shop round the corner. Well, it's more like an antique supermarket. Aladdin's Cave. Do you know it?'

Well, of course I did.

'I collect old postcards. Daft, I suppose,' said Justin, shrugging.

'Let me see.'

He held them out. He used his Sleeve hand but Sleeve seemed dazed by his spell in the paper bag and stayed silent. I looked at the Edwardian man, an 1880s lady with severe eyebrows and a bustle and a very fat baby in woolly rompers.

'Do you like babies?' I asked, surprised.

'No, I hate them. But they come in useful. I use the postcards to make collages, you see,' said Justin, growing pink.

'Collages?'

I simply didn't know the meaning of the word, but Justin thought I was knocking him. He was carnation by this time.

'I know it's a pretty wet sort of thing for a boy to do.'

'No, I don't know what they are, that's all. Collages.'

'You don't know—? They're pictures made of scraps of all different things. I make mine as surreal as possible.'

'As real?'

'*Sur*real. Look, I'll show you if you like. Come round to my house and see them.'

'I can't leave my stall.'

'After. When the market closes. Come to supper.'

'Well. Won't your mother mind?'

'Of course not. Anyway, I'll cook you supper. I'm a good cook.'

'*I'm* the cook and I don't hold with that foreign rubbish. I'm a chappie for good plain English cooking and very tasty it is too,' said Sleeve, bobbing out of Justin's pocket.

I sighed and Justin quickly rolled up his Sleeve to his bony elbow.

'There, he's gone again. Say you'll come, Amber.'

So I did.

Chapter 6

THE Smallwoods have gone out for an afternoon walk. Jay's gone with them, thank goodness. I'm so sick of her. She goes on and on about personal freedom and alternative life-styles but she can't leave me in peace. I'm not free and she ridicules my alternatives. I knew she'd comment on my newly dyed night-dress but I never thought she'd burst out laughing. I hate her. *She's* the one who wears fancy dress, the tart who trailed after pop stars, the druggie who overdosed, the commune flower child who wilted when her men left her. She's thirty-two, practically middle-aged and she's still scrounging. All her worldly goods fit into a battered knapsack tritely appliquéd with 'Make Love Not War'. She makes love with everyone else but she wages war with me. I'm the one who should be laughing at her, only she's not even funny any more, she's pathetic. She said she was sick of having such a loony lump for a daughter just because I wouldn't change out of my black robe and go downstairs for Sunday lunch with the Smallwoods. If she's sane I'm glad I'm mad, and I won't be a lump much longer because she won't give me any food. Not even any breakfast. She thought I'd be so starving at lunch-time that I'd give up and get up. She knows how I love Wendy's lunches. I missed onion soup with cheesy *croûtons* and buckwheat chicken pancakes with green salad and apricot compote and coffee with tiny chocolate fudge brownies. Jay spitefully told me every single ingredient as she put on her boots ready to go out. I pretended to be asleep and I'm still pretending now.

That's the lavatory flushing downstairs. Perhaps she didn't go with them after all. No, that's not Jay's footsteps, she struts in her boots. Oh God, don't let it be Leonora. She'll laugh at me too.

If only I could find a real anchorage and live on my own. I used to play with a little girl called Julie when we lived in the seaside chalet. Julie had a Barbie doll with twelve different outfits and we used to spend hours dressing her up and parading her about on her little pointy toes. I wanted to make Barbie a real person and talk to her and make her have adventures but Julie tapped her head with her forefinger and said, 'You're nuts.' Julie was a tough little girl with short hair and sores under her nose and I was scared of her, so I agreed I was nuts and we went on with the fashion parade. I used to get so bored I'd yawn and yawn and sometimes Julie would get cross and pinch me, but just occasionally she'd stuff Barbie and her twelve outfits into her miniature plastic wardrobe and tell me stories about The Children's Home. Julie had spent most of her life in care. It didn't sound very caring. Perhaps Julie had an imagination after all and made it all up. It sounded like a Grimms' fairy-tale. The children had to wash their own wet sheets in stone cold water in winter. They had to eat up every scrap of food on their plates and once when a child was sick it was even made to eat that too. They had to wash out their mouth with soap if they said bad words. If the little boys were caught fiddling with themselves they had to wear a placard for the next twenty-four hours declaring 'I am a dirty boy'. One little boy really was dirty and kept deliberately messing his trousers so he was put in the cupboard. This was the worst punishment of all. Julie shuddered as she said it.

I asked her what was in the cupboard, thinking of rats and spiders, but Julie said, 'You're nuts. They just left you alone.' It didn't sound so awful to me. If you were safely shut up in the cupboard then the other children couldn't tell you off and you didn't even have to do any lessons. You just sat by yourself in the dark. I'd give anything to be in Julie's cupboard now. Someone's coming up the stairs. High heels. So it must be Leonora. Go away, go *away*.

A soft tap at the door. Leonora would never dream of knocking.

'Who is it?' My voice sounds stupid, cracked. I suppose it's because I haven't done much talking this week. Talking out loud. I've talked inside my head almost all the time.

'It's me, Polly. Can I come in?'

Well, that's a surprise. She comes in with a tray, tipping it precariously because she's wearing Leonora's Oxfam stilettos.

'Hello,' I say, sitting up. I comb my hair with my fingers. At least it's clean now. I've decided anchoresses have a daily bath and I do it in cold water as an extra penance.

I smile nervously at Polly. I wish I didn't always feel so shy.

'I've brought you this. Mum told me to,' Polly says, holding out the tray.

Onion soup! Oh joy. And there's a great hunk of Wendy's wholemeal bread.

'I heated it up again. But it's all right, you don't have to eat it. I won't tell,' Polly says earnestly.

'No, I want it! Please. Oh, the smell!' I hold out my arms for the tray. Polly stares at my hands but I'm too hungry to mind. I spoon and munch. 'It's so good.'

'I think it looks utterly disgusting,' says Polly. 'Brown smelly scum. And a big brown lump like—'

'Polly!'

She can't put me off it. It tastes wonderful.

'There's still some left downstairs,' says Polly. 'I'll get it for you if you like. And you can have my apricots. *And* my pancake, although I'm not sure how to heat it up.'

'I'll have it cold,' I say quickly.

'Why didn't you come down at lunch-time then if you don't mind eating? Jay said you didn't want anything.'

'I didn't want to get up.'

Polly nods seriously as if she understands. Perhaps it's because she's so eccentric herself. She totters off and returns with a loaded tray. She shuffles now because she's kicked off Leonora's shoes in case she trips. She's wearing black socks that flap several inches at the toes. They obviously belong to Gordon. Polly won't wear her own clothes. I don't know why. I think they're wonderful and if only I were little enough I'd beg to borrow them. Polly's wearing a pinafore dress that Wendy wore when she was expecting Naomi. The grooves of the corduroy have worn smooth with age and the purple has faded to a dingy grey. Perhaps Wendy also wore it when she was pregnant with Polly. It hangs ludicrously on Polly now, making her stick arms and legs look odder than ever.

'Why are you wearing Wendy's old pinafore?' I ask, tucking into my second bowl of soup.

Polly shrugs her skinny shoulders. Her collar-bone looks as if it's going to poke right through her papery skin. 'It hides my fat stomach.'

She isn't joking. She honestly thinks she is fat, even though she's down to six stone something and is diminishing day by day. It won't be long before I'm literally twice her size. I feel such a pig beside Polly. She's watching every mouthful that I take. If I'm so ravenous after a few days what must it feel like to starve yourself for months?

'Do you really hate to eat now, Polly?'

'Well. I make myself hate it.'

'Why?'

'So I won't get fat.'

'Do you *really* think you're fat?'

'Not as bad as I was. But I still don't look quite thin enough. And anyway, I daren't start eating again or I'll get really fat.'

'But you do still eat some things? Your cottage cheese and your slimming biscuits?'

'I've cut the biscuits out, they're much too fattening, and I've cut down on my cottage cheese. I was getting through two cartons a day which was ridiculous, so now I eat ten teaspoons each mealtime, level teaspoons of course.'

'Do you measure absolutely everything you eat?'

'How else am I to know what my calorific intake is? Of course it's still much too high and I'm having problems cutting it down. Mum's making such a fuss each mealtime, nagging and looking reproachful all the time, so I've increased my activity to burn up the extra calories. I do an hour's aerobic exercise when I get up and another hour in the evening, and I swim in the school pool as many lunch-times as I'm allowed and I walk to school now instead of busing, I walk everywhere—'

'So why aren't you out walking now with the others?'

'That sort of walk isn't much use. They don't go anywhere near fast enough, and Naomi keeps stopping to look at flowers or feed the ducks and Leonora can't walk fast because she wears such stupid shoes. And they wouldn't let me come anyway. I'm in disgrace.'

'Why?'

'Because I ate some soup and some green salad just to stop Mum moaning, and it made me feel sick so I went to the loo and put my fingers down my throat and Mum heard me vomiting and told Dad and he got furious and now they're scared I've got Bulimia as well as Anorexia.'

'Bul—?'

'When you eat and then make yourself sick.'

'Well don't do that. It's revolting. No, *pretend* to eat and hide the food in your lap and then smuggle it up to me.'

Polly suddenly grins.

'O.K. Honestly. We are a pair. Jay's really worried about you, Amber.'

'No, she's not. She couldn't care less. Look at the way she won't give me any meals. You should think yourself lucky you've got a mother trying to feed you up. It's far worse having a mother who's doing her best to starve you,' I say, munching a large mouthful of cold buckwheat pancake.

'Peter would say it's significant we're discussing our mothers. He says that's why I'm anorexic. It's my way of manipulating Mum, making her notice me.'

'Do you think that's true?'

'Not really. I just don't want to be fat. Although I quite like it when he goes on about Leonora and Naomi and how horrid it must be for me, being stuck in the middle. I'm not the eldest or the littlest, I'm not the cleverest or the cutest, so . . . . '

'So you're going to be the thinnest?'

'Mmm. Well, that's what he thinks. And I go along with it because he's so nice to me and he lets me do anything. He specialises in child psychiatry so he's got all these toys in his room and I can play with them if I want. He doesn't tease and say I'm too old. There's a doll's house. So when I run out of things to say to Peter I play with the doll's house dolls. There's a mother and a father and lots of children and a baby. Peter pretends to read his paper or write up his notes but he's watching like a hawk.'

'To see if you stuff the big sister down the toy toilet and boil the baby on the toy cooker?'

Polly laughs. 'You watch out. You might be going to him too.'

'What?'

'Mum and Dad told Jay how good he is and said he could maybe sort you out too.'

'But there's nothing wrong with me! Look, I'm eating like a pig,' I say, scraping up the crumbs.

'Yes, I know you eat, but you won't get up, will you? Dad says that means you're trying to escape from something.'

'*He's* not a psychiatrist. He's just making that up.'

'He's read all these books on adolescent troubles because of me. And Leonora too. When she went on the Pill and kept talking about her sex life. Then she had some thrush thing and Mum was scared it might be V.D. and had the doctor examine her and it turned out Leonora's a virgin.'

'She's not!'

'Well, she mightn't be now, but she was last year.'

'Good heavens!' I'm so surprised I stop eating. 'But she told me—'

'She told me lots too. It was all lies.'

'Why don't they send Leonora to this psychiatrist then?'

'She did go once, but said it was so boring she couldn't bear to go again. I suppose it is a bit boring, especially if you don't like playing with dolls' houses.'

'Jay isn't really going to send me, is she? Well, I won't go either. She can't make me. Anyway, it's private, isn't it? She couldn't afford it.'

'Yes, it costs a fortune, but Dad said this psychiatrist is doing his own book on adolescent behaviour and he's specially interested in ex-commune children, so he might see you for nothing.'

'Oh God. Well, I'm not going and that's that.'

'It's all right, Amber. You're right, they can't make you go. And you're not seriously disturbed like me, are you? I mean, anorexia can actually kill you, I know that, but you don't die if you just lie in bed and paint your hands black.'

'I didn't paint them black. It's dye.'

I got black dye on them when I was doing my night-dress. Not my embroidered night-dress of course, my old white winceyette one. I borrowed Leonora's dye yesterday afternoon when she was out. I knew I ought to wear rubber gloves but I couldn't find any. I tried wearing old woollen ones but of course the dye seeped right through. I've scrubbed my hands raw but they've stayed as black as beetles. They've dyed much more successfully than my night-dress.

'They're not supposed to be black,' I explain.

'Oh. Gordon thought—'

'Go on. Tell me.'

'Well, do you know Lady Macbeth? Leonora's doing it for her O level and she's always Lady Macbeth and I have to hear her say her lines. Lady Macbeth has murdered someone, I think, so she goes a bit crackers and keeps washing her hands because she thinks they've got blood on them. So Gordon thought you might be repressing some sort of murderous desire and so you've painted your hands the symbolic colour of death.'

He's the one that's crackers! 'Who does he think I want to murder?'

'He didn't exactly say. But your mother looked very worried.'

'Honestly! He's not serious, is he?'

'He doesn't think you're really going to murder anyone. Although he did say that murderers are often very timid and repressed.'

'What rubbish!'

'Yes, it is,' says Polly, but she's fidgeting, hitting her puny thighs. 'I'm trying to break down the fatty deposits,' she explains. 'I'm sorry if I'm jogging the bed.' She pauses, hitting harder. 'Although actually, I tried to commit a murder once. And I'm timid, aren't I?'

'Who did you try to murder, Polly?'

'Leonora,' says Polly, pummelling.

'Did you have a fight with her?'

'I knocked her unconscious.'

I stare at her.

'I did, really,' says Polly, slapping now. Her legs must be scarlet under her skirt. 'I hit her with a saucepan and it was a cast-iron one and I caught her on the temple. She fell in a heap and just lay there and didn't move and I was positive I'd killed her. Of course, I was only little. Mum and Dad pretended it was all an accident, but it wasn't. I wanted to kill her.'

'Why? I mean, I can see why, I couldn't stand having Leonora for a sister, but why in particular? What had she done?'

Polly stops slapping and stares at her lap.

'She betrayed me. We were still living with the commune people although we'd moved to a farmhouse in the country and it was much nicer, we even had a donkey in the paddock.

Anyway, I fell in love with someone. It was real love, I thought he was wonderful and he was so nice to me, although he didn't know about it. Not then. I hardly said anything to him but I wrote down all the things he said to me in a special notebook and I made my own secret casket. Do you remember Miranda? I made my casket out of a chocolate-box and I stuck Rowntrees Fruit Gums on it for jewels and I kept the notebook inside and all sorts of other . . . mementos. There were some really silly things, a tissue he used, one of his socks, I stole that, and a few hairs I picked secretly from his shoulder, but there were some really special things too, drawings and stories. And Leonora found them and showed them to everyone and told *him* and I couldn't bear it and so I tried to kill her.'

I know who it was. Davie. I loved him too.

Chapter 7

DAVIE'S the first person I can remember. Long before Jay, although I know that's not possible. When I was born she lived in this old-fashioned Mother and Baby Home and then there were all sorts of places, bed-sits and squats I suppose, and then she met an artist called Zap or Pow or something equally improbable and he was living in the commune so we went to live in the commune too. I was about two and a half. I was not an appealing little girl. I was fat and timid and my face was permanently obscured by a nappy. A clean nappy—although it was probably grey because I'd never let it go long enough for it to be washed, and Jay was not likely to insist on laundering it. My nappy served as a cuddle blanket-cum-shawl: I nuzzled my nose into it and wound the fraying ends round my neck and up over my head. No wonder the other children teased me.

The commune children came and went but Leonora and Polly were there from the start. Polly was a baby and Leonora was a pretty little girl who pinched me until I cried. I huddled in a corner, knees against my chest, nappy over my head. And then I heard some music. I was used to heavy rock or strummed guitars. This was so delicately different that it made me shiver. I peeped out from under my nappy and saw Davie playing his penny whistle, a perfect Pied Piper. He even looked the part, because he always wore odd socks, one day red and green, another blue and yellow, and he had a long patchwork jacket of black and purple hexagons. He nearly always wore a big black battered hat with a purple feather, even indoors.

I can't work out which girl Davie was with at the commune. It could have been any or all of them. They certainly all loved him. The men liked him too, which was surprising. We were all supposed to love each other and the adults freely expressed that love, but it often seemed to end with the women crying and two of the men fighting. But no one ever fought with Davie. The children loved him the most. All the adults in the commune were supposed to spend one day a week in the children's room looking after us. It didn't matter whether they were parents or not. Commune children were supposed to belong to everyone. There were quite a few adults we didn't really want to belong to. Some were so stoned that they just slumped in a corner and let us do what we liked—or didn't like—so the big ones tormented the little ones and the few toys got broken and once Polly crawled into a sack of lentils and tried to eat her way out and almost choked to death. Others were fine for a little while, full of ideas for games and fun, but then they quickly got bored and irritable. Jay was like that. Zow or Pap or whoever he was had no patience either, but he bribed us with illicit Smarties and Golden Wonders. We were only supposed to eat the commune wholefoods so we were passionately fond of sweets and crisps. Most of the others liked Pappy old Zow but I still didn't think much of him, even though he gave me more than my fair share of sweets so that I wouldn't pester Jay when he wanted her to himself.

Davie didn't need to bribe anyone. The days he was in charge were better than birthdays. He played with us all day long and he seemed to be having as much fun as we were. He played his pipe while we danced, he told us stories, he drew pictures for us in chalk on the bare floor-boards, he filled a big trough with sand so we could play seasides, and he made giant balls of dough from flour and salt and water so that we could make necklaces and pots and little animals. Davie made little dough people called Dodies. He baked them until they were solid and then he introduced them. They all had distinct personalities and their own special voices: Doleful Dodie and Dim Dodie and The Divine Dodissima and the Dreadful Destructive Dangerous Dodie who went round biting everyone with his ferocious dough fangs.

The only thing that spoilt those wonderful Davie days was having to share him with the other children. I wasn't cut out for commune life. I disliked my extended family, all those surrogate sisters and brothers and fathers and mothers. I didn't even always like my own particular mother. I just wanted Davie.

I don't think he singled me out more than any of the other children but he had the knack of making me feel special. He'd play his pipe and then catch my eye so that I'd feel he was playing just for me. He'd tell a story and there would always be one little girl in it who seemed exactly like me. When I was sad Davie would know straight away and lift me up on to his lap for a cuddle. I can see now that he somehow did the same for all the children. Of course he did. But I don't want to think about it. I don't want to discuss him with Polly. Davie is mine.

We've always kept in touch. He sends me little presents: a cowrie shell, a bead bracelet, a paper-knife carved from a piece of driftwood, a lump of unpolished amber very nearly in the shape of a heart. I've kept them all of course. In a secret casket. I made mine at primary school from a Kleenex tissue box. I made a hinge for the lid with sellotape and then I painted it inside and out with white paint and covered it with Christmas silver glitter. It was supposed to be a present-making session for our parents but I hung on to my silver casket, hiding it from Jay. It was so precious I had to keep it for myself.

I've still got it now, although it's so battered I have to keep reinforcing it with tape to stop all the treasures falling out.

He sends me postcards too, from France and Italy and India and Israel and all over America. He's travelled a lot since the commune broke up, but he comes back to England every so often and then we always see him. The last time was when we were camping up in the Black Mountains waiting for the magic mushrooms.

Jay was with Tim. He was as hairy as a yak and he smelt like one too. I couldn't see how Jay could bear to share his sleeping-bag. I didn't want anything to do with him—or her either. I knew some of the other children camping but most of the time I went off by myself. I walked down from the mountains into Hay and wandered round the town. Tim gave me money 'To go get myself a snack'. He wasn't American, I think he came from Birmingham, but he wore cowboy clothes and sang hill-billy songs and affected an American accent most of the time.

He only gave me 25 or 30p which wasn't enough for the cafés, so I usually bought myself a sticky bun for lunch and then saved the rest for books from the cheap rack outside the Cinema Bookshop. Well, sometimes. Other times I was too greedy and bought two or even three sticky buns or a bag of chips. Once a man noticed me hanging around hungrily outside the fish and chip shop and he came out with a parcel of cod and chips and pressed them into my hands. 'Go on, give yourself a treat' he said. My mouth watered at the smell, my hands cupped the paper parcel automatically, and I so wanted to take them but I was scared there was a catch. He looked silly but harmless enough in his shorts and stout walking boots, the top of his balding head burned strawberry by the sun, but there was something about the way he was looking at me that reminded me of Tim, of Zap, of all the other men who messed Jay about. I became painfully conscious of my tight T-shirt and shorts. He was looking at me and I hated it, I hated him, so I thrust his fish and chips back into his hot horrid hands and ran away from him. I ran right through the town and up the road to the mountains, running until I was soaking wet and sobbing for breath. I still felt hot and horrible when I got near our camp. I saw Jay and she was looking different, prettier, in her crimson skirt and the white peasant blouse with little puff sleeves that made her arms look so delicately thin, and her hair was piled up girlishly into a knot on the top of her head so that her face looked more elfin than ever. I stared at her, surprised, and then she spotted me and smiled and told me the reason for this transformation.

'You'll never guess, Amber. Davie's here.'

There he was, over by the stream with Tim the Yak, and before I could shut her up Jay had shouted to him and I had to go and meet him still in my old tight hot and hideous clothes. I hung back foolishly but Davie waved and came running over and hugged me and he wouldn't let me stay stiff and shy, he cuddled and coaxed until I felt I was the old Amber again, the little girl who loved him unselfconsciously.

He stayed three days and they were beautiful, even though Jay and the Yak and their idiotic druggie friends hung around Davie most of that time. But the last day Davie went down into Hay with me. We went to the Cinema Bookshop because I'd shown him my small library and he said he wanted to contribute to it. I hovered by the cheap bookshelves outside but Davie took me into the shop. It was the first time I'd dared go right inside and we wandered around slowly, upstairs and down, our footsteps loud on the bare floor-boards, and my eyes ached with looking at all the books and my hands trembled as I turned the dusty pages and my heart banged like a gong behind my new bosom because it was such a special place and Davie was so special too and I badly wanted to find one very special book—and I couldn't choose. I changed my mind a dozen times and ended up almost in tears. Davie saw the state I was in.

'Shall I choose for you?'

He took me to the Craft section because he wanted to find me a special book on needlework but they didn't have any that pleased him. He browsed through the illustrated books instead and found a selection of old French fairy-tales. He nodded when he saw the black and white illustrations and showed them to me. I wasn't sure if I liked them at first. They were too dark and detailed, strange and sinister. There was a cat with savage claws dressed in a feathered hat and ornate boots, a slavering wolf attacking an ugly old woman, an ogre with swivelling eyes slitting the throats of little sleeping children.

'They're too frightening.'

'Look at the princess and the moonlit castle and the shepherd girl,' said Davie, turning the pages.

I looked but I still wasn't sure. The princesses had lovely clothes but they were all too plump and they had silly soulful faces.

'I don't think she's very pretty for a princess,' I said, pointing.

'I do,' said Davie. 'She looks like you, Amber.'

I shook my head, feeling awkward, almost wishing he hadn't said it. Now I wanted the book with all my heart and Davie knew it and bought it for me.

Chapter 8

'Do you intend to lie in that bed for the rest of your life?' Jay asks, poking me viciously.

She was all sweetness and light yesterday after her walk. She brought me back a Whippy ice cream, the biggest size 99 with extra chocolate sauce, my favourite treat. A lot of it had melted messily up Jay's arm but I ate the remains with relish. Jay was vaguely irritated when she found out I'd eaten all Polly's offerings too, but her voice stayed stickily sweet and her tone light as she sat on the end of the bed and talked to me. Wendy and Gordon had obviously advised her to try new tactics. She wouldn't give up when I answered in monosyllables, if at all. She chatted on determinedly and she kept it up, on and off, throughout the evening. I've no idea what she said because I didn't bother to listen. I tried to read the Bible like a good anchoress—it was Sunday, after all—but after a chapter the words wouldn't make any sense so I started sewing. I didn't feel like making anything for my craft stall. I scrabbled in my remnants bag instead and found an old white blouse from a long-ago school uniform. I cut the back into a large handkerchief and started hemming.

I reach for it now, needing its distraction, but Jay tweaks it out of my hand and throws it on the floor.

'Do you have to? That floor's dirty.'

'Then clean it instead of complaining.'

Where's the Sunday sweetness now? It's Monday morning and Jay is in an appropriate mood. She is dressed and breakfasted and all ready for work so why doesn't she go?

'Look at the time.'

'You look at it.'

'You're late for work.'

'You're late for school.'

'Why are you being so childish?'

'Why am *I* . . . ?'

She looks so ugly when she's angry. Her eyes are pink and peepy at the best of times but now they're scarlet slits and her face is screwed up into a simian expression. I bet she thinks she's *sexy* in her skin tight jeans and, oh God, why doesn't she wear a bra, who wants to see her going wibble-wobble inside her green velour? She's spilt something down it, several things, she is one great mess from head to foot.

'You make me sick,' says Jay.

She makes *me* sick, but I'm not stooping to her level. I'll just lie here and shut my eyes and pretend to sleep and sooner or later she'll get bored and go to work. Please make it sooner. What's that noise she's making? She's crying. Jay doesn't cry. She's just pretending, playing one of her stupid tricks. I give her a quick glance. Real tears. Well, so what? But my heart thumps and I feel hot.

'What are you thinking about?' Jay sobs.

'Nothing.'

'Don't you care that you've got me into this state?'

'I haven't done anything.'

'Exactly! Look, are you *ever* going to get up? Answer me!'

I shrug, although it's hard to do it effectively lying down.

'Don't just lie there ignoring me!'

Her hand whistles through the air. There's a sharp crack and my cheek stings and I bite my lip in shock. I can taste the blood. I put my hand to my face. She's panting above me, tear-stained, runny-nosed, disgusting. I take my hand away. Only a little smear. I bite harder under the cover of the bedclothes and then wipe the blood triumphantly on the back of my blackened hand.

'Look.'
'Well, answer me.'
'I can't even remember what you were asking.'
'When are you getting up?'
'I don't know.'
'That's not an answer.'
'It's the only one you're getting.'
Her fist clenches again but she checks it. 'Look, if you've got fed up with school then bloody well go out to work.'
'I'm not old enough.'
'You're nearly sixteen. And anyway, you can work in the craft market.'
'It's only there at week-ends.'
'There are other markets. Or you could help Wendy at Aladdin's Cave. You could do heaps of things.'
'I don't want to.'
'It's not a question of wanting! Why should I work every bloody day in that boring health food shop while you laze around in bed?'
'You didn't work when you were my age. You dropped out. So why can't I?'
Jay glares at me. 'You think you're so clever, don't you. I'm sick of you sneering at me all the time. You think you know it all, Amber, but you know nothing.'
I want to know nothing. I want all the worries flickering inside my head to burn themselves out. I want to be left with nothing, black and bare, nothing, nothing, nothing.
I hear Jay crying and then I hear her talking and then she gives up and goes and I strain to hang on to the idea of nothing. My head is empty, scoured of thought, as black as the darkness behind my eyes, and I hide there, thinking of nothing. No, all right, thinking of anything, but not that, not him. Tick tock, think to the clock, click to the ticks to stop yourself thinking, click clock with my tongue against my teeth, his tongue, let loose in my mouth, wet and wiggling—
I sit up, scrabble out of bed for my handkerchief and stitch.

I finish the hem and start sketching out a design, and then I stretch the material on to my embroidery frame. My needle makes little plicking noises on the taut cloth, plick and plock in time to the clock, my hand moves rhythmically up and down, up and down, faster and faster, no I'm *not* going to think about it. Think of the embroidery. I'm sewing a holy picture. I'm an anchoress locked into my little cell and I'm sewing the Virgin Mary—'Are you a virgin?'—I'm chain-stitching Mary's golden hair and soon I'll be ready to use the sapphire thread for her long flowing robe, with the darker blue for the folds and the inside of her sleeves. There are folds in her sleeves because she's cradling Jesus and I've got a special pale pink for his skin. No, I don't want to do a baby, I hate babies, she's not holding a baby at all. She can be praying instead. How can I make it obvious she's Mary if she hasn't got a Jesus? She doesn't look much like a holy woman, she looks more like a fairy princess with her long golden curls. So she'll be a fairy princess, it doesn't have to be a holy picture, and anyway, I'm not much use as an anchoress. I daren't remember and there's no way I can do a proper penance for my sin. She can be one of the princesses in Perrault. I reach for Davie's book and flick through the pages although I know every picture by heart. I stare at the Sleeping Beauty and then I turn my embroidery round so that Mary is lying on her back. She will make a splendid Sleeping Beauty and I can do her bed too, and embroider delicate cobwebs trailing from the bed-posts, and perhaps there's even room for a handsome prince. There are no handsome princes. Justin and I agreed. Romance is Rubbish. Love is Lunacy. Sex is Stupid. Our three golden rules.

We talked about it the first time I went to his house. He hung around until I packed up my stall at the craft market and then I went home with him. I rushed into Aladdin's Cave to tell Wendy I'd packed up because my stall's officially in her name. I knew she was surprised to see me with a boy at long last, but she just smiled in her winsome-Wendy way. I wished

Justin was shorter, sexier, saner—but at least he had Sleeve temporarily under control.

'I bought my postcards from her,' said Justin when we were outside.

'I thought so.'

'Is she your mother?'

'No. We just live with her.'

'What, you share a flat or something?'

'My mother and I have a room in her house.'

'So she's your landlady?'

'Not exactly.'

But Justin needs to know everything exactly. 'What do you mean?'

'She's a *friend*.' I was beginning to be irritated. Did Justin fancy her or something? So many men think Wendy's wonderful, with her long silky hair and her big blue eyes and her sweet little simper. Her Serene Highness. Jay calls her that sometimes and I'm not sure if she's being catty or not. She must be at least forty but she still looks very young, years and years younger than Jay. One of Leonora's boy-friends developed an overwhelming crush on her, much to Leonora's disgust.

'She's very attractive, isn't she?'

'Attractive?' Justin sounded astonished.

'Of course, she is quite old now. She's got a daughter my age.'

'I think she looks a mess,' said Justin, speaking with Sleevish authority. 'I hate that jumbly gypsy look, all those scarves and smocks and clanking bangles.'

'I agree,' I said happily.

'She's stuck in the seventies.'

'*Yes*.'

'That hippy hair hanging all round her face—honestly! I like the way you always pin your hair up in that neat little bun thing.'

Justin held out his arm awkwardly as if he'd like to

touch my hair, but his hand suddenly tucked into his sleeve.

'Excuse the lad's personal remarks, young lady,' said Sleeve. 'He doesn't mean to cause offence. He's got no social graces whatsoever.'

'Justin.' I stood still. 'Justin, please make Sleeve go away.'

'You prefer conversing with a callow youth to a Sleeve of such style and sophistication?' said Sleeve, sounding pained.

I wouldn't laugh. 'You promised to keep him under control.'

'O.K., O.K.' said Justin, unwrapping his hand and waggling his fingers at me. 'He's gone.'

It was a long walk to Justin's house and I began to wonder whether suppressing Sleeve was such a good idea after all. At least Sleeve was a fluent conversationalist. We were often stuck without him. Justin carried my big bag of stall goods and they kept banging awkwardly between us. We trekked to the north end of the town, near the park. We walked through the Neo-Georgian estate of town houses where I bought my bed. I looked for my imaginary Elizabeth Ann. I was impressed that Justin lived in such a posh area. I didn't know the half of it. We left the new estate behind and walked up the hill along an avenue of large Victorian houses. Some of them had been turned into Old People's Rest Homes or luxury flats but Justin's house was still a family house although it was huge. I stared at the white stucco, the red gables, the arched hedge, the shrubbery, the sloping lawns.

'Do you really live here?' I said stupidly.

'Mm,' said Justin, matter-of-factly, as if it was an ordinary two-up and two-down.

He stalked up the stone path, ignored the imposing front door with the brass lion-head knocker, and walked round to the back of the house. I tagged along behind him. We walked into a domed conservatory with ceanothus climbing up to the glass roof and a potted palm shading the Lloyd loom easy chairs. Justin paused by a pile of wellington boots, kicked off his dusty shoes and padded on in his socks. I wasn't sure whether I ought to take my own shoes off too. I wondered if his mother was very houseproud. However, there were little bits of dust and fluff on the quarry tiles and when Justin went through into the kitchen it was in upper-crust chaos, food and dirty dishes all over the scrubbed pine, an overflowing wicker laundry basket on the floor by the Automatic, and the Miele hanging open, untidily stacked. A man was leaning against the fridge gnawing at a large stick of French bread and a woman was sitting at the table sipping from a pottery mug. They beamed at me in a bewildered fashion.

'These are my parents,' Justin mumbled. 'This is Amber. My friend.'

Justin's parents were a surprise. I'd imagined them elderly and eccentric, but they were only mildly middle-aged and trendy in a very dated sort of way. Mr Popper wore a cream safari jacket and had an Indian scarf knotted at the neck; he sported a little goatee beard and gold-rimmed granny glasses. Mrs Popper wore a long Liberty printed skirt with a contrasting smock. Several tortoise-shell bangles clanked on her wrists and large tortoise-shell slides tucked her long greying hair behind her ears. They were the seventies couple of the century.

I caught Justin's eye in a moment of perfect understanding. I felt very nervous of his parents all the same. They invited me to muck in and join their messy meal so I sat down obediently. Justin glared at me.

'We'll fix ourselves something after you've gone,' he said, rudely stressing the last word.

'Right you are, old fellow,' said Mr Popper, abandoning the French loaf. There was a sprinkling of crumbs in his little beard. 'We've got to get cracking anyway, haven't we, Clara?' He smiled at me. 'We're going to the National and we like to catch the free concert in the foyer first.'

I smiled back knowingly although I didn't have a clue what the National was. He fetched a patchwork quilted jacket for Mrs Popper. I sold similar jackets at the craft market. I wondered about telling her but I felt too shy.

'Well, cheerio, kids. Have fun,' said Mr Popper. He gave us a wink that made Justin wince. 'We won't be back till midnight because we'll go and have a proper meal after the play. And Jonty's out with . . . . Who is it this time, Clara? Emma or Anna?'

'Oh darling, why are you so hopeless at keeping track of Jonty's girls? It's Louise now, has been for at least three weeks,' said Mrs Popper, doing up her toggles.

' 'Bye then, Amber. Lovely to meet you.' She glanced at Justin. 'You will remember to walk Amber home, won't you, darling? Or shall I leave some money for a taxi?'

'Mother!'

'Sorry, sorry!' said Mrs Popper, pulling a silly face.

Justin pulled a face too when they had finally driven off in their Volvo. It expressed extreme disgust. His hands clutched an imaginary machine-gun and he peppered the carpet and his parents with bullets.

'They're not a bit like you,' I said. 'And who's *Jonty*?'

'Jonty! Quite. My brother Jonathon. And he's not a bit like me either. What a *mess* this is,' he said, banging the table irritably. He picked up the French bread. 'Teeth-marks! I ask you.' He inspected a lump of Stilton gloomily. 'It's a wonder he didn't sink his choppers into the cheese too. We're not eating in here, it's a total rubbish tip. Come upstairs to my room at once.'

I blinked at him. He blushed. Sleeve bobbed out.

'The boy should make himself clear. You need not fear a fumbling sexual approach. The lad simply means that his room is a little oasis of order in this derelict desert. Oh I say. I do have a fancy turn of phrase when I put myself out.'

'Put yourself back, Sleeve,' I said. I looked at Justin. 'You won't try anything, will you?'

Justin looked offended. 'I just *said*. You don't have to worry about sex when you're with me. I think it's stupid.'

'Do you really?'

'Yes. And Romance and all that hearts and flowers stuff. Romance is Rubbish.'

'And—and Love is Lunacy?'

'Exactly!' Justin grinned. 'Our three golden rules, O.K.?'

Chapter 9

'HI. I've brought you these.' Leonora bursts into my room and balances a squashy bag on my chest. I squint at it warily.

'Grapes,' says Leonora, helping herself.

'Thank you. Thank you ever so much.' My mouth is watering. I sit up and start on them. 'They're lovely. But you shouldn't have.'

'Relax. I nicked them off a barrow,' says Leonora airily.

I'm not sure whether I believe her. Did she steal the paper bag too?

'And anyway, you're supposed to be ill,' says Leonora. 'Although actually what *is* the matter with you, Amber?'

I shrug, embarrassed.

'Jay was crying about you this morning. It was weird, I've never seen her cry before. You haven't got anything *serious*, have you?'

'No.'

'So you're just quietly going off your head?'

'Something like that.'

'Oh well. I'm used to nutters. Look at Polly Pudding.'

'You shouldn't call her that. You'll make her think she's still fat.'

'She's got eyes, hasn't she? She's a positive skeleton, it's disgusting.' Leonora crams a handful of grapes into her mouth. 'What have you been doing with yourself all day then?'

'Nothing much.'

'Don't you get bored?'

'Yes.'

'Don't you mind?'

'Not really.'

'God!'

Leonora is beginning to find me boring too. She prowls around the room for a few minutes, spitting out grape pips, and then wanders off, mumbling something about homework. I eat what's left of the grapes. The ones at the bottom of the bag are sour and slimy. I eat them nevertheless and then lie down. I want to go to sleep before Jay gets back.

I don't manage it.

'Hello Amber.'

She looks subdued. I hope she isn't going to cry again. She comes and sits on the end of my bed.

'Sorry I slapped you this morning. I just got so mad. You know how it is.'

I don't know. I get angry but I can't fight or shout. I just think the words inside my head. Sometimes I'm surprised they don't burst out like bullets.

'I can't stand it when you won't talk to me, Amber. I've always tried to be open with you.'

Too open. She's sobbed and shrieked so many things when she should have shut up.

'I could never talk to my mother,' says Jay. 'We lived in completely separate worlds.'

How I'd love Grandma's planet of peace and politeness. She hasn't written back to me.

'And now we can't seem to talk either. I don't know what to do. You can't go on acting like this. You'll make yourself really ill if you don't watch out.' She looks at me. 'You're not ill, are you?' She feels my forehead. 'It does feel hot. I wonder if you *have* got a temperature. You do look funny. And you're so pale. How do you feel?'

'Odd.'

'What sort of odd?'

'Tired. A bit sick. Just odd.'

'Someone at the shop was saying there's a really nasty flu bug going round. Maybe you've been sickening for it, and that's why you've been all odd and depressed.'

I think about the flu. I hadn't even thought I might get it too. Perhaps Jay is right.

She borrows a thermometer from Wendy. My temperature is barely 99 but she still clings to the belief that I am ill. She makes me a special invalid supper: two boiled free-range eggs (she cracks the odd half-dozen at work so she can get them half-price); fingers of yesterday's wholemeal bread and an apricot yoghurt only two days past the sell-by date.

Tuesday is even better. There's a huge wholemeal pizza from the health food shop (it fell on the floor but it was a clean floor so it just got a little squashed) and Jay *buys* a bag of Jaffa oranges so all that vitamin C can charge me like an electric current and liven me up a bit.

Justin made a weird Jaffa orange salad that first day I went to his house. He chopped up the oranges with almonds and sweetcorn, and we ate it with Stilton sandwiches and sticks of celery. After a hunt in the cupboard for a likely pudding he found some sponge finger biscuits and a tin of condensed milk. You can't be shy of someone when you're dipping into the same tin of condensed milk, even if you're sitting side by side on a bed. Justin's room was more a study than a bedroom anyway. There were books everywhere, even piled in the middle of the floor, and two old filing cabinets and a desk and all sorts of charts and maps and newspapers crackling in corners. I asked about his collages. He kept them in a large black folder tied with tapes.

'They're not very interesting,' he said nervously. 'It's terribly childish, all this cutting out and sticking.'

His collages were anything but childish. There were claustrophobic parlours with pumas lurking behind the potted palms and huge woodpeckers drilling holes through the heads of staid Victorians and severed limbs bleeding on silver salvers. They were so cleverly composed that I fingered the edges of the cut-outs to make sure they'd been stuck on. I struggled to think of an appropriate comment.

'They're . . . brilliant.'

Sleeve squirmed into view.

'Now, now, young lady, don't bandy words like brilliant, you'll turn the laddie's head. They're neatly put together, I grant you that. He's a dab hand with the Evostick, although they're convinced he's a glue-sniffer down at the newsagents, but what about his subject matter? Tut tut! A psychiatrist would have a field day. Evidence of a very warped personality. Ghoulish. Grotesque. I'd beat a hasty retreat if I were you. Ugh! Look at that horror.'

I'd come to the last picture. Sleeve wasn't exaggerating. Justin had cut up a book of Flemish paintings of the Crucifixion and various martyrdoms and reassembled them into one horrific collage of carnage. All the heads of the painted people had been replaced by Polyphoto babies. I looked at them closely. I thought they were all different babies at first, but then I sorted them into two. The torturers were all one baby, the tortured another. The torturing baby had an anxious frown and his hair waved in wild tufts. Justin. I peered at the other immensely suffering infant. He always had an incongruous smile on his face. He was the cute cooing sort of child you see in advertisements.

'Can't you guess?' Sleeve demanded. 'Dear, dear, you're not very bright. Haven't you ever heard of sibling rivalry? It's his *brother*. Jonty the Jaunty. Jon-boy the original Con-boy.'

I didn't know what to say.

'I suppose it's a bit sick,' Justin murmured in his own voice. 'I wish I hadn't shown you now.'

'I once made a doll of my mother,' I said. 'It was when I found her with this man that I thought really wonderful. I couldn't bear it that he wanted her. So I made my little rag doll. I made it very carefully with embroidered features and woollen hair and a full set of clothes. I put patches in all the right places and rubbed tiny stains all over the dress. I've never taken such care over any other doll. It was a perfect miniature of my mother. And the moment it was finished I took my big dressmaking scissors and I chopped it up into tiny little pieces.'

Chapter 10

I DON'T know what to do about night-time. Jay's alarm ticks and tocks relentlessly and the hands play tricks on me. I lean out of bed and look at the time and lie down again and turn one way and turn another and plump up my pillow and murmur prayers like an anchoress and chant the few hymns I learnt at school and think about golden crowns and glassy seas and plan a magnificent tapestry as big as a wall, a tapestry to wind round these four walls, a tapestry without seams so that I stitch past windows and doors, stitch myself into safety, only there's no safety, it's an illusion, my delusion, and something's tearing through the stitches, don't, you're hurting, it's hurting, and I sit up, sweating, and look at the clock again and one minute has ticked by, a minute the length of an entire night, and I have to endure fifty-nine more to make one single hour and it isn't even midnight yet.

There are clicks as well as ticks. Jay lies literally at my feet, her mattress at the end of my bed against the wall, and as she breathes she makes a clicking sound somewhere at the back of her throat. The ticks and clicks are not co-ordinated. Tick and click, and I count them and make bargains; if I can count to a thousand before Jay turns over, if I can hold my breath for twenty, if I can time my breaths to hers and block my ears for five minutes and then still be in time, if, if, then it will be all right. I struggle and strain but Jay conspires against me even unconsciously. She turns over immediately, she burrows her head under her covers so I can't hear her breathing, she outmanœuvres all my magic spells. She stays smugly sleeping while I lie with my eyes achingly open.

Night after night. Day after day. I count them too. I count them until I lose count because they are all the same. But today is different. Jay is holding a letter.

'It's for you.'

I sit up, rubbing my eyes. Jay's slipping another letter in the pocket of her jeans, a blue airmail letter.

'Who's that from?'

Two letters in one day! We don't get letters. We move around too much.

Jay shrugs. 'Just a bloke.'

So she's starting again. It's been so peaceful recently because there have been no blokes. What a stupid ugly word and yet it's one of Jay's favourites. She sounds at her most middle-class when she says it too, pronouncing it with such precison. Perhaps it *is* appropriate. Nearly all Jay's blokes have been stupid and ugly.

'What about your letter?' she says, holding it out to me.

I stare at the envelope. It's long and cream and it rustles because it's lined with tissue paper. The handwriting is elegantly illegible. The postmark is Marylebone, Marylebone, Marylebone.

'It's from my mother.'

'Yes, I think so.'

'Why is she writing to you?'

'I don't know.'

We both wait.

'Well, open the bloody letter and find out!'

I hold on to the envelope. Still waiting.

'Amber. Open it.'

'It's addressed to me.'

'Yes. I know. I just want to— She's my bloody mother.'

She always swears when she's excited.

'She's my grandmother,' I say calmly. And win.

'Oh Christ, as if I care about your stupid letter,' Jay yells.

'You can stop clutching it to your chest. I'm not interested, O.K.? I'm off to work.'

She pulls on her ancient awful jacket and swaggers away in her down-at-heel boots, slamming the door.

I wait five whole minutes, till I'm certain she's not coming back, and then I carefully slide my finger under the edge of the envelope and ease it open. I can't bear the thought of tearing it, it's so beautiful. The tissue-paper lining is dark brown, such style! I take out the letter and unfold it. I look at the bottom at the signature. It isn't 'Grandma'. Or 'Grandmother'. Of course it isn't 'Granny'. She's signed her name, 'Cicely Elliston'. 'Yours sincerely, Cicely Elliston'. At least she's started 'Dear Amber'. Its a wonder it's not 'Dear Miss Elliston' or even 'Dear Madam'. But perhaps it's polite. Perhaps it's the way it should be done.

It takes me another five minutes to decipher the letter although it's short to the point of being curt.

Dear Amber,

I suggest we meet at 10.30 on Saturday morning at the W . . . . . . C . . . .

Yours sincerely
Cicely Elliston

Next Saturday. This Saturday. But what is the W . . . . . . C . . . . ? I can only think of water closet which is ridiculous. I peer and peer at each letter but they're blurred into a meaningless swirl of royal blue Quink. Westminster Cathedral? No, it's an Abbey, isn't it? There's a silly pop song Jay used to sing, 'Winchester Cathedral'. Is there such a place? But why would my grandmother want me to go all the way to Winchester? And would you say '*the* Winchester Cathedral' anyway? Perhaps it's the something college? Yes, there are definitely two l's, they loop up unmistakably. But *which* college? I don't know any colleges.

Justin might. Sleeve seems to know that sort of thing. He's

very partial to Radio Four, particularly the quiz programmes: he bobs about during the *Brain of Britain* contest and punches the air in pride whenever he gives the right answer. They nearly always are the right answers even though Justin's so hopeless at lessons.

'It's Sleeve who knows, not me. He absorbs information the way other sleeves absorb fabric conditioner. He's a brainy old bit of Botany wool. He could say the alphabet backwards when he was just a weeny skein.'

Oh Justin, I do miss you. Why did I have to ruin everything? No, I'm not going to think about it, I'm not going to worry, not now, W . . . . . . C . . . . , think about that, puzzle it out. Only I can't. And it's Saturday tomorrow. There's no telephone number on Grandma's letter. I get up and pad downstairs and try to look her up in Gordon's telephone directory but there are no C. Elliston's in the book. She must have a telephone. I can remember it. Old-fashioned, black, and the receiver had pointed ends. It gleamed, like everything else in her flat.

I dial Directory Enquiries but they can't help me. She's ex-directory. So that people can't get in touch with her. Me.

No, she *wants* to see me, at this elusive and infuriating W . . . . . . C . . . . I'll have to ask Jay when she comes home from work. It's probably a place she knows well, and even if she doesn't, she'll know Grandma's telephone number. I don't want to ask Jay. She'll see the letter then. Maybe she'll even come with me. Then I won't stand a chance. Grandma hates Jay and no wonder. I have to show her that I'm not the same.

Yes, you are, tarred with the same brush, I clench my black hands, no, stop it, think, W . . . . . . C . . . .

Wendy might help. I wait until I hear her coming home in the afternoon, chatting to Naomi, and I run down the stairs, wanting to grab her before Leonora and Polly come home from school. I run too fast and the stairs turn into a switchback and I stagger.

'Amber!'

Wendy sounds alarmed. Naomi stops clamouring for Ribena and edges away from me.

'Are you all right, Amber?' Wendy asks. 'Here, sit down.'

She gets a kitchen chair and eases me on to it. She's treating me as if I'm really ill. I feel ill. Neon lights are flashing in Wendy's pale pine kitchen and the quarry tiles are tap dancing and there are two little Naomis nodding at me, two Wendys murmuring at my side.

She makes me a coffee and Naomi shakes the biscuit tin at me. My teeth clink against the mug and it's hard to stop it spilling, but by the time I've drunk my coffee and eaten two chocolate fudge brownies I feel better. Wendy settles Naomi at the sink with a bowl of water and her plastic tea-set and then turns to me.

'You can't go on like this, Amber. You're worrying us so. Poor Jay is in a terrible state. I think you ought to see a doctor, don't you?'

'I'm all right.'

'You're not all right, Amber. You need help.'

I stare at her and I want to laugh. She really thinks I'm crazy. Yet I feel a bit crazy sitting shivering in my weirdly dyed night-dress. I pluck at it with my black trembly hands. How can I meet Grandma looking like this?

'Do you know what W.C. stands for?'

Wendy stares at me. 'It's what some people call the loo.'

I burst out laughing and can't stop. Wendy lifts Naomi down from the sink and tells her to go and play in her bedroom for a little while. Naomi protests and pours a teapotful of water down her dress. Wendy has to bribe her to her bedroom with another brownie. Does she think I've gone so stark staring mad that I'll seize the bread-knife and slice Naomi's head open? I laugh and laugh, wrenched with laughter, drenched with it, sweat bursting out all over my large lumpy body, and I'm getting larger and lumpier every day, in every way. Am I laughing? I'm crying and Wendy has her arms round me and I cling to her for comfort.

'What's the matter, darling?' Wendy murmurs. She's stroking my straggly hair as if she really cares about me. 'What started this off? Can you tell me, you poor love?'

'I think I'm . . . '

'Mmm?'

I want to tell her, the words are twitching on my tongue, but then she'll tell Jay, it'll all start, I can't, I'm too much of a coward.

'I can't,' I sob. 'I want to but I can't.'

'Never mind,' Wendy soothes, and she sounds as if she really understands. 'Never mind, Amber. I know. Growing up's so horrible and worrying and lonely. But everything will work out for you. You're a lovely girl, did you know that? I think you're a bit like my poor Polly. It's so hard for her having a sister like Leonora, who's always so chirpy and confident. In a way, Leonora's almost like a sister to you too, isn't she? And I know it must be maddening seeing her rushing around, making all these new friends and having such fun when you feel too shy to join in.'

I pull away, unable to *believe* what she's saying. She hangs on to me determinedly.

'But you can have fun too, Amber. You're so pretty in your own special way. If you can only learn to like yourself then everyone else will start to like you too.'

I stiffen and suffer while Wendy rocks me backwards and forwards and believes she is comforting me.

'There now,' she says at last, wiping my eyes with the tea-towel. 'Better?'

Of course I'm not better, but I nod nevertheless. Wendy looks as if I've given her a wonderful present. Oh how she loves being Mother Earth. No, more Mother Hen clucking over her chicks, even the ugly duckling.

'Why don't you go and have a lovely long hot bath now?' she suggests.

Oh God, do I smell? Wendy runs the bath for me as if I've

shrunk down to Naomi's size. She shakes in Naomi's bubble bath too but doesn't actually try to pull my nightie over my head and lift me into the bath. I almost wish she would. It's such a stupid effort. The steamy air makes my head throb. I can feel a pulse in my eyelids and I close them as I clamber into the bath, so I won't see myself in the mirror-tiles. I sink under the scented water and it's beautiful, I'd forgotten how wonderful, I was mad to opt for those ice-cold plunges—and anyway, aren't hot baths meant to be helpful? Boiling baths. I run the hot tap until the water brims the edge and lie there. My whole body pulses, throb throb, a steady rhythm, I can feel it all over, I can feel, 'You feel so soft', no, NO. I jump out of the bath, water splashing everywhere, and I scrub with the towel, dizzy and disgusted.

I'm still as pink as a prawn when I'm back in bed in my clean petticoat. No more black night-gowns and acting like an anchoress. My hands are elephant grey now and the hot water has wrinkled them appropriately. I leave faint finger-marks on Grandma's letter as I stare at W . . . . . . C . . . . White Cross? Woolworth's Corner? Winston Churchill? This is getting ridiculous.

The door opens, banging back against the wall, making me jump. Leonora, who else, back from school, her school tie slung round her neck like a scarf, a Vice Head Girl badge jokily pinned to her bosom.

'Hi. What's up with you now, scarlet fever?'

'I've had a hot bath.'

'About time too. My ma's just had a word, says I've got to be ultra tactful with you and ask you to go out with me and my mates this evening. So I'm asking.'

'No thanks.'

'Yeah, I didn't think you'd want to come somehow. I don't know what Mum was on about. You don't want to join in, do you? I mean, you're quite happy being the neighbourhood nutter, aren't you? Hey, who's the letter from? Your weirdo?' She grabs it before I can stop her. '*Cicely* Elliston? Oh, your grandma, you wrote to her, yeah. Well? Are you meeting her at the Wallace Collection tomorrow?'

Chapter 11

TWENTY-SEVEN minutes past ten. I stand here outside the Wallace Collection, staring at the deep red bricks as if there is some meaning in their pattern. The wind is cold and I'm shivering. I do hope there is a lavatory. I need to go so badly I have to hop about. And I feel so sick. I couldn't eat any breakfast and then I felt so faint that I bought a Cadbury's Flake and a packet of Hula Hoops and ate them on the tube. And now little shreds of flake jump through each hula hoop, jumping higher and higher until I can taste their sourness at the back of my throat.

I shall greet Grandma dramatically: I shall either wet myself or vomit. Oh God, it's twenty-eight minutes past ten, she'll be here any minute, and what if I don't recognise her? I thought she was fixed like a photograph in my head, but now when I try to remember exactly what she looks like she blurs until she's barely there at all. Smart, slender, silvery hair—but here come two women in navy suits and they're *both* thin and elegant with white bobbed hair. Could one of them be her? They pass me without a glance, talking in high haughty voices, and they make me feel so shabby and so scared.

Twenty-nine minutes. I really am going to wet myself. There's a man in uniform standing just inside the door. Shall I ask him if I can use the loo? He gives me a little nod every now and then, he looks quite friendly, but I *can't* ask him, he'll think me such a baby, and what if Grandma comes while I'm in there and then goes away before I can get back?

It was such luck that Leonora knew all about the Wallace Collection.

'It's a museum place in Marylebone. I went there last summer with Peter and Andy. They think the Wallace Collection is too chic for words but I didn't go a bundle on it myself.'

'What *is* the collection? Does it cost much to see it?'

'I don't know. There was heaps of armour and a lot of paintings of simpering ladies with great pink bums,' said Leonora. 'I don't think you had to pay though.'

'So it wasn't terribly posh?'

'I don't think so. Just boring. You'll probably like it.'

I'm sure I won't. It all looks impossibly elegant and it's gone half-past ten and I'm sweating under my arms even though I'm still shivering. I catch sight of myself in the window at the entrance and I look even worse than I'd imagined. My hair's coming out of its slides already and there are great wisps dangling down my neck and my jacket looks cheap and crumpled and my skirt's a mess, I scrubbed and scrubbed but I couldn't get rid of that stain and she'll spot it straight away.

It's twenty-eight minutes to eleven now and I'm in such a state that I walk up and down, my steps as stiff as a soldier's, left right, only I don't know what to do with my arms. It's mad, but I seem to have got out of the habit of walking and my shoes hurt; my feet feel so tender after being tucked up in bed all this time.

What am I going to say to her? Hello? Good morning? What *do* people say to their grandmothers? Wendy's mother is dead I think, but Gordon's mother comes on a Sunday sometimes and I don't think Leonora and Polly even bother to acknowledge her. Naomi rushes at her and goes 'Gran-gran-gran' but I can hardly do that. It's twenty-seven minutes to eleven and I fish out her letter and peer at W . . . . . . C . . . . for the five hundredth time. I'm sure it is Wallace Collection, and it's in Marylebone, she lives near here, I have to be in the right place, unless there's another entrance—oh God, did she mean meet me inside? At the Wallace Collection. Does that mean inside or out?

I go up to the entrance, grin foolishly at the attendant, and peer inside. There doesn't seem to be anyone waiting, not in the hall, not by the huge staircase. It's so *grand*. Oh, trust Leonora to get it wrong.

'Can I help you, Miss?'

It's the attendant. He's being nice, I know he is, but I can feel myself blushing like a fool.

'No thank you. Well, I'm looking for someone, my grandmother, I just wondered—but she isn't here yet.'

'You can go in and look if you like.'

'No. I—I'd better wait outside.'

So I pace around, up and down, bladder clamouring, I should have asked him, it's gone twenty-five to now, she's not coming. She's not coming. I clench my grey hands into fists. (Pearl grey now: I immersed them in bowl after bowl of near-boiling water and scoured so hard the skin nearly peeled away). She's thought better of it. Maybe she had no intention of coming at all. She's played a trick on me. No, that's silly, why on earth would she do that? Could something have happened to her? Perhaps she went hurrying out to meet me, stepped off the pavement and went smack under a car. I'll never know. Yes, of course I will, I've got her address. I can go round there. I can give her another ten minutes—twenty to now—perhaps I'd better make it another twenty, and then at eleven I could find my way to her flat; I can always ask someone the way, I'm not completely helpless.

But that's the way I feel. I don't know what to do. I think I might cry. Yet I can't cry here, it's far too grand and the attendant is still watching me, and someone's coming. An odd old lady. She's wearing an old-fashioned black suit that has obviously been stored in a trunk for years. I can see all the creases where it's been folded. It's much too big for her now. The hem droops around her sad stick legs. She's not wearing stockings so they look painfully white. Her cracked black patent shoes slip from her heels at every step. She's stopped stepping. She's standing looking at me and I'm looking at her. It can't be.

'Good morning. I believe you're . . . Amber?'

'Good morning. I—I believe you're Grandma?' I stammer, trying to be equally polite.

She flushes under her thick powder and her mouth puckers. Lipstick slides up all the wrinkles.

'Are you making fun of me, young woman?' she says sharply.

'No! Honestly!' I'm so horrified she realises she's made a mistake.

'You copied what I said,' she explains, pulling a torn lace hanky from her pocket. Her eyes are watering in the wind and she dabs at them impatiently. Her blue eye-shadow smears down one cheek but I cannot possibly tell her.

'You're much bigger than I expected,' she complains. She sniffles and dabs. 'This wretched wind! We'd better go inside. Do you like museums?'

'Yes,' I say, trying to sound enthusiastic.

'The Wallace Collection is one of my little haunts.'

She totters in her ill-fitting shoes through the doors. I realise too late that I should have held them open for her. She's talking to the attendant now. He wants to inspect her handbag, presumably to make sure she isn't hiding a bomb. It isn't a proper handbag. It's a padded sponge-bag from Boots. She unclicks the gilt fastener and I'm sure she's going to produce a tooth-brush and flannel and then we'll all know my grandmother is loopy, but she displays a perfectly ordinary purse, another crumpled lace hanky, a lipstick and my letter, neatly folded.

'I hope you didn't mind me writing to you,' I say, as we start up the sweeping flight of stairs.

She doesn't answer but I think it's because she's concentrating on the climb. Her mouth has almost disappeared and her eyes bulge with effort. I wonder if I should take hold of her arm. I don't dare. I hover ineffectually until she reaches the top of the stairs at last. She aims at a seat and almost topples as she sits down, but she manages to right herself, her knuckles white as she clings to her own knees. Her hands are twisted into slopes, as if she always lies on them the wrong way at night. They are speckled with liver spots. Her three rings hang loosely, the diamonds twisting round the wrong way.

How did she get to be so old? She smells a little bit too. She's struggling for breath. She puts her hand on her slipped chest and closes her eyes. She's not having a heart attack, is she? Oh God, what shall I do? I clear my throat and her eyes snap open. She frowns.

'Don't look at *me*. Look at the paintings,' she commands.

I hadn't even noticed them. I stare at the sugar pinks and baby blues. I've never seen these paintings before and yet I feel I know them. These soft shepherdesses and naked nymphs are fairy-tale people. I look at their little pink mouths, their round breasts, their marshmallow flesh. I'd like to be draped in wisps of silk, garlanded with rosebuds, free to fly up with my own flock of white doves into the great gilt frames.

'I think these paintings are beautiful.'

She looks surprised. 'You like Boucher?'

I nod, although I hadn't even heard of him before.

'Come and see what you think of Watteau,' she says, and as she hauls herself up from the seat she reaches out and clutches my arm. I think she might like me a little after all.

Perhaps she thought I'd be like Jay. She once sat cross-legged on the floor for a whole hour in a room of great black and red canvasses. Black paint and red paint, great washes of it. Nothing else. I asked her what it was supposed to represent and she got irritated and said why did I always have to be so literal, it wasn't boring old representational painting, it was about mood. She breathed in deeply and gestured towards the baffling canvasses and said, 'Don't try to analyse, Amber, *feel*.' I got terribly embarrassed because people were starting to look at us, and I didn't ask any more but pretended

I needed to go to the loo to get her away from the paintings.

I'm not pretending now, I need to go so badly that I have to concentrate on each step, because if I stop clenching everything just for a second I know it's going to come streaming out all over the polished floor. I shall have to tell her, and yet it sounds so childish and I'm scared of irritating her.

We press on, peering at the French paintings, and I want to impress her and say all the right things but I just keep up a witless chant of 'How beautiful'. I think I'm supposed to like Watteau more than Boucher and I pretend I do, but his people look so sad in spite of their frivolous fancy dress. And Grandma keeps getting muddled. She can't read the labels underneath the paintings and thinks pictures by people called Pater and Lancret are all by Watteau too. She's got a very clear voice and I hop from one foot to the other, praying no one will realise she's getting it all wrong. She shows me some miniatures in a cabinet—'Aren't they charming, Amber?'—but when I press my nose against the glass I see they're also rather rude. One pretty pearly little lady is actually peeing into a chamber-pot. Oh, I'd give anything for a potty myself. It's getting worse and my whole stomach is hot and heavy with the pain of it. Jay and I once lived in a squat where the loo was blocked up and so filthy anyway that we couldn't even walk in there so we had to use a bucket. We had to go in front of each other and I hated it and couldn't go unless Jay shut her eyes and put her hands over her ears. I shut my own eyes now and shake my head to stop thinking about it.

'What *are* you doing?' Grandma asks.

'Nothing.'

'I presume you're bored.'

'No! No, honestly. I love it here. I think it's . . . beautiful.'

Oh God, why can't I think of anything else to say? I can't think because the pain in my stomach is so bad. It squeezes at every step. The pain. That pain? Oh please, please let it be, let it be, let it be . . . I'm not muttering, am I? Grandma is still looking at me.

'I'll show you the porcelain,' she says grandly, as if this is her own private house.

We edge slowly round a big glass cabinet of china, turquoise and green and royal blue and rose pink. I wish Davie was here with me, we could make up such wonderful stories of fairy-tale feasts. There's another cabinet with a set of solid silver plates, with matching knives and forks; it could come straight out of *Sleeping Beauty*. Shall I say that to Grandma? I rehearse the words in my head but they sound silly now. I'm not sure she does like me. I keep catching glimpses of myself in the glass cases and clock faces and I look bigger and blowzier every minute, and the minutes tick by, there's a clock in every room, a clock in every corner, and they're all ticking steadily, time is slipping away and I am here with my grandmother but I can't seize the opportunity, I can't say anything, I'm trapped inside myself, I think I'm going to be trapped in here for ever, I'm a fly in my own Amber.

'Perhaps it's time for a cup of coffee,' says Grandma, as the clocks start chiming one after another. 'Come along, Amber.'

I accompany her down the stairs. She steps down with one leg and then down with the other and rests before attempting the next, like Naomi. Her face is absorbed in the effort so I can stare at her. We don't look at all alike. I suppose she's a little like Jay. It's her cheek bones and the way she juts her chin. Will Jay look like that when she's old? We haven't mentioned her yet.

Grandma pauses for a minute at the foot of the stairs, eyes shut, composing herself. She rearranges the white silk scarf at her neck. It isn't really white any more and she's scorched it with her iron. She repins her brooch, a china bunch of flowers. I remember it from her jewellery box, but she must have dropped it, because all the rose petals are chipped. I can't bear it, she's falling to bits. I don't want this frail fumbly old lady, I want Grandma the way she used to be.

'I will take you to *Maison Sagne*,' she announces mysteriously.

I'm obviously expected to be grateful so I mumble thanks. Even though I'm in 5e I know that *maison* means house so we're probably going to another posh place full of French paintings. Maybe it's because I said I liked Boucher. Well, I do, but I've seen heaps of paintings since we came in, and my tummy hurts and I'm scared I'm really going to wet myself the minute we get outside in the cold wind. Ask her, tell her, find the loo yourself, you fool. Why do you always have to be so hopeless?

'I think I'll visit the Ladies Room first,' says Grandma. 'Do you want to wait here for me?'

'Oh no, I'll come too.'

We walk through halls of gleaming armour, through a door and down a flight of steps. Grandma takes so long, shuffle step, other leg, shuffle step, little pause, and then she starts the next step. Oh God, we'll be here hours, and now I'm actually near the loos my bladder's at bursting point and I have to keep squeezing upward and I can't stand still.

I leave her half-way down the stairs. It's no use, I can't help it, and I'm in a loo and fumbling with my clothes, sitting, oh the relief! And then I dare look, hoping against hope, I've still got the pain, has it happened?

No. Nothing. I'm suddenly so scared I sit shivering, wondering what I'm going to do. I can't pretend any more. I've got to think about it. I'm five days late and I've been like clockwork ever since I started. And I keep needing to pee and I feel sick and dizzy, I have every single one of the symptoms. I looked them up in *The Ladies' New Medical Guide*. I am going to have a baby.

I whisper the words. They sound preposterous. And it's so undignified, sitting here with my knickers round my knees. I lift my skirt right up and peer at my stomach. I know it's mad, but it actually looks bigger already. It'll be a lot bigger soon. I watch it as if I expect it to blow up like a beach-ball right before my eyes.

'Amber?' Grandma calls.

'Yes. Sorry. I'm coming.'

I sort myself out and reappear. Grandma looks agitated. She hurries past me and slams the door. I listen. I wait, my heart thumping. I wash my hands, running the taps loudly. After a long time Grandma emerges. I can hardly bear to look at her although she seems perfectly calm and in control. But the door swings open behind her and although I hate myself for looking I stare at the puddle on the floor. I glance at Grandma, terrified, but thank God there's nothing to see. She washes her hands and then gets out her lipstick. She applies a shaky smile to her face. Our eyes meet in the mirror. I smile back at her uneasily.

Chapter 12

I CAN'T make up my mind what I want to eat. The cakes are displayed behind glass, like the treasures of the Wallace Collection. They're all so perfect that I can't choose.

'We will have coffee,' Grandma says grandly. She's not at all cowed by the superior waiter standing at our table. 'And a cake, Amber? Or perhaps a scone?'

'Yes please.'

I suppose I've ordered scones. I don't even like scones. Jay brings them back from the health food shop, the brown burnt ones that no one will buy. They lie in the stomach like stones. I could have had the pink fancy cake, the cherry tartlet, the green frog with the chocolate grin. I could have had my pick and I've ended up with a scone.

Two scones. And they're pale and delicate, definitely upper-class scones, and there's real butter too, none of your sunflower substitute here. They taste as good as they look. A cake would have been better, of course, but the scones are still a treat. Perhaps I can choose a cake next time? I think there will be a next time. She likes me, I'm sure she does, so there's no reason why we shouldn't start meeting regularly now. She might even invite me to live with her.

I can't. Oh God, I can't, not now. I'm already bigger than she expected. I'm going to get bigger and bigger now. I'm Jay all over again.

'Are you enjoying your scones, Amber?'

I take a big bite although I'm not hungry any more. 'Yes,

thank you,' I say, spraying crumbs. Trust me to speak with my mouth full.

'The scones are always very good at *Maison Sagne*.'

I wonder why she hasn't ordered any for herself. There were two. Was one for her? I've already eaten one and a half. Shall I offer her what's left? But I've chewed at it, she'll be disgusted.

I put it back on the plate and sip coffee in shame. Grandma sips too. We can't seem to think of anything more to say. People talk all the time at the elegant tables around us. It's easier for them because they know each other. Why doesn't she want to know me? I'm her only granddaughter after all. Why doesn't she ask me questions, ask about school? Well, I'm glad she doesn't want to know about that. She could ask me what subjects I like though, enquire about my hobbies. Shall I tell her about my sewing? Or would that sound a bit like boasting?

'Do you have any particular hobbies, Grandma?'

She stares at me. 'What?'

I repeat it, blushing.

'Well, I don't collect stamps or play the violin, if that's what you mean,' she says crisply.

'No, I meant . . . do you sew?'

'Buttons. Hems.'

'Oh.'

'I can't do more nowadays.'

We both look at her crooked hands. I feel terrible.

'I used to sew quite a lot. I made this blouse as a matter of fact.'

'Did you!' I can't see much of it because of her suit. I lean over the table as decorously as I can and peer at the faded material. It's peach crêpe-de-Chine. The collar is fraying at the corner and it needs a good wash but I concentrate on the stitches.

'You've done it beautifully. It's hand-sewn too, isn't it?'

'There's embroidery on the pocket,' she says, pulling back her jacket to show me.

'Oh, it's beautiful. Satin stitch. And you've done it so smoothly.' I hesitate and then open my mouth to tell her about my night-dress.

'I embroidered all your mother's baby-clothes, you know. And smocked every little dress. People used to stop me in the street to admire Joyce. I made her look a picture.'

'I sew, Grandma. I'm quite good at it. I've done a night-dress, I—'

'Of course, she did her best to make a mess of herself even in those days. I had to put her in two clean pairs of socks each day, sometimes three. She'd rub her shoes on them, if you please. And mealtimes! Do you know, that child had to wear a bib until she was *six*?'

'The sewing teacher pinned—'

'I sometimes think she did it deliberately to spite me. It's always been her way. Do you know she failed her eleven plus? The brightest girl in the class, always top. We'd drummed it into her, it's no use coming second or third in this life, it's number one or nothing. And yet she failed it when she should have passed with flying colours. She couldn't have tried. Oh, she passed it the second time round, and we got her into a decent girls' day-school without too much bother, but it wasn't the same. We'd promised her a new bike if she passed and her father still bought it for her because he said he couldn't bear her to be disappointed. He thought the world of her, you know. And yet just look at the way she treated him. She broke his heart, and I mean that literally—and then she didn't even bother to turn up at his funeral.'

'She didn't know about it.'

'Well of course you'll stick up for her,' says Grandma, glaring.

'No, I—' I don't know what to say.

The waiter is hovering. I think he wants us to go. People are staring. Grandma's voice has been getting louder and louder.

She sighs impatiently and shakes the plate so that my half-eaten scone topples over.

'What a waste! Come along.'

She opens her sponge-bag, takes out her purse and pops the scone in its place. Then she fumbles for her money. She takes out a pound note and slides it under her saucer. A pound? It'll be much more than that. Oh God, what are we going to do? I haven't got any money, I had to borrow from Leonora for my fare here. That waiter's looking at it. Perhaps he thinks it's his tip. Grandma's standing, hanging on to the table and rattling the teacups until she gets her balance. She fiddles with her scarf, her little claw hands shaking.

She's handed a bill and she stares at it, puzzled, squinting. Eventually she passes it to me. 'Do you want to keep it as a little souvenir?'

I look at the total. 'I'm sorry but I think you have to pay a bit more, Grandma.'

'What do you mean? I have paid.'

'No, it's *more*'. I hiss the amount in her ear.

She glares at me as if it's somehow my fault and peers in her purse. Her hands scrabble inside the shabby leather. It's empty. Everyone's staring at us now. I'm burning all over. And Grandma's cheeks are carmine but I'm not sure whether it's rouge or embarrassment. She's stirring the contents of her sponge-bag now. She takes out the grubby lace hanky. It's tied in a knot; it bulges and clinks. It takes her six hours to undo it.

'Shall I try?'

'I can manage. I'm not quite in my dotage yet.'

She tugs violently and the handkerchief gives way. Coins spill everywhere. They're not pound coins. They're mostly coppers. I crawl round retrieving as many as I can while Grandma counts out the exact amount. She has to do it twice to check. I wait for the sarcastic comments as she hands them over but she's treated with scrupulous politeness. Somehow this makes it worse. Even when we're outside Grandma still examines her sponge-bag, picking out odd coins and muttering. As she fumbles she finds a letter, my letter.

'Did she put you up to this?'

I stare at her.

'She did, didn't she? Joyce got you to write it.'

'No! She doesn't even know I'm meeting you.'

Grandma doesn't look as if she believes me. The wind is cold and she puts her chin in her scarf. I wait, wondering where we will go next. Grandma holds out her hand. I'm not sure what she wants me to do with it.

'Goodbye, Amber.'

She can't just go, not yet!

'Couldn't we—?' I don't know what to suggest.

'I shall get a chill if I stand around on the street.' She snaps it unpleasantly but she really is shivering. She looks so small and shaky that I stop being so scared of her.

'I'll walk home with you, Grandma,' I say, and I hold out my arm so that she can tuck in if she wants.

She doesn't want. She looks appalled. 'Oh no, dear. No. That's out of the question.'

'I don't mean I want to come and *live* with you—like I wrote in my letter. I was being silly. I know it wouldn't work out. I just want to see you home safely.'

'There's absolutely no need. You go that way, down towards Oxford Street. You can get a tube at Oxford Circus.'

'But I'd like to go with you, Grandma.'

She looks at me, her eyes watering in the wind. 'It's been very pleasant meeting you, Amber.'

This time there's no mistaking her hand. I shake it limply. She says goodbye and then, before I can reply, she's off. I stand, dismissed, staring after her. I wonder if there's an even darker patch on her dark suit and then hate myself for being vulgar. Then I hate her, because how can she shuffle out of my life like this? Her shoes slop at every step. It must rub her bare feet terribly. Well, I don't care. She doesn't care about me. So I walk away.

It's only half-past eleven. I can have a lovely day out in London all by myself. I haven't got any money but I can window-shop. I can go to Selfridges' haberdashery department and see if they've got anything interesting. I can plan a new line for my market stall—no, I've lost that now, I'll never get back in because there's a long waiting-list and the man was never that happy having me because I'm under age, and anyway, the only sewing I'll be doing now is baby-clothes.

It's still not real. As soon as I start thinking about it the pain starts in my stomach and I start hoping, but when I get to the Ladies in Selfridges it's another false alarm. I don't think I want to wander round any more, I'm worn out already. So I go home and I don't even bother with lunch. I take off my clothes and crawl into bed. The sheets need changing but I don't care. I pull them right up over my head.

Jay wakes me up when she gets home from work. She sits on the end of my bed. 'Well? How did it go?'

She looks scruffier than ever. She dyed her hair yesterday and made a mess of it. Those are not auburn highlights, they are more like aubergine floodlights. It makes her face whiter than ever, and her orange T-shirt clashes terribly. And those khaki dungarees—oh God, I'm so sick of those ugly idiotic garments. She's a mother, she's thirty-two years old, surely she can see she looks ridiculous? If she wants to dress like a teenager why not try to be fashionable? People haven't worn her sort of clothes for years. All right, she hasn't got any money but neither have I and I manage, and anyway, it's all her fault; if she'd got herself a proper job years ago we wouldn't have to live like this. She hasn't got any training but that's her fault too, she was at a posh school, she had all the chances, she could have stayed on, got her A levels, gone to university . . . . But what about me? How could she do all that with me?

'Amber? Oh God, you're not starting this nonsense all over again, are you? Look at me.'

So I do. 'Why didn't you get rid of me?'

'What do you mean?' Jay sighs. 'Is this going to be one of your poor-little-me conversations? Because I haven't got the patience. I've had a bloody awful day, all the bread was burnt and I dropped a dozen eggs and this nutty old man with a Father Christmas beard stood at the counter and spoke for a solid hour on *ectoplasm*. What do you *mean*, why didn't I get rid of you?'

'When you knew you were pregnant.'

'What's she been saying to you?'

'Nothing.'

'You did meet her though, didn't you?'

'Have you been reading my letter?'

'No I haven't. I don't snoop, you know I don't. It was obvious. I mean, you've slummocked in bed for weeks and then suddenly you're up before anyone else, bathed and in your best clothes. I'd have to be daft not to realise.'

'I want to know, Jay. You always make out I can ask you anything at all and you'll tell me.'

Jay fidgets, running her fingers through her livid hair.

'Why do you dye your hair?'

'Is that a burning question too?'

'No.'

'I feel it brightens me up a bit. O.K.?'

'O.K.'

'And about you. Well, I wanted you, didn't I?'

'You couldn't have done. You were sixteen. You were still at *school*.'

'I was desperate to leave anyway, you know I hated it. I'd never have gone into the sixth.'

'But it wasn't even as if you had a proper boy-friend. I mean, my father—you didn't know him, did you?'

Jay shrugs. She's not looking at me.

'How could you have messed about with all those men you didn't even know?'

'My God, you've *obviously* been chatting with my mother, you're beginning to sound like her. "All those men". You make it sound like six each night, seven on Sundays. I wasn't a *whore*, Amber. I wasn't even a proper groupie. I didn't know much about sex. I mean, the idea of a groupie getting pregnant! If I'd known a bit more about it then I'd have realised that was ridiculous.'

'Didn't you even think about having an abortion?'

I hate that word. It hangs in the air between us. I think of a great hook probing bits of bloody baby.

'I didn't want one. I hated the idea then.'

Her voice is muffled. We both remember the Wales baby.

'Didn't your parents try to make you?'

'It was a bit late in the day when they found out.'

'Were they terribly angry?'

Jay pulls a face, not bothering to reply.

'Why didn't you get rid of me afterwards, Jay? When I was born? Why didn't you have me adopted?'

'They wanted me to.'

'Your parents?'

'Not just them. The women in the Home. They kept saying, "Think of the baby, if you really love her then don't you want the best for her? Give her the best gift in the world: two loving parents and a decent family home." There was one woman like a P.E. teacher, very brisk and bossy, and another who was soft and sweet and very gentle. She was the worst. She always made me cry. But I wouldn't sign the bloody forms.'

'What was it like, this Mother and Baby Home? Did they keep you locked up or could you walk around wherever you wanted?'

'Of course you could. It wasn't a prison. Although it felt like it at times. That food. And we really did have porridge in the morning, grey lumpy muck made with water. I don't know what happened to our milk allowance. Yes I do! We had mugs of hot milk every morning. And every evening too, or was that cocoa? It was all disgusting, with skin on top. I used to bribe one of the other girls to drink mine for me. They were a smashing lot of girls. My mother was so rude about them. She came to visit me once and looked at my special friend and whispered that it was a pity she Wasn't Quite Our Class. Ugh!

What did she say to you, Amber? I bet she went on about me, she always does.'

'No, she didn't. She talked about me. About my sewing and what I'm doing at school, that sort of thing. And she took me to this posh place with a waiter for scones and morning coffee and we went round the Wallace Collection and looked at all the Bouchers.'

Jay fidgets, gets up, wanders across the room and looks out of the window while I'm telling her. 'What a lovely morning,' she says.

'There's no need to be sarcastic.'

'I'm not.'

There's a sudden lull in the conversation. I lie here. She stands at the window.

'Oh well. Tea? You might have got it ready and waiting for me. Or are you full up? I suppose she treated you to lunch as well? Did you go back to her flat?'

'Mmm. Jay. Did you *really* want me?'

'Yes.'

'But you don't like babies.'

'I liked you.'

I can't believe her. Although she doesn't lie. 'Rubbish,' I mutter, feeling stupidly embarrassed.

'You were a good baby anyway. You were quiet most of the time and you slept between feeds.' Jay laughs. 'You haven't changed.'

'So you kept me because I was good?'

'No, because you were mine.'

I turn over, thinking about it. Thinking about me.

'I'm going to have a baby.'

'Yes, of course you will. I can imagine you with lots. Although shut up about it, I don't fancy being a granny just yet.'

'You're going to be.'

'What?'

'I told you, I'm having a baby.'

Jay whips round from the window. She bursts out laughing! She stands there *shrieking* with laughter.

'What's so funny?'

'Oh Amber. You. Of course you're not pregnant.'

'I *am*.'

'You don't think you're another Virgin Mary, do you?'

'Of course not.'

'Well, you've been so funny recently, pretending you're a nun and—'

'An *anchoress*. Look, stop making fun of me.'

'Well stop being so silly. What on earth makes you think you're pregnant?'

'I'm five days late.'

She laughs, scornfully. 'I'm often—'

'But I'm not. You know I'm not. And I've got all the symptoms. I've got sore breasts and I keep—'

'That's pre-menstrual tension, you idiot. You don't get any pregnancy symptoms for months. What's brought all this on? Is it because I was talking about having you?'

'I'm not *competing*. Stop sneering at me.'

'Well honestly. You don't mean to tell me you and that funny boy from school have actually gone to bed?'

'Oh shut up. I don't want to tell you now.'

I'm crying and I hide my face, but she comes over and tries to pull my hands away.

'I'm sorry. I didn't mean to upset you. I didn't think you were serious. Amber, do you really think there is a chance Justin could have made you pregnant?'

I take my hands away myself. 'There's no chance at all. I didn't sleep with him. I slept with his brother.'

Chapter 13

'COME round to my place,' said Justin.

I was always going round to his place. It got so that I went there every day after school. We did our homework together. Well, we got out our textbooks and our exercise books and our pens, but no one did any work, not even Sleeve. We sat and talked and wrote silly messages and played paper games and drank cups of coffee and ate chocolate and crisps and when it was so late that I really had to go home we packed our unused books and pens back into their tattered carrier-bags. Sleeve sometimes gave us little lectures.

'Don't you want to get on in life, young lady? How are you going to get a job without any qualifications? You're a bright girl. Get stuck in to your lesson books and show them.'

'Well, what about Justin?' I'd argue. 'He's cleverer than me, and it's worse for him because all his family are clever too, so why doesn't he work harder and show *them*?'

'Absolutely!' said Sleeve, bobbing up and down. 'I've always thought this dyslexia tag a mite suspicious. If you ask me it's just an excuse for laziness. The boy doesn't try. Now look at his brother. He'll be closeted in his study at that splendid school of his, attentive under his Anglepoise, his Parker pen gliding along the lines. There's a six-side essay, a perfect translation, a five hundred word prose. He's like a little computer, press the button and he performs, well done my boy, seventeen out of twenty, nineteen out of twenty, *twenty* out of twenty. The little Wonder Word-Processor. *Jonty* can do it, Justin.'

'Shut up Sleeve,' Justin said and suppressed him.

He didn't want to see much of me in the Christmas holidays. It was a while before I worked out why. Jonty was home from school.

I waited for ages and then I received a postcard. It had a picture of a large woolly sheep on the front and a message from Sleeve on the back.

> 'Hope you like this pickture of The Grate Providor. All hail to the Gloreus Sheep say the little wooly peeple. Can you come round Wensday? The boy is distraut with greef he is missing you so much. Wensday, any time after 10 am. Please come. Your obedient servent Sleeve. (Excuse scrawl and spelling. My seckratry is a defecktive.)'

I arrived at one minute past ten. Justin was at the door waiting. He went pink when he saw me coming. Sleeve bobbed into view, waving at me, but then Justin controlled him. He spoke to me himself:

'Come on, come on, you're *late*.' He pulled me inside and up the stairs. 'Everyone's out,' he explained jubilantly. 'You can stay all day, can't you? I've got a special lunch planned, a special tea, special everything.'

'Left-over turkey and Christmas cake?' I said. I was hurt that he'd ignored me for so long.

Justin was too bouncy to be snubbed. 'You guessed!' he said. 'And I've got you a left-over Christmas present too.'

It was a collage. He'd made it specially for me. He'd covered a sheet of white cartridge paper with golden cellophane. Parts of it were opaque. Parts were delicately patterned. Parts were transparent and you could see a girl peering through. You could see her face, a shoulder, one hand. There was a little dark creature nestling in this cupped hand. I wasn't quite sure what it was at first. It was elongated and ugly and it had protruding eyes that looked comically like spectacles. It was obviously some kind of insect. Of course. A fly.

I looked at the amber collage while Justin waited.

'Do you like it?' he burst out, unable to wait any longer.

'I think it's . . . . ' I couldn't find the right word but my face must have expressed it because he grinned.

'Coffee? And *that's* special too, I nicked their Gold Blend, and actually I was going to offer you Christmas cake, there's heaps left in the tin. It's oozing brandy, two bites and you're drunk.'

'I only really like the icing.'

'O.K., coffee and a slice of ice, anything to please Madame,' said Justin, bowing and scrabbling at my shoes.

'What are you *doing*?'

'Scraping.'

'Idiot.' I gently kicked him away and fumbled in my bag. 'I've got your Christmas present too.'

I gave him the parcel. He held the shiny patterned paper uncertainly, fingering the red satin ribbon.

'It looks very pretty. Sorry I didn't wrap yours up.'

I took the paper from downstairs. They always wrap everything up with Paperchase paper, even Naomi's things, and then they tear it off and leave about ten pounds' worth crumpled in the corner. I sifted through it and saved all the best bits.

'Open it,' I said, my tummy tight with nerves in case he didn't like it. It had taken me weeks and the wool was really expensive. I could have found an old sweater in a jumble and washed it and unravelled it but I wanted this present to be brand new and perfect.

Justin opened the crackly paper carefully and took the knitted pullover out, stroking the soft wool as if it were a pet. He unfolded it.

'Does it fit? Hold it up against yourself. Here, let me.'

I held it up to his chin and smoothed it down. It had been difficult to gauge the right length. I'd kept adding another few rows and then another, remembering how tall he was, until it looked like a jumper for a giraffe. I was scared I'd made it much too long now, but it fitted neatly to his hips. It was French navy with a vee neck and I'd knitted an elaborate Fair Isle pattern in blue and jade and marigold.

'Oh Amber. It's lovely. Here, it's not a girl's, is it?'

'Of course not! I knitted it specially for you.'

'I just thought as it's so bright and pretty—it won't make me look . . . ?'

'I think you'll look smashing in it. But you don't have to wear it if you don't want to.'

'I want to! I want to very much. I'll put it on now, shall I?'

I shrugged. Justin took off his old threadbare sweater and wriggled into my pullover. He poked one long spindly arm through, then the other. He looked at his arms in their flannel grey shirt.

'No sleeves,' he said.

I smiled. And he smiled too.

'Thank you,' he said. 'Thank you ever so much.'

'Thank you for your collage.'

We stood and looked at each other, our smiles becoming just a little fixed. I wondered if Justin was going to take me in his long arms and kiss me. I think Justin was wondering it too.

'Thanks,' he said again. 'So. Coffee and icing?'

We gnawed at choice chunks of icing and marzipan all morning. The cake began to look as if mice had got at it but Justin insisted no one would notice. I contributed to the feast: I'd brought two crystallised pears in a paper bag.

They were part of my present from Jay. They came from her health food shop. The wooden box they were in got broken so Jay bought the fruit inside very cheaply. Maybe they even gave her it for nothing. I'd asked for new knickers and a fountain pen. God knows where she found those red nylon wisps. They certainly weren't the set of three plain white cotton bikini briefs from Marks that I wanted. The green Pentel pens were O.K., but I had asked for a Sheaffer fountain-pen on a special

£1.50 offer in Smiths. Gordon and Wendy gave me a dress from Aladdin's Cave. It was an old seventies Afghanistan dress covered in embroidery and little mirrors, the sort of dress I once thought beautiful back in the commune days. It had slight sweat marks under the arms and the embroidery round the hem was coming unstitched. Leonora gave me a very rude mug in the shape of a woman's breast. Polly gave me a calorie counter. Naomi gave me a crayonned picture of the house with all of us in it. I wasn't sure which purple squiggle was meant to be me.

The only present I really loved was from Davie. He sent me a little tin Father Christmas with a hole in his red hood. You were supposed to hang him on a Christmas tree but I threaded a narrow ribbon through mine and wore him round my neck. But then Polly copied me. Her Christmas charm wasn't the same, it was a little wooden fir tree, but I still couldn't bear seeing her wear it. I pulled my Father Christmas charm off and stuck it in my old magic casket. There wasn't anything magical about that any more either: it was just an old cardboard box falling to bits containing a few odd items of junk.

It didn't matter now that Davie's present had lost all its point. I had my Amber collage and no other present could be as perfect.

I kept looking at it and giving it pleased nods as I sucked my crystallised pear.

'You like it, don't you?' said Justin happily, sucking his pear too.

'Mm. You know I do. Don't get sticky sugar on your new pullover.'

'No Mummy. Has yours shrunk any yet?'

We compared the softening pink sections. They nearly fitted together to make an odd sugary heart.

'We're rotting all our teeth, I hope you realise,' I said, nibbling my pear. 'All this sugar and think of all that icing.'

'Aha! I am prepared for every possibility,' said Justin, rummaging in a drawer.

He brought out a narrow box still in its Christmas wrapping-paper. He shook it free and produced it with a flourish.

'Oh Justin!'

It was an electric tooth-brush.

'A present from my grandma. Honestly! What a weird present to give a grandson. She obviously thinks I'm Halitosis Harry.'

'What did she give Jonty?'

'Oh, he got one too. People always had to give us the same when we were little or else I'd whine and grizzle and want his presents as well as my own. I was a right little charmer as a child. You'd have taken great delight in kicking me in the teeth. Which I can now clean. Have you ever used one of these gadgets? I'm a bit scared to switch it on. I expect blue flashes and gyrating jaws and a mouthful of bloody molars.'

'Idiot. I'd quite like an electric tooth-brush. They had one at Elizabeth Ann's. I saw when I went to the loo.'

'Who's . . . ?'

'You know, that house where I got my bed. It's quite near here. And I thought it was so posh. I never realised you were one of the real nobs, Justin.'

'Oh, that's me, I'll show you the aristocratic strawberry mark on my right buttock if you don't behave yourself.'

'What else did you get apart from the tooth-brush?'

'Nothing much.'

'Don't be so maddening. You must have got something from your mother.'

Justin sighed and poked the presents still in his drawer. 'Have a look yourself then. Honestly, you're meant to be interested in my person, not my flipping presents.'

It turned out he got a fountain-pen from his mother. Not a Sheaffer on a special offer in Smiths. A big black magnificent Mont Blanc fountain-pen.

'Do you know how much they cost?' I whispered, handling it reverently.

Justin shrugged. 'She's loaded.'

'Justin!'

'Well, she is. She doesn't even work for it. It's money she inherited from her father.'

'But it's still a beautiful present.'

'Not if you have difficulty even writing your own bloody name,' said Justin. It was the first time I'd heard him swear.

'Perhaps she thought it would help.'

'Perhaps.'

'She thought you'd take special care with such a lovely pen. Have you tried it yet?'

'No.'

'Oh Justin, honestly. Give us a bit of paper. Do you mind if I have a little go?'

'Help yourself.'

I wrote: 'I am Amber and this is Justin's pen and it is simply beautiful. He really is a fool. I would be over the moon if I had a pen like this.'

'So you have it then,' said Justin, reading over my shoulder.

'No! Oh goodness, I wasn't hinting, I promise I wasn't. And you can't give your mother's pen away, she'd be so hurt.'

'Then take it at once.'

'You are an atrocious son.'

'Don't you want to be an atrocious daughter?'

'That's different. Jay's different. She's the one that's atrocious. Your mother's nice.'

'Why don't you take her along with the pen? She'd be tickled pink. She thinks the world of you.'

'Does she?'

'She can't believe that her subnormal son has actually got himself a girl-friend.' Justin shifted uncomfortably, licking sticky pear syrup from his wrist and cuff. 'I mean, friend who is a girl. You know what I mean.'

'It's a good job I didn't knit you sleeves, you slobby thing. Did she actually *say* she liked me?'

'Yes. I said.'

'Do you like me, Justin?'

'Mm. Yes. You know I do.'

'Then why don't you want to call me your girl-friend?'

'What? Oh. It just sounds a bit . . . silly.'

'No it doesn't.'

'Well. All right. You're my girl-friend. O.K.?'

'What else did you get for Christmas?'

'Nothing.'

'There's more things in the drawer.'

'It's just boring stuff.'

It was: socks and handkerchieves and plastic puzzles from endless old aunties.

'Half of them don't keep track of how old I am,' said Justin, exhibiting a Mickey Mouse jigsaw. 'Or maybe they've had a word with the parents and they think Mickey Mouse is about my intellectual level.'

'I quite like doing jigsaws,' I said. 'I used to do a patchwork bag like a giant jigsaw, the little pieces all interlocked. It sold really well but it took too long to make so it wasn't economical.'

'You're a boring little business woman at heart, aren't you? Never mind the creative satisfaction, just pass her the pennies if you please.'

'Some of us have parents who are loaded. Some of us haven't.'

'Ouch. O.K., O.K. So how come you're so good at talking back to me when at school you hardly open your mouth?'

'Well, if you're going to bring up school then you're not exactly relaxed there, are you, busy doing the Mad Professor Act all the time?'

'No, you're not meant to say that. You're meant to flutter your eyelashes and tell me that you feel you can say anything you like to me. That you feel you've known me all your life. That you—'

'Are you practising for when you write your Mills and Boon?'

'My charm does not seem to be fatal today. Got any more crystallised pears, that was absolutely delicious.'

'Not on me. I'll bring some more next time. If you ask me round again that is.'

'Aha. I detect a faintly peevish tone.'

'Well. You didn't ring or anything. Not even at Christmas.'

'And you sat hunched over the telephone, hoping?'

'No. But I did wonder why that rude pig Justin didn't get in touch.'

'That rude pig was stuck here in the sty with the Hog and the Sow and the Sibling Pigling, that's why. But thank God they've all gone off to Market today so that this little Piggy can invite his little friend around. *Girl*-friend.'

'Where have they gone?'

'Another old aunt. And the Boy Wonder is seeing some girl. Don't let's waste time talking about them. And leave those boring old presents alone.'

'These aren't boring,' I said, finding books. They were lovely old boys' books, Henty and Rider-Haggard. I looked inside and raised my eyebrows. 'First editions! They must have cost a fortune. Who are they from?'

'My dad. But *he* collects Henty, not me. These are *his* boyhood favourites.'

'So he wants you to like them too. That's not a crime, is it? Well, I'd be thrilled if Jay gave me . . . I wonder what she read when she was little? *Lady Chatterley's Lover*, knowing her. And what are these?'

I pulled out the last present. It was a pair of hand-knitted socks with special toes, each having a little embroidered face. It was the sort of thing I make myself. I decided I might pinch the idea for my stall, I could see at once they'd be popular.

'Aren't they smashing?'

'No.'

'Oh Justin, you really are being obstinate now. They're the perfect present for you. You won't wear proper slippers so these are beautifully cosy, and you can wiggle your toes and give each one a separate personality. Lovely company for Sleeve. Who gave them to you?'

'I don't know,' said Justin sulkily.

I found the label on the paper. It was written in elegant italic. '*To Justin from Jonathon.*'

'What did you give him?'

'Nothing.'

'Don't be silly.'

'Well, nothing much.'

'Do you have to be so irritating!'

'Well, you're beginning to irritate me, if you must know, harping on about these boring presents,' said Justin, flinging them all back into the drawer and slamming it shut. 'I gave them all boxes of chocolates. Not very nice chocolates as a matter of fact. I got them cheap in the market. And if you want to point out that I give rotten presents then I'll agree with you. O.K.?'

He threw himself down on his bed. His head jerked back and he banged it painfully but he seemed determined not to care. I sat still, staring at my lap. There was a silence. It went on for a long time.

'Ouch,' Justin said eventually, and he rubbed his head.

'You do give lovely presents. To me.'

Justin bowed. 'Sorry about the little tantrum.'

'Sorry if I was a bit nosy, going through all your things.'

'Feel free. Do you want another coffee? There's some Stollen cake too, you know. Stolen Stollen, how about it?'

'After all that icing and the pears?'

'This is going to be the day of the Great Gorge, my girl. Shall I show you some of the goodies I've got hidden away? Listen and lick your lips. Turkey pâté. Cranberry sauce. Bath Oliver biscuits. Satsumas. An entire packet of strawberry Angel Delight plus the requisite milk. A bottle of sparkling apple juice. We might even nick some wine, although my father gets a bit funny about that. But mother barely blinks if she finds the fridge completely ransacked. Which it is. I've taken some chocolate mousse too. We'd better eat that soon, it seems to have gone a bit runny.'

'What celestial food.'

'And I've selected a special video too, in case we run out of conversation.'

'Which one?'

'Something so shocking and spine-chilling you'll never be the same girl again.'

'You haven't got *Driller Killer* or *I Spit On Your Grave*, have you?'

'Worse, far worse.' Justin waved it in front of me.

'*The Hundred and One Dalmations!*'

'Cruella de Vil will give you the creeps.'

'Who?'

'You mean you haven't seen it?'

I shook my head.

'Great! It's my favourite film. I used to go and see it twice a week every Christmas holiday. You have an enormous treat in store.'

But it wasn't an enormous treat. And the feast was a failure.

Jonathon came home.

Chapter 14

THE front door banged downstairs. We heard someone whistling and then footsteps on the stairs.

'Oh *God,*' Justin whispered.

'What—?' I began, but he shook his head at me frantically, putting his finger to his lips.

'Sh, sh, *sh*!' he mouthed in hysterical pantomime.

The footsteps were approaching. The jaunty whistle grew louder.

'Greetings, Little Brother,' Jonathon called.

Justin said two terse words.

'What's up?' Jonathon asked, sounding amused.

He was right outside the door.

'Don't come in!'

Justin screwed up his long legs and bit his knuckle in despair. I stared at him, beginning to be irritated.

'Aha! So you're lying there playing with yourself, are you?' Jonathon said.

'Don't be disgusting,' Justin hissed.

Why was he making such a silly fuss? Was he that ashamed of me?

'Well, hands off, I'm coming in,' said Jonathon, and he opened the door.

'Get *out,*' Justin screamed.

Jonathon took no notice. He was staring at me. And I stared back. I suppose I'd imagined him like Justin, lanky and awkward, with the same preposterous hair. And the glasses, because he was brainy. But Jonathon was glamorous. Justin always looked as if he was trying on the wrong size of body, let alone the wrong clothes. Jonathon was certainly in command of his body and his clothes were exquisite. He had a Crolla shirt and trousers but he was too clever to be a complete dandy. He wore shabby tennis shoes and thick grey grandad socks. A long white scarf was slung casually round his neck. No, there was nothing casual about Jonathon. He knew the effect of that scarf, that style, that smile.

It was a studied sardonic smile, lips barely parted, one eyebrow slightly raised. He must have practised in front of the mirror for hours. His long straight shiny hair was flopping into his eyes and he shook it back so that it became attractively ruffled. He smelt of an expensive citrus aftershave that I would have hated on anyone else.

I wanted to hate him. Not just for Justin's sake. Jonathon obviously loved himself so much he deserved to be disliked.

'Hello, Amber,' he said, as if we'd known one another years.

'Hello Jonathon,' I said.

I wanted to sound bored but I knew I was blushing. Justin looked as if I'd slapped him. Jonathon's smile switched from sardonic to sexy.

'I've heard a lot about you.'

'Shut your face, Jonty,' Justin squawked.

'Hey, look at all this food. Good, I'm starving.'

'It's *ours.*' The years seemed to be slipping away from Justin. He was starting to sound like a shrill six year old. Jonathon ignored him. He selected a Bath Oliver biscuit and dipped it in the turkey pâté.

'This is good,' he said, nibbling appreciatively.

'No more!' said Justin, when he reached out again. He snatched the tub of pâté away, guarding it ridiculously.

Jonathon raised his eyebrows. He looked at me. 'Why don't we all go downstairs and have a proper lunch in comfort?'

'No bloody fear,' said Justin.

'Wouldn't you like to, Amber?' Jonathon said softly.

'I—I'm all right here,' I stammered.

'Right, did you hear that? She wants to stay here with me. So get lost, Jonty. Go on, push off.' Justin stood up and tried pushing literally. He was taller than Jonathon, but it was obvious who was stronger. Jonathon stood smiling. Justin's pushes hardened into punches.

'Don't, Justin,' I mumbled.

'You're embarrassing Amber,' Jonathon said. 'Do grow up a bit, Justin.'

'Then get out of my *room*,' Justin panted, nearly in tears.

'O.K. Don't get in such a state. See you again, Amber.'

Jonathon shook hands with me. I was surprised by this oddly formal gesture and scared my palm was damp. Jonathon's fingers lingered momentarily, and then he strolled out of the room.

'Good riddance!' Justin shouted, as if he'd won.

He wiped his hands together, his chin tilted. Our eyes met and he looked panic-stricken. He started strutting round his room, swearing. I waited. Justin's clockwork ran out and he flopped on to his bed. He banged his head again and rubbed it, pulling a face. He looked like a gangling baby. I wanted to shake him. I understood, of course. But that didn't help. I couldn't bear his hopeless defeat. And he couldn't bear that I'd witnessed it.

I should have gone home there and then but I sat it out senselessly. Justin sulked on his bed, scarcely saying a word. I talked for both of us, skimming sentences over the silence. I spoke loudly, hoping that Jonathon might hear. If only Justin would try too we could manufacture conversation, laughter, a private party atmosphere, and then it would be Jonathon's turn to feel excluded. We could hear him down in the kitchen getting himself some lunch. He had the radio on and he was singing unselfconsciously. He couldn't even keep totally in tune, but it didn't matter. His voice was light and lilting. I gabbled on, sweating with the effort. Justin made no effort at all. He sprawled on the bed, his new pullover wrinkling up over his stomach, his trousers flapping back from his socks, exposing legs like mushroom stalks. His feet smelt, scenting the whole room with their staleness.

We tried eating our own lunch but neither of us had any appetite. The feast became a childish mess of melting food. The mousse was a dark drink and the pâté seemed to have flavoured everything else. I picked miserably and Justin gobbled at random. Down in the kitchen Jonathon seemed to be heating soup. That smell was unmistakable, Heinz tomato soup. I heard him tearing crusty bread. I was suddenly hungry again, longing for homely soup and bread. We could all be sharing it down in the kitchen if Justin hadn't been so silly. We could still go, couldn't we? There was no *need* for us to be besieged in Justin's bedroom.

We stayed stuck there. We stopped eating. We stopped talking. So we watched *The Hundred and One Dalmations*. I wondered why we were watching it. It was a sweet film. Absolutely gripping if you happened to be under ten. I wondered what Jonathon would think of us. Justin stared fixedly at the screen, his chin digging into his hands. He was biting his lip, nibbling the skin compulsively. It made him look uglier than ever. He went on staring at the screen after the film finished.

I went and knelt beside him on his bed. We weren't used to sitting so close together. Justin didn't look at me.

'Justin?'

It was only a whisper but it made him jump.

'Mm?'

I wasn't sure what I wanted to say. There was no point asking what was the matter because we both knew. In desperation I took hold of his hand. It lay limply in my clasp, the fingers curved, as if it had recently died.

'Is Sleeve sleeping?'

Justin shrugged.

'Wake him up.'

'There's no point.'

'Yes there is. Look, put your grey jersey back on. Make Sleeve come and talk to me.'

'You hate it when he does.'

'No I don't.'

'Yes you do.'

'I hate it when we argue so stupidly.'

'So let's stop it.' Justin snatched his hand away. 'Why don't you go home?'

So I did. I didn't see Justin for the rest of the holidays. I avoided him the first day back at school. It was my turn to sulk. Justin caught up with me on the way home.

'Why aren't you coming round to my place?'

I tried to ignore him but he capered round me, his hands a megaphone, bellowing my name.

'Justin!'

'Ah! She can hear again! A miracle. Fling away your hearing-aid and ear-trumpet, my child.'

'Do you have to be so idiotic?'

'I'm an idiot, aren't I?'

'Yes.'

'I was an idiot the other day.'

'The other week.'

'Yes. Well. I'm sorry about that. So. Come back with me now, eh? I have invented a new pudding in your honour. Amber Supreme. Yellow meringues with peaches and a big blob of cream, smothered in butterscotch sauce. There's a huge bowl in the fridge, waiting, made specially for you.'

'You told me to go away last time.'

'And I'm asking you home now.'

'Justin—'

'Look, I *said* I was sorry.' Sleeve bobbed up between us. 'Shall I apologise on the lad's behalf, young lady? Do give the silly young whipper-snapper a chance. And by the way, you don't happen to have any of that excellent wool left? I am revealed in all my fleshly nakedness whenever the lad wears his new pullie.'

I laughed and decided I was tired of sulking. I went home with Justin and we shared the huge bowl of Amber Supreme and talked non-stop until ten o'clock. There was only one thing we didn't talk about. One person.

Justin walked me back all the way home and as I put my key in the door he caught hold of me and kissed me. He took me by surprise so that our noses knocked and our teeth clinked together. We straightened up awkwardly. Justin grinned with embarrassment. I giggled. We waited, neither of us sure whether to try again. We didn't in the end. We didn't kiss the next night or any other night. Sometimes I worried that it was my fault, that I wasn't pretty or sexy enough, or I had bad breath or some equally repellent complaint. Other times I thought it was Justin's fault. He didn't know how to go any further and he was too frightened to try.

Then one afternoon Justin fidgeted and fussed and at four o'clock blurted out some excuse about a dentist. The next afternoon it was a visit from an aged aunt. And the next afternoon I asked him outright.

'What excuse is it going to be this time, Justin?'

'What do you mean? What excuse?' Justin blustered.

'Oh come on. I don't want to hear any more rubbish about dentists and aunts.'

'All right. Although today's excuse was really inventive. Swimming lessons? And I suppose you wish I'd take a running jump. I've been acting like a big berk, I know. Come home with me, Amber.'

Jonathon was there. He'd been home from school for a long week-end and had developed gastric flu. Even Jonathon could not look decorative under such circumstances. I caught one glimpse of him dashing to the loo, his face white and unshaven, his hair lank, the effect of his cream pyjamas marred by his ancient guernsey sweater. I don't think he even noticed me.

'We're going to give him a little leper's bell,' said Justin cheerfully.

But next Monday Justin wasn't in school. Or Tuesday. So I borrowed some money from Leonora and bought a pineapple and a box of man-sized tissues and a pot of Vicks VapoRub and walked up to his house. I was nervous, not sure he'd want me to come.

Justin's mother came to the door, in large Laura Ashley and ethnic jewellery. She threw up her hands in surprise, her tarnished silver bangles clinking up to her elbows.

'Amber! How lovely! Do come in.'

'I came to see how Justin is. I take it he's got flu now.'

'With a vengeance, poor darling. He's been very much under the weather, but he'll certainly perk up now he's got a visitor. I'll just dash upstairs and spruce him up a little. You know what slobs these men are in their sick-beds.'

She showed me into her living-room meanwhile. Justin's father was there, in a fisherman's smock and baggy cords, sitting cross-legged on a cushion reading a Penguin. To my dismay he shut his book with a snap and started to make conversation. He kept making silly jokes with a dead-pan expression and my jaw ached trying to smile politely at the right moment.

There was no sign of the other invalid.

Justin's mother returned, looking pink.

'Up you go then, Amber. It *is* good of you to come. You don't know what it means to Justin to have you for his friend. He hasn't found it very easy to make many friends, you know.'

My jaw ached on. How poor Justin would writhe if he could hear her.

'Take care you don't catch his rotten flu bug,' said Justin's father. 'Put a curb on the kissing for tonight.'

I giggled uneasily and hurried upstairs with my pineapple, tissues and VapoRub. I knocked on Justin's door. He didn't answer. I knocked again and then called his name. I heard him groan inside.

'Oh come on in then,' he mumbled thickly.

I don't know what he can have looked like before his mother

spruced him up. He was sprawling in his bed, one hand and both feet sticking out of his duvet. His face was grey, although his nostrils were crimson and crusted. Even his hair had lost its spring. It lay limply on his pillow like unravelled knitting.

'How are you?' I asked foolishly.

'In the pink,' said Justin.

'Sorry. It was a silly question. Here, I've brought you these.'

I produced the pineapple, the tissues and the VapoRub. I was proud of them but Justin wasn't in an appreciative mood.

'I was reading an article about pineapple enzymes the other day,' he said. 'They're incredibly powerful. These starving soldiers in the last war came across a pineapple plantation and had a feast. A few days later all their teeth dropped out.'

'It's got lots of vitamin C,' I said determinedly. 'It's very good for colds.'

'I haven't got a cold. I've got gastric flu. Which means I was spewing all day yesterday and half the night too.'

'And I got you tissues and some of this Vick stuff. You put it on your chest. Or you can try inhaling it.'

'Goody goody. It sounds a sensual delight.'

'Why are you being so nasty? I was only trying to help.'

'All right. It's very sweet of you. But I really just want to be left on my own. I *told* Mum not to let you up here.'

'O.K. I'll go then.'

'Now don't get in a huff,' Justin whined. His nose bubbled and he fished out a grubby handkerchief and blew it noisily.

'Why don't you use your tissues? It'll be horrid for your mother, washing that.'

'Tissues make your nose sore.'

'Then good. I should try sandpaper,' I said, flinging my spurned presents on to his bed.

'Do you mind. Look, I'm *ill*. You're meant to nurse my fevered brow, not pummel me with pineapples.'

He sat up to shift them over, and groaned. 'Oh God. I still feel so *sick*. I think it's the smell of that thing.'

'I'm sorry. I think pineapples smell lovely.'

'Can you take it away with you? You'd really better go now, Amber,' said Justin, fumbling under his bed for a washing-up bowl. 'Unless you want to stay and see me spewing.'

'No, I—'

'Do go *away*.'

He started retching before I was out of the room. I wondered whether to get his mother but he seemed determined to be left alone. I held my pineapple awkwardly, not sure what to do with it. I heard the bathroom door open along the landing. I started blushing as soon as I saw it was Jonathon.

'Hello Amber.'

'Hello. Are—are you better now?'

He certainly looked better. He was still in pyjamas, black ones this time, with a black and cream Japanese happy coat over the top. His hair was newly washed and shining and he smelt of soap and Eau Sauvage.

'Much better now,' said Jonathon. His smile was in full working order again. 'How sweet of you to come and see how I am. And you've brought me a pineapple, how perfect!'

I hesitated, smiling foolishly.

'You can have it,' I said, holding it out to him.

'Thank you.' He held it like a trophy.

I wondered if he could see my scarlet cheeks in the dim light of the landing.

Justin was still making disgusting noises from behind his bedroom door.

'Come away and let's leave the poor sod in peace,' said Jonathon. He held out his hand and I hesitated stupidly and then took it. I thought he'd lead me down to the living-room. We went upstairs instead.

'Where are we going?'

'My room. I've got the attic. I'm dying to know what you think of it. I just did it all up at Christmas and I'm rather proud of it.'

I felt it would look too feeble for words to refuse, so I went with him. It was only to admire his room, after all. And I did admire it. He left me alone for several minutes while he went to get us both a drink. I wandered around, almost on tiptoe. It was a sophisticated room for a sixth-former: black walls and ceiling and carpet, with cream silk cushions and rugs. He had an Art Deco lamp and clock and a posturing china lady with two long lean dogs, but he didn't seem to have any personal clutter at all. I dared open a little black lacquered cupboard and was reassured by the jumble of old *Face* magazines and albums and ancient annuals stuffed inside. I thought I shut them up properly but when Jonathon came back into the room the cabinet door creaked open again, spilling several *Beano* annuals.

'You've been having a little pry,' said Jonathon, shoving them inside with his bare foot.

'No I haven't,' I said too hastily.

'I'm glad you want to know all about me,' said Jonathon.

He'd abandoned the pineapple and had a tray with two black cocktail glasses instead. I thought he'd meant coffee when he'd asked if I wanted a drink.

'Pina colada,' he said. 'With slices of your fresh pineapple.'

I didn't see how I could refuse. I think I drank it too quickly. But I wasn't drunk when Jonathon sat beside me on the arm of his cream chair and kissed the nape of my neck. I had never thought of being kissed there before. I couldn't believe it could feel so beautiful. Then his hand touched my breast and that felt so beautiful too that I shivered. I saw Jonathon's smile and I tried to wriggle away. I nearly spilled pina colada on the cream upholstery. Jonathon took my smoked glass away from me.

'Everything matches in this room,' I said shakily. 'Even you, with your natty happy coat.'

He didn't wear his happy coat much longer. Up in my head I still hated him but my body was acting with a compliance that astounded me. I'd thought it would all be so awkward and uncomfortable. I'd had no idea it would be overwhelming.

Jonathon was much less worrying out of his black pyjamas. His body wasn't quite as perfect as I'd thought. He was a little too skinny and he had spots on his back but I didn't mind at all, I found it comforting. I was far more concerned about my own imperfections but Jonathon seemed to find me exciting. I couldn't quite believe what we were doing. It hurt at first but then it started to get much better, although it was still sore. I had just begun to want it to go on for ever when it stopped abruptly. Jonathon became much heavier, his chest squashing my breasts uncomfortably. He was panting.

'Was it good for you, Amber?' he whispered.

It wasn't as good as I'd hoped but I said it was lovely. Jonathon laughed triumphantly. Then the door of his room opened. Justin stood there, greyer than ever, staring at us.

Chapter 15

JAY is asking me all sorts of awful questions.

'I don't know. I can't remember. Anyway, it's none of your business.'

'I'm not just being nosy, you fool, I want to know if you can really be pregnant,' Jay snaps. 'Now, you're sure he didn't use a sheath?'

'*Yes*.'

'He didn't fumble with himself a couple of seconds before . . . Oh God, you're making me go all coy now,' says Jay, giggling nervously.

I glare at her, but then my lips quiver and I start giggling too. We laugh hugely and hysterically.

'This is ridiculous,' Jay gasps.

'You started it.'

'Well, did he?' she asks eventually, taking deep breaths.

'No.'

'And he didn't withdraw? You know, before he—'

'I bet Grandma didn't ask you all these questions when you told her you were having me.'

'True,' says Jay. 'She just kept calling me a dirty little slut. Over and over. Would you sooner I called you that?'

'No.'

'Then stop nagging at me. You know what withdrawing means, don't you?'

'Yes, but—'

'You're not making all this up, are you?'

'No!'

'I just find it so hard to take in. And with this boy's *brother*. Why him and not Justin?'

'It just happened,' I mumble.

'How old is this brother?'

'Eighteen. Maybe seventeen. I don't know.'

'Did you know what he was doing?'

'Of course I did, I'm not stupid.'

'Did he talk you into it?'

'He didn't rape me. *Please* stop going on about it, Jay.'

'I gather it wasn't a great success? It's never much good, the first time. But don't let it put you off. It gets fantastic with practice.'

'You've certainly had enough.'

'You sound just like my mother.'

I pull my face into Grandma's pucker. 'You dirty little slut,' I say, trying out Grandma's cut-glass tone.

Jay grins. 'Hey, that's good. You sound just like her. Actually practice doesn't always make perfect. Let me tell you . . . . '

She does tell me, in explicit detail. This is ridiculous. I don't want to talk about her stupid sex life. Why do we always have to talk about her? I'm the one that's having the baby.

'What am I going to do?'

'I don't know.'

'You're supposed to tell me.'

She's laughing again, although I think she's forcing it this time. 'We don't have much luck, do we? First me and now you.'

I pull up my knees and rest my head on them. 'I feel awful.'

Jay reaches out and puts her arm round me. 'It'll be all right. We'll sort something out.'

'I don't just feel awful about the baby. It's Justin.'

'Oh. So he knows about you and his brother?'

I wriggle, not wanting her arm. I remember Justin's face and I start crying.

'Don't,' says Jay. 'Oh Amber, it's not the end of the world.' Her arm tightens round me. 'If you must know, I'm quite relieved.'

'Then you must be mad,' I say, pushing her away.

'I thought *you* were. Mad. I really thought you'd gone nuts.'

'You're the nutty member of the family.'

'I had myself convinced. I never dreamt you were pregnant. No, I had it all worked out. Schizophrenia. I even found out about mental homes, modern ones where they counsel you and don't drug you into submission. Only the best ones are all private and cost a fortune.'

'You didn't!' I hadn't realised she'd taken it that seriously.

'I did. I was so desperate I even wrote to Davie.'

'About me?'

'Asking if he'd come.'

'*Why*?'

'Because he's the only one you've ever been close to. I thought he might be able to—I don't know—talk you out of it.'

'And is he coming? How did you know where he is? I bet he hasn't written back.'

'Yes he has,' says Jay.

Of course. I remember the airmail letter the day Grandma replied to me. 'Let me see it.'

'No. I don't know what I've done with it anyway. It doesn't say much. He's going to come to England soon, maybe next week. He's in Amsterdam at the moment so it's not really that far for him.' She's gone pink and I sense some sort of conspiracy.

'Why can't I see the letter? It's about me,' I say, and then a thought enters my head and taps inside like a woodpecker. It's too insistent to ignore. 'Jay, is Davie my father?'

She stares at me and it's no use hoping. I can see she's amazed at the idea.

'Davie? Of course he isn't. What ever made you think that? Look, you know all about your father.'

'Yes, but that story always sounds so . . . .'

'It's the truth.'

I don't want it to be. I'd give anything for Davie to be my father.

I dream it when I eventually get to sleep. Jay and I talk endlessly all evening but we don't get anywhere. I beg her to tell me what to do but she's useless.

'You've got to decide, Amber. It's your baby.'

I'm the baby in my dream of Davie. Not an infant, a small girl of two or three, the age when I first went to the commune. Davie is there in his black and purple jacket, playing his penny whistle. The other children don't exist. We live in the house all by ourselves. I listen to his music, so close to him I can feel the force of it as it flutters from the end of his pipe, and then he finishes and takes me in his arms instead. I nestle there while he strokes my hair and plays with my ears and my nose and my chin. I grow sleepy and he kisses my eyes shut. I lie safe in his arms, very nearly asleep, sleeping inside the sleep of my dream, but there's something stopping me, something tickling my foot.

It can't be Davie because I can feel both his hands holding me. It's tugging now, not tickling, and I shake my leg to stop it, but it clings determinedly. I don't want to open my eyes. I want them to stay safely sealed by Davie's kiss, so I kick out blindly but it's got me by both legs now. I put my hand down and touch another hand, tiny, with scrabbling fingers. I have to look. It is a naked baby. It starts climbing up my body, its little limbs surprisingly efficient. I try to push it off but it's as strong as I am. It climbs right up until its face is hanging over mine, saliva dripping from its empty mouth. I beg Davie to rescue me but I've somehow slipped out of his arms and he's not there any more. The baby drools. Its eyes are empty as well as its mouth. Its head is like a Halloween pumpkin and it's growing bigger all the time. It's squashing me, right over my face, smothering me. I shriek until Jay shakes me out of the nightmare. Just for a second, maybe mixing her up with

Davie, I cling to her as desperately as the baby clung to me, but then I smell her stale patchouli and push her away, pretending I'm still asleep.

I don't want her. I don't want anyone, not even Davie. He won't come anyway. Why should he? I'm not his problem.

But he arrives next Monday—and I'm all alone. Jay is at work, the Smallwoods are all out, I am here waiting and we can be together.

I don't even recognise him at first! He looks too old and too ill. And he's not wearing his black and purple jacket and the huge hat. Of *course* he isn't, he'd look bizarre still trailing round in ancient seventies fancy dress, he could get away with it in Hay but not here, and yet he looks so oddly ordinary in his jeans and bomber jacket. And he's cut his hair. His face looks uncomfortably exposed and his ears much too large. He needs a shave and his eyes are red-rimmed: he looks as if he's been up all night. Perhaps he has, on the boat from Amsterdam. Coming specially to see me.

'Hello Amber,' he says, and he wraps his arms round me and gives me a hug. He smells just the same, of warm wool and toast, and he's still the same too, he's Davie and though I still feel shy my arms go round his neck and I hug him back. Then he unwinds me so that he can look at me.

'You look blooming even in the midst of your dramatic nervous breakdown.'

'I'm not having one. I was just acting stupidly and Jay got into a panic. I'm sorry, Davie, she shouldn't have written to you.'

'I'm glad she did. It was about time I had a holiday,' says Davie, yawning and stretching. He takes in the house and raises his eyebrows. 'Gordon's obviously gone up in the world since I saw him last. Which bit do you live in, Amber?'

'Up at the top. Come and see.' I want to take his hand the way I always did but I haven't quite got the courage. I show him upstairs.

'What work do you do, Davie?'

'This and that. More that than this,' Davie says vaguely. 'Maybe I should have gone into advertising.'

He whistles at the Hockney lithograph on the wall and dodges the low Tiffany light on the landing.

'This is our room,' I say, pulling him in, and he looks round and laughs.

'It's just how I imagined it. I see Jay still sticks to her old mattress.'

'You imagined it? Our room?' I say, pleased. I can't imagine Davie's room at all. I've never thought about him having a domestic life. He's always been like a character in a fairy-tale, living in a different dimension. 'What's your room like, Davie?'

'I haven't really got one. I share with various friends.' He's looking in his knapsack. 'Here, Amber.'

He hands me a little paper bag, tied at the top with a scrap of ribbon. I undo it and discover a miniature marzipan flower in a little waxed container. It has red and yellow marzipan petals and a slim green marzipan stalk. A tulip from Amsterdam.

'You always give perfect presents.'

'Gobble it up then.'

'No, it's far too precious to eat.'

Davie smiles and sits on the edge of my bed. He smooths my old quilt admiringly. 'Did you do this? It's beautiful. I always remember you sewing little bits and pieces when you were tiny. You once got some old cotton curtains and said you were going to make me a shirt.'

'I didn't know what I was doing then. The sleeves wouldn't go right. I tried to do them four or five times. And I didn't have enough material anyway, it was all bits cobbled together and it looked a mess so I ripped it up.'

'You should have given it to me. I'd have treasured it,' says Davie, stretching, and then lying down on top of the bed. He carefully kicks his shoes off because of the quilt. He groans appreciatively as he stretches out. There are large holes in both his socks.

'I could make you a proper shirt now,' I suggest. 'Or a jacket. Anything you like. What would you like, Davie?'

'I'd like . . . to sleep for half an hour.'

'All right then. Shall—shall I go downstairs or—'

'I'm not serious,' says Davie, sitting up with an effort. 'I've come here to see you, Amber, not to go to sleep. Are you free today? Shall we go out somewhere?'

'Yes please!'

'Doesn't Jay come home for lunch?'

She said she'd rush back in her lunch hour in case Davie came. But I shake my head firmly.

'I'll see Jay this evening then. Now. Where will we go?' He spots the Perrault fairy-tales beside my bed. 'Do you still like bookshops?'

'Yes, very much. You bought that book for me, Davie, remember?'

'Of course I do.' He flicks through it. 'You look even more of a Sleeping Beauty now.'

He really does remember. I love him, I love him so much, even though he's yawning again and the skin showing through his socks isn't very clean. He sees me looking and waggles his feet, pulling a face.

'New book for you. New socks for me,' he says.

We get the tube to Oxford Circus and go to Marks and Spencer for the socks. They're all rather dull, brown and black business men's socks. Davie has small feet so we try Women's Hosiery and Davie buys himself a natty navy pair with red stripes. I wish I'd got the money to buy them for him. I shouldn't have been such a fool and stayed away from the market. I've lost the chance of making all that money—and it hasn't made any difference. I've still betrayed Justin. And I'm going to have a baby. No. I'm not going to think about it today. I'm not going to let anything spoil being with Davie.

'Let's have a picnic lunch,' says Davie, as we hover near the food hall.

'Can we! Oh good, I love picnics.'

I don't mean Jay's limp pitta bread picnics, I mean old-fashioned Jane and Peter picnics with a blue and white check cloth and square sandwiches and boiled eggs and fairy cakes and orange squash in red and yellow beakers.

'What sort of picnic shall we have?' says Davie, as we inspect the cabinets of food.

Marks is much more modern than the Jane and Peter world. Pâté, prawns, pizzas . . . . I dither helplessly, unable to decide. Then I spot the blackcurrant cheesecake in the frozen foods. 'I wish they did smaller ones.' I reach out and touch the icy packet wistfully.

'Is it your favourite?' Davie asks, amused.

'I've only had it once, when I went to buy my bed.'

I tell him all about it and he understands. I even tell him about the imaginary Elizabeth Ann. I send myself up, saying that perhaps Jay is right, I must be crazy playing imaginary games when I'm nearly sixteen, but Davie says he still does it now.

'Really? What sort of imaginary games? Tell me,' I beg.

He shakes his head, smiling. 'Shall we have the cheesecake for our picnic?' He grins. 'Let's see if we can eat it all.'

It's the most wicked wonderful idea. We deliberate a little over the cherry and the gooseberry but decide to stick with blackcurrant.

'We'll have to wait a couple of hours for it to thaw,' says Davie. 'So we'll have a good wander around first.'

We go to Liberty's and play the 'if I had all the money in the world' game and I end up with an amber ring on my finger and real silk stockings on my feet, swathed in six metres of every single material in the store. Davie's not so good at playing, he obviously doesn't want things the way I do. I have to bully him before he chooses, and then they're extra presents for me: a long white broderie anglaise Victorian night-dress, a cake of snowdrop soap, a box of white chocolate creams.

'I think I could just about afford a couple of the chocolates. Let's try them,' says Davie.

I'm *longing* to try them but I'm not sure you can buy them two at a time. I worry when Davie asks the girl and just for a moment I notice his jacket is grubby and his sweater is fraying at the neck, but the girl calmly puts on a little transparent glove and selects two chocolates without any fuss.

'This is the most sinfully expensive chocolate I've ever eaten,' I say, licking it in delight.

'Let's eat them in a sinful setting then,' says Davie, and we go out of the back of Liberty's into Soho.

I gaze with great interest at all the sex clubs and shops. Davie puts his arm round me protectively. He won't let me pause and look properly at the sex places, but he shows me a Chinese supermarket and Italian pasta shops and French patisseries. I see Patisserie Valerie at last and peer in past the wonderful cakes in the window.

'Do you want to go in?' says Davie. 'We could have a coffee there. And a cake.'

'We've got our blackcurrant cheesecake,' I say, tapping the cold packet. 'I just wanted to see what it was like. Leonora goes there a lot.'

Davie nods. I grit my teeth, waiting for him to ask all about Leonora. But he doesn't seem interested and talks about cakes instead. It makes me love him more. We wander on through the back streets fancying ourselves cake connoisseurs, admiring gateaux and brioches and pastries, passion cake and syrupy strudels and strawberry tarts top-heavy with cream. I tell Davie about the cakes in *Maison Sagne* and how I was in such a state I settled for a scone. I even tell him about Grandma not giving the waiter enough money.

'Do you think she could be going senile, Davie?'

'Maybe. Though it sounds as if she's simply short of a bob or two.'

'She's not poor. She lives in this really posh flat in Marylebone and she's got stacks of money. She sent Jay to a private school and a daily woman came to do all the housework and—'

'Then. What about now?'

'Well. She's still rich. She must be.' But I'm not quite so sure now. I think about her and frown.

'Do you have a grandmother, Davie?'

'No.'

'What about your mother? Tell me about yourself.'

Davie shakes his head. 'There's nothing to tell.'

'You mean you won't tell it.'

'Maybe.'

'You're like . . . have you read *The Hobbit*? You could be Gandalph. You pop up as if by magic and then pop off again. Don't you ever want to stay anywhere?'

'Sometimes.' His arm is still round me. 'I'll stay with you, Amber, O.K.?'

O.K., O.K., O.K. It's only a joke, but if only, if only . . . .

Chapter 16

DAVIE suggests the second-hand bookshops of Charing Cross Road but when we get there we find that most have disappeared. Half of Charing Cross Road has disappeared too and become a monster building site.

'I've been away longer than I realised,' says Davie, and he sounds at a loss. But it's only momentarily. 'I bet Cecil Court's still there,' he says, taking me by the hand.

Cecil Court is a little alleyway leading off Charing Cross Road and almost every shop in the alley sells books. Davie squeezes my hand proudly as if he's personally manufactured them just for me.

'Come on. You have to choose one special book.'

'You can't keep on buying me things, Davie,' I say, hoping he'll insist.

We're both taken aback by the prices. There are no 10p bargains here. Most of the books are well over ten pounds.

'Never mind. We'll pretend instead. And I've *got* my special book from you, the Perrault fairy-tales,' I say quickly, but he darts away from me.

'There's children's books here, come and look,' Davie calls.

I'm not a child any more but I go and look. The shop-window is enchanting, an elaborate arrangement of picture-books and paper cut-outs and pink-cheeked Dutch dolls.

'Let's go in,' says Davie.

We find ourselves waist high in books and have to wade through them, but they're all as decoratively ordered as a page of Victorian scraps. The owner stands on a sort of rostrum at the back of the shop, peeking at us through his spectacles, but he's gravely benign and doesn't mind in the least when we thumb through half his stock. Davie finds a big red edition of *Robinson Crusoe* with hundreds of detailed illustrations. He turns the pages very carefully, nodding. I find a *Girl's Own Annual* over a hundred years old, with a serial called 'Our Gallant Girl'. The Gallant Girl supports her feckless family by her skilful sewing. I flick through the episodes to the end, past sepia paintings and soppy poems and tartly unsympathetic correspondence pages—'You shouldn't waste our time with such a trivial problem. You are an inconsiderate girl. We feel your chances are nil'—and find that the Gallant Girl gets taken up by a Kind Gentleman who sends her to a Ladies' College and the feckless family fizzle out of the story and the Gallant Girl grows up and marries her Kind Gentleman.

I want the *Girl's Own Annual* terribly but it's twenty pounds, and Davie's *Robinson Crusoe* is thirty, so we have to put them back on their shelves. But there are little books too, old and new, and we browse through them. I find a facsimile of a little Victorian novelty book on babies. It's in the shape of a baby, and there's a different one on every page, smiling babies, solemn babies, sleeping babies. I flick through the babies again and again, mesmerized.

'Would you like the baby book?' Davie asks, looking over my shoulder. '£1.95. I can manage that. It's cheap at the price, just under 20p per baby.'

I can't smile. I stare at the babies. The sweet smiling one floats off the page and holds out her chubby arms. I reach out for her, but she's gone in a flick of the page and now there's the fat cross one, a real piglet of a child with slit eyes and a square mouth. It's screaming and I hide it hurriedly and find the sleeping one and it's so still and silent it might not be asleep at all, it could be dead.

'I don't know,' I whisper. 'I don't know, I don't know, I don't know.'

Davie stares at me and shuts the book. He can't know why I'm in such a state but he seems to understand. He tucks it behind some other books and shows me a little shelf of doll's size poetry paperbacks. He distracts me with them, reading out a line here, a verse there, until the babies recede.

' "Swart-headed mulberries,
Wild free-born cranberries,
Crab-apples, dewberries,
Pineapples, blackberries,"
Blackcurrant cheesecakes—'

'It doesn't say that!'
'Of course it doesn't.'
'But I like it. The fruit.'
'It's "Goblin Market". Haven't you heard it before?'
'No, I don't think so. Read some more.'

' "Buy from us with a golden curl."
She clipped a precious golden lock,
She dropped a tear more rare than pearl,
Then sucked their fruit-globes fair or red.
Sweeter than honey from the rock,
Stronger than man-rejoicing wine,
Clearer than water flowed that juice;
She never tasted such before,
How should it cloy with length of use?
She sucked and sucked and sucked the more
Fruits which that unknown orchard bore;
She sucked until her lips were sore;
Then flung the emptied rinds away
But gathered up one kernel stone,
And knew not was it night or day
As she turned home alone.'

I take it from him and look at the illustration on the cover.

There's a girl with her hair spiralling down her back, her neck and arms and ankles circled with chains of cherries, her dress a brocade of berries. Little goblin men dance around her, holding out her heavy skirts and smoothing her hair, and more goblins delve into huge wicker baskets and tempt her with great globes of fruit. They are ugly gnarled little goblins, but there's something familiar and endearing about their tousled locks and big pointed ears.

'They look a bit like you, Davie. *Please* can I have it? It's a special book, better than any others.'

It's thirty-five pence, probably the cheapest book in the whole shop, but now it is the only one I want. Davie buys it for me and the man puts it in a bag and gives me a pretty paper bookmark with a picture of a Kate Greenaway girl.

We walk down the Charing Cross Road hand in hand and whenever we pass a window I stare at our reflection and see a large girl with her fair hair flying in the wind and a small man with goblin ears. The girl is quite a bit taller than the man. I don't believe the reflection. Davie towers above me the way he's always done.

We go in the National Gallery and I look at all the religious paintings and arrange my face in a reverent expression. Then I realise all the Marys are young, some only my age, and I look at all the infant Jesuses and they shake their little haloed heads at me.

'Let's find some landscapes. We'll choose the land we want to live in,' says Davie.

We slip in and out of Italian fairy cities and tropical forests and fields of waving corn and eventually find a small painting of a blue mountain. A path winds gently to the top and there's a snug cave half-way up. A little man already lives there, but he looks as if he'd be neighbourly.

'Here,' I say.

Davie nods too. 'Here.'

We stand in front of the painting, imagining, but then a party of school children troop into the gallery and sit down cross-legged on the floor for a lecture and we have to pick our way through them.

'Come on, it's lunch-time,' says Davie, fingering the damp paper bag. 'I'm not sure it's thawed yet, but we'll try giving it a little gnaw.'

We open the packet in Trafalgar Square. Davie breaks me off a mouthful. I munch slowly and appreciatively, savouring the sharp taste of the currants and the sweet taste of the cheese. It is still so cold that it shocks my mouth but it's too good to wait any longer.

'It's wonderful. Let's eat it now.'

We're pestered by pigeons in the square so we go through Admiralty Arch to St. James's Park. We walk along the little path, green grass and grey water on either side. It's so still and quiet that it's almost as if we're really in our own private painting. We sit on a bench and Davie balances the cheesecake on top of its cardboard packet.

'It's still frozen,' he says, tapping it.

'But it tastes marvellous, honestly. Try a bit.'

'It's more like ice lolly than cake,' he says, biting gingerly.

'But it's lovely, isn't it? Let's eat it now, Davie. I can't wait, I'm starving.'

'You're like Laura in the poem,' says Davie.'Are you going to cut off a precious golden lock for me?' He plays with a straggly curl and then snips with his fingers. I jump, almost believing he's cut it, and he laughs.

'Cheesecake,' I insist.

He breaks off a huge chunk of cheesecake for me and another rather smaller for himself.

My hands are already mottled because I don't have any gloves and now they quickly become numb. It is very chilly sitting still on the bench nursing the icy cake and the wind is making my eyes water. I eat on determinedly but perhaps the cake isn't quite so wonderful now I'm on the second chunk, with the first clenched like a cold fist inside my stomach.

'You don't have to finish it,' says Davie.

He takes my frozen hands and rubs them until they tingle. One finger stays obstinately white and drained. He lifts it to his mouth and sucks it. His lips and tongue are wet and warm and my finger throbs to life. Our eyes meet and I can feel the thawed blood beating all over my body and I know it's beating in Davie too because I can see the pulse at his throat. I wonder if it's all right for a girl to kiss a man's neck. He suddenly drops my hand and jumps up.

'Come on. Let's give the sparrows the meal of their lives,' he says, scattering large crumbs of cheesecake.

I follow him, wiping my wet hand on my jacket. 'We could feed the ducks,' I suggest. 'The sparrows are only going to get chronic indigestion.'

So we walk by the water's edge, throwing cheesecake at the ducks. They look surprised but peck at it eagerly enough and then swim along after us, obviously wanting more. Their quacks attract moorhens and Canada geese and they set up a clamour. There isn't going to be enough cheesecake to go round.

'I feel like Jesus trying to feed the five thousand,' I say, spraying crumbs. 'And they'd probably prefer loaves and fishes. You don't think cheesecake really could upset them, do you?'

'Of course not. They're London birds with sophisticated palates,' says Davie, but then we come to a stern notice:

PLEASE DO NOT FEED THE PELICANS. DEATH HAS BEEN CAUSED BY UNSUITABLE FOOD.

'Oh Davie. We've probably poisoned them! I'm sure cheesecake is unsuitable.'

'They're not pelicans. They're ducks, give or take a goose or two.'

'Some of them might be pelicans.'

'You idiot, you can't possibly mistake a pelican. It's got a huge beak with a flappy thing underneath.' Davie gestures to show me.

'What, those birds that look as if they're carrying handbags in their beaks?'

'Those birds. That's it.'

'I can't see any,' I agree. 'But we'd better stop feeding this lot all the same.'

'Maybe. There's a little house up here and I think the man who looks after the wildlife lives there.'

'Oh help.' I cram cheesecake into my own mouth and then throw the empty packet into a waste-paper basket. I munch and then choke.

'Amber!' Davie pats me on the back, and then rubs while I cough and splutter. I'm his little girl now, not the big girl that took us both by surprise. 'Spit it out.'

'No!' I protest through the great purple sludge in my mouth. 'It would be a wicked waste.'

I carry on coughing dramatically.

'Are you quite sure you haven't got any pelican blood?'

I laugh and choke some more.

'Chew at it.'

I chew until my jaws ache and at last it disappears. I am beginning to feel very full indeed.

'I've eaten half an entire cheesecake. More than half, because you didn't have a very big slice and we didn't give the ducks that much. Two thirds,' I say, awed.

'You'll remember this day for ever. The day you ate the blackcurrant cheesecake,' says Davie.

I'll remember this day for the rest of my life but it's got nothing to do with the cheesecake. I wish I was bold enough to say it to him. I wish I could manage 'I love you'. Jay would say it. Leonora certainly would. Even Polly would whisper it. But I'm still stuck inside myself and I can't get the words out.

We walk past the little house by the water. It's a small Swiss chalet, cream with brown tiles, all carvings and crevices. It's such an unlikely dwelling that I almost expect the roof to lift off to beguile all the lurking pelicans with tinkly music.

'Is it a real house?'

'Yes. There are curtains at the windows, look.'

I want to get closer, to stand on the little bridge and peer in through the curtains, but there's another notice: PRIVATE. NO ADMITTANCE.

'Do you like it?'

'I'd give anything to live there.'

'So we'll abandon our detached cave with no mod. cons. in the mountain and come and live in a cottage in St. James's Park?'

'Yes please.' I glance at him. I swallow several times. I feel as if the cheesecake is still gumming up my mouth. 'With you.'

Has he heard?

'Would you like that?' I mumble.

'You know I would,' says Davie, and he takes hold of my hand.

We walk on through the park. We don't talk. I think we're both scared of breaking the spell. We glide over the grass and circle the trees. It's a magic park and we are enchanted. It's getting colder but it doesn't matter. My legs ache and my shoes have started rubbing but who cares about something as silly as sore feet. The cheesecake is curdling in my stomach but I'm not going to let myself feel sick.

'Are you all right, Amber?'

'Yes, I'm fine.'

'Let's have a little rest.'

We go back to our bench but we've only just sat down when a vagrant in a greasy rain coat sidles up to us and starts muttering. He's glaring. We're not sure if he's muttering to us or about us.

'Isn't it a lovely day?' Davie says.

The vagrant disagrees. He tells Davie what to do with himself.

'O.K.,' says Davie cheerfully. 'Come on, Amber.'

We walk on, hand in hand. There's another vagrant stretched out on the cold grass, and two more on the next bench, passing a bottle of cider back and forth.

'Where have they all come from? Didn't we notice them before?'

Davie shrugs. He doesn't look quite so cheerful. 'Maybe I'll end up like them.'

'Oh Davie.'

'No, I mean it.'

'Of course you won't! You're not a *vagrant*. You couldn't ever be.'

'They didn't start off looking like that,' says Davie.

I stare at the one drinking cider. His shoes have soles that flap open. He has no socks. His toes stick out of the gap, swollen and purple, the nails like claws. His hands shake as he lifts the bottle to his lips. He drools as he drinks, spilling down his whiskery chin. His skin is grey with grime which makes him look more than ever like a being from another planet. I try to imagine him thoroughly scrubbed and dressed in decent clothes; I shave him and fit him with shoes and give him a haircut. For a moment he gives me Davie's smile, his head on one side—but then he's a drunken vagrant again, an alien whose smell makes me feel sick.

'Come on,' I say, tugging at Davie. I wish he'd managed to have a shave today. And I know he can't help it, but his jumper is fraying and his jacket is stained. 'You don't drink,' I say quickly.

'I do. Sometimes.'

'Yes, but not like that.'

'I do all sorts of stupid things, Amber,' he says seriously.

'I don't care what you do.'

'I wish I hadn't made such a mess of my life.'

He looks so unhappy that I can't bear it.

'I love you.'

He looks at me. There are tears in his eyes.

'I love you too.'

He kisses me. It's a little soft kiss with closed lips. It only lasts a second but I can still feel his mouth long after it's over.

'I've loved you ever since I was a little girl.'

'You're still a little girl.'

'Of course I'm not.'

'Fourteen.'

'*Fifteen*. I'm nearly sixteen actually.'

'You're still much too young.'

'For what?'

'For me.'

'No, I'm not.'

'Amber, look at me.'

'I like the way you look.'

'It's not just age anyway. You're all young and fresh and innocent and I'm—'

'No I'm not.'

'You're still—'

'I'm going to have a baby.'

It shuts him up for a moment. I'm out of breath. Davie seems winded too.

'Does Jay know?'

'She didn't until the other day.'

'Are you in love with the boy?'

'No. I hate him. It was the first time I ever did it. Trust me to make a mess of things.'

'What are you going to do?'

'I don't know.' I don't want to talk about it. I should have kept my mouth shut.

'What do you *want* to do?'

'I don't know.' I shrug. 'Jay says I should have an abortion.' I hate that word. It sounds so ugly. It's an ugly act. I don't know exactly how they do it. I imagine myself strapped to a bed, my legs splayed, while a masked man cuts me open with huge steel scissors.

'It's all right, Amber. You don't have to have an abortion. Nobody can make you. You can keep your baby.'

I wasn't even thinking about the baby. My eyes are watering in the wind. Two or three blinks and I'm crying.

'Amber,' Davie whispers.

He puts his arms round me and holds me close. I can feel his heart beating. Mine is pounding too. I can feel all the pulse points in my body. I feel as if I'm going to spring a dozen leaks and spout scarlet fountains. I don't want to cry, but I'm afraid he'll let go of me if I stop.

'Amber,' he whispers. 'It's all right. Don't cry. It'll be all right, I promise. You can have the baby.'

'I can't. I don't know how,' I wail.

He doesn't laugh at me or get cross. 'There's no need to feel so frightened. Think of all the people in London, in England, in the whole world. They've all been born. So it must be the most ordinary event ever. You don't need to know how, it just happens. Although you can go to classes in childbirth if you want. It doesn't matter if you don't. Your body takes over and does all the work.'

'It'll hurt so.' It isn't just the pain. I can't bear the thought of the position, the indignity of the whole performance. I don't want to gasp and grunt.

'Of course it will hurt. But it will be worth it. Wait and see how you'll feel when you have your own baby in your arms.'

'I'm frightened.' I don't want them to put the baby straight in my arms, all slimy from inside my body. I don't even want it washed and powdered and pristine.

'I don't like babies,' I mumble against Davie's jumper.

'You'll like your own. And I'll like it too, especially if it's anything like you. A funny little girl with curls like dandelion fluff,' says Davie. He gently combs my hair with his fingers.

'You won't be here,' I say. I hold very still.

'I could be,' says Davie.

'You won't. You'll be back in Amsterdam.'

'I could come over. Or I could stay here now. Maybe it's time for a big change. I could stay here with you, Amber.'

'How could you? With Jay?'

'Not at Gordon's place. We could get our own room somewhere. In a squat. We could live there together and you could have your baby.'

'With Jay?' I repeat. 'Or just us?'

'Just us.'

Is it still a game? It must be. I'd give the whole world for it to be real. Why must he play games with me? I jerk away from him, pulling my hair. 'That hurt,' I say, rubbing my scalp, as if it's his fault.

'Wouldn't you like to live with me, Amber?'

'Don't. It's silly. We can't.'

'Yes we can. If you want to.'

If I want to. I see us curled up on a sofa, Davie at one end reading aloud to me, me at the other, sewing. The baby is tucked up in its cot, fast asleep.

I start shivering. Davie rubs my arms through the thin sleeves of my jacket. 'You poor little thing, you're freezing,' he says.

I love the way he calls me little, even though I'm bigger than he is. And fatter too. His wrists look about to snap and his clothes hang on him. We'll have to be careful cuddling when I'm big with the baby. If I leant on him I could knock him over.

'Come on, let's go and have a coffee to warm ourselves up,' says Davie, fingering the change in his pocket. 'Yes, I've got heaps.'

How can he look after me and the baby when he has to count to see if he can afford two coffees?

'I could get a job,' says Davie, as if he's heard me. 'An ordinary nine to five job with a wage packet every Friday. It's time I stopped playing Peter Pan. Look at Gordon. It's time I settled down too.'

But he's still out of touch. How can he get a job just like that? I don't think he's got any qualifications, he certainly hasn't got any training. He could work in a shop like Jay. Perhaps he could be a barman in a pub—but he doesn't mean that sort of job. He's talking now about going into advertising like Gordon which is nonsense, or even writing a novel or a travel book. He's just like a kid playing at what he's going to do when he grows up.

We walk past the little house again. We look for the pelicans. Maybe they're hiding inside the house. Ducks flap and quack excitedly. I look to see if any are foaming blackcurrant froth from their beaks, but they seem to have digested their unsuitable meal without mishap. Which is more than I have. My tummy aches badly now. I slide my hand under my jacket and rub it surreptitiously. We come out into the Mall and Davie points at an art gallery place across the road.

'The ICA. We'll get a cup of coffee there. I used to go there a lot.' When we're inside he peers round, looking relieved. 'It hasn't changed much anyway.'

But Davie doesn't seem to fit any more. There are no seventies people in sight. The people here look sharp and smart and street-wise.

We sit at a table and sip coffee. Davie feels for my hand underneath the bright oilcloth.

'What is it?' he whispers.

I shake my head.

'Are you still worrying about the baby, Amber?'

'A bit.'

'It'll be all right, I promise. I'll look after you.'

I nod and squeeze his hand, scared to say any more in case I start crying and make a fool of both of us. I don't know why I'm nearly in tears. This is the happiest day of my life. I've got Davie at last.

I'm still shivering. I drink my coffee down to the bitter dregs. Two gay men in black leather are toying with cakes: when they get up to go one of them leaves almost all his chocolate gateau. Davie sees me staring at it and before the gays are even out of the restaurant he nips across to their table and seizes the cake. He brings it back to me triumphantly. I don't want the cake at all. I remember the man's soft lips and gleaming teeth. I'm sure I can see saliva shining on the brown icing. I don't even like chocolate gateau very much and I'm still overwhelmingly full of blackcurrant cheesecake. My tummy is hot and hard with pain, pressing against my waistband, shifting me uneasily in my chair. But I know it will hurt Davie if I don't try the cake. I manage two bites and nearly gag. I'm really scared I'm going to be sick.

'Is there a Ladies anywhere?'

Davie tells me where it is. I rush off and thank God there's nobody in there. I lock myself into a cubicle and sway over the stained porcelain. I gasp and gulp helplessly but I'm not actually sick. I wait a while and then sit down on the lavatory, doubled up with stomach ache. I sit there, shaking my head, bleeding into the bowl.

Chapter 17

I FASHION myself a makeshift pad out of a wad of toilet paper. It prickles and feels uncomfortable. So do I. I'm such a fool. Jay's been right all along. I've been making a tremendous fuss over nothing at all. And it is nothing. It hurts but it's the same squeeze it always is. The blood flows but it's only blood, there's no baby. I almost wish I was having a proper miscarriage. I could keel over, flooding the floor with a crimson lake, and get whisked into hospital. They would rush to my bedside and hover over me and tell me how much they love me and beg me not to die. They? Davie? He's already told me he loves me. He wants to look after me. Only he needn't now. I have to tell him.

I don't announce it immediately when I walk awkwardly out of the ladies' lavatory. I wait until we're wandering again. We go in the National Portrait Gallery because it doesn't cost anything and it's warm inside. We start up at the Elizabethans on the top floor and walk down through history. I feel as if all those painted eyes are peering at me instead of the other way round.

'Amber?' says Davie. 'You look as if you're going to cry again. I promise you, it'll be all right. I've been thinking, working things out. I'm going to look after you and the baby and—'

'There isn't a baby.'

He stares at me. 'What?'

'*There isn't a baby.*' I'm almost shouting.

An attendant looks at me anxiously. Davie's face is puckered and he's obviously not sure what to say next. I don't know what I'm going to say either. I feel as if I've been tightly sewn up and now someone has cut the stitches and pulled me painfully free. Words, tears, blood. I can't staunch any of them.

Davie bundles me out of the gallery and tries to soothe me. I cry all the way home. It must be awful for Davie on the tube with everyone glaring at him accusingly. A middle-aged woman comes over to us, bends her grey perm down to my wet face, and whispers, 'Would you like to come and sit with me, dear?'

I don't want to sit with anyone. When we get home I lock myself in the bathroom for a long time. Davie knocks on the door and asks if I'm all right. I let him lead me upstairs. I lie on my bed and he eases my shoes off and pulls the covers up over me.

'I'm sorry, I'm sorry,' I splutter.

'It's all right. Don't worry, Amber, I understand,' Davie says, sitting down beside me.

'It's so stupid. I'm spoiling everything but I can't stop crying.'

'Don't try to.'

'I really did think I was going to have a baby before.'

'I know you did.'

'Jay *said* I was just—'

'Never mind Jay.'

'Oh Davie, what am I going to do?'

'Curl up. Cry some more if you want. And then go to sleep. I'll stay sitting here.'

He holds my hand and I clutch his.

'What am I going to do about Justin?' I wail.

I tell him all about Justin and he listens to my great gabble.

'You're being so nice to me and yet, can't you see, I'm wicked. I did the very worst thing in the world to Justin.'

'You didn't do it deliberately.'

'I think I did.'

'You thought he was ill in his own room.'

'Yes. So how could I have gone off with Jonathon like that? And we didn't even lock the door.'

'So what did you say to poor Justin?'

'It was so awful. I didn't say anything. And neither did he. We just all looked at each other. It was like the end of a film when it suddenly freezes into a still. Then I think Jonathon said something, I can't even remember what, and Justin just turned and walked out of the room. And I got up and went home. Jonathon wanted to go with me but I wanted to be by myself. I went straight to bed when I got in and then the next morning I couldn't bear to get up.'

'And you haven't seen either of them since?'

'No.'

'And I take it you don't want to see Jonathon any more?'

I shake my head violently.

'What about Justin?'

'I don't *know*. I suppose I've got to see him and yet I *can't*.'

'You still like him?'

'Yes, of course I do. But he'll hate me now.'

'Maybe.'

'How did they cope at the commune? I mean, people slept with all different people, didn't they?'

'People still got hurt, even if they didn't show it,' says Davie softly.

'You always managed to stay everyone's friend.'

Davie smiles. He tucks the covers round me in a fatherly fashion.

'My tummy hurts,' I whine.

'Try to go to sleep.'

'I wish you still had your pipe. Then you could play me a lullaby.'

'I only used to fool around. I can't really play properly.'

'You can. I can remember you playing, remember all the tunes.'

I can hear them in my head even now. I think about them and shut my eyes and fall asleep still holding Davie's hand.

It's dark when I wake up. I know Davie's still there even though I can't see him. He hears me stirring and bends over me and kisses me very gently. He wants it to be like the fairy-tale.

'Someone's just come in the front door,' Davie whispers. 'Will it be Jay?'

It's Wendy and Naomi. He switches on the light and calls to them. Then Leonora and Polly come home—and then Jay. We're all crammed into this room, *my* room, six females fluttering and flirting, even Naomi is at it. She climbs on to Davie's knee and wriggles around on his lap, tilting her head right back to stare up at him, giggling infuriatingly and clinging when Wendy tries to unhook her. Naomi is a hefty child and Davie looks tired out but he gives her a cuddle and keeps her quiet by playing some complicated finger game with her. He smiles wryly over Naomi's head to Wendy to show a) what a lovely intelligent child but b) my God, doesn't she wriggle about and you have to cope with her every day, aren't you marvellous. Wendy gazes at Davie adoringly, glaring at Leonora every now and then because she is doing her best to hog the limelight, standing up and talking at the top of her voice and roaring with laughter at her own jokes. Davie laughs too, egging her on, and yet he does his best to draw Polly into the conversation as well. His voice softens when he talks to her; he soothes her with it and she whispers several replies, the first time she's ever contributed to a conversation when Leonora is in action. Jay is oddly quiet. She's slumping on her mattress, her back hunched. She was probably fed up when she came home at lunch-time and we weren't here. She livens up whenever Davie turns to her, tossing her sparse coppery curls like a middle-aged Shirley Temple. It is Wendy's house but Jay invited Davie, he is her guest, and although the others don't know it he is here on my behalf. Davie makes sure I remember it though, he looks at me and says things like 'Amber and I had a lovely walk in the park' so that we will both remember its misty magic.

Was it really magical for him? Would he have looked after me if I'd had a baby? I don't know. I only know that he's not staying now. Wendy asks him how long he's in England, telling him he can always have a room at her house, Leonora and Polly can share, they'd *like* that, and Leonora and Polly actually nod, and Davie thanks them all but says he's just over here for a day or so. He looks at me as he says it, sounding wistful, as if he wishes it could be for ever. I don't know whether to believe him or not. I know what he's doing, I'm aware of his gentle guile, and yet it still works. If only I had him to myself again. If only I hadn't wasted so much of today behaving like an idiot.

Jay is staring at me. Wendy invites us downstairs for supper (which is just as well, as the grey broccoli quiche and cold kidney beans Jay has carried home from the Health Food shop seem inadequate in every respect). I get out of bed and step into my shoes.

'Are you all right?' Jay whispers.

'Mm.'

'Why were you in bed?'

'I was just tired.'

'You've been crying. Did you tell Davie about the baby?'

'Jay! Leonora's listening. Do shut up.'

I don't want to tell her that there isn't going to be a baby. She'll probably make a joke of it, tell everyone, turn me into a party piece. I feel enough of a comic turn as it is. My clothes are horribly crumpled from lying under the bedcovers and my stomach is so swollen I can't do up the zip of my skirt. I'd sooner stay up here by myself but I follow Davie downstairs.

Gordon comes home when we're half-way through supper (wonderful honey chicken with sweetcorn and peppers and there's more than enough for everyone although Wendy couldn't have known she'd be entertaining). There's plenty left for Gordon but he's a bit sulky at first, annoyed that we didn't wait for him. Davie can handle him too. He asks him all about his boring advertising job, behaving as if he's really interested, his fork poised half-way to his mouth, his eyes intent, and Gordon calms down and eats his own chicken and tells Davie all about it, going into all the latest campaigns, acting the adverts out himself whilst Davie laughs appreciatively. He must be fooling now, he can't find *Gordon* fascinating. I'm wedged between Leonora and Jay and I wonder about commenting on Davie's charming little act but I don't think they'd have a clue what I meant. Justin would know. I still can't think about him without shivering. I can't blot him out any more. It's as if he's standing at my side all the time, looking at me. I shut my eyes and shake my head to try to blur him a little and Jay tenses beside me.

'What are you doing?'

'Nothing.'

'*Do* try to—' She pauses helplessly. Then she bends her head nearer. 'What did Davie say about . . . it? What does he think you should do?'

I take no notice of her and chew a mouthful of chicken.

'Amber!'

'I'll tell you later,' I hiss.

I have to. After supper I need to go to the bathroom to sort myself out and Jay's waiting for me when I come out of the door.

'Have you been sick?' she asks anxiously. 'I was sick a lot at first, all the time, not just in the mornings and it was hell.'

'I haven't been sick.'

'Are you sure? You look awful.'

'I feel it.' I struggle. 'I'm not having a baby after all.'

'Amber!' Her arms are round me and she's hugging me. 'Oh Amber, I'm so glad.' She clings to me. She's so stupidly small and skinny, not a bit like a mother. Not that I'd have been much good at mothering either.

'Jay.' I push her away.

'You didn't—?'

I stare at her.

'Did you get rid of it?' she whispers.

'No!'

'You would tell me if—'

'*Yes.*'

'So it was all a mistake?'

'Yes. You were right. You said I was just late, didn't you?'

'Did I?' says Jay vaguely. 'Oh Amber, the relief! I was so worried. But you're not pregnant, you're not schizophrenic, you're not anything. You can go back to school tomorrow, can't you?'

'I'm not going back. I've sort of left school now.'

Jay might have let me get away with it. She's not the sort to fuss about school leaving ages and local authorities. But Davie insists. He comes up to our room in the morning and mutters with Jay. She goes downstairs to the bathroom or somewhere. He comes over to my bed where I'm pretending to sleep. He sits down beside me and waits. I keep my eyes closed.

'Shall I go through the Sleeping Beauty routine again?' Davie whispers.

I open my eyes, giggling foolishly.

'Hello Amber.'

'Hello.'

'How do you feel?'

'Better.'

'Good. So. Back to school?'

I close my eyes again.

'Amber?'

I stay closed. Davie doesn't get cross. He just laughs at me. I can't help laughing too. I look at him.

'Davie. Did you really come all the way over from Holland just because of me?'

'Just because of you,' says Davie, but he's still laughing. 'And also because there are some people I've got to see. But mostly you.'

'What did Jay say about me in her letter?'

'Ask her.'

'When we talk it's like a game and you always end up winning,' I say, sitting up. I rub my eyes and smooth my hair, hoping I don't look too much of a mess. Davie smells of fresh air and his hand is cold when he takes hold of mine.

'Have you been out for a walk?'

'Yes. A long walk up to the park. I climbed over the railings and went through the woods. I've never seen so many birds. Jays, magpies, woodpeckers. And pelicans.'

'Did you feed them?'

'I didn't need to. They feed themselves from their great shopping-bag beaks. Are you getting up?'

'No. You must have been up for ages. Couldn't you sleep?'

'Not properly.'

'Why?'

'I was thinking.'

I fidget hopefully.

He laughs. 'About you.'

'Really?'

'Some of the time. Thinking that you've got to go to school.'

I pull my hand away in disgust.

'Look, I dropped out. And where has it got me?'

'You're free to do whatever you want. You can get up at dawn and walk in a park and look for pelicans.'

'Gordon can go to Harrod's zoo and order his own personal pelican. He could even have the beak gold-plated.'

'I'd sooner be you than Gordon and so would you.'

'Do you want to be Jay?'

I glare at him.

'I'm not running her down. But you do. You don't want Jay's sort of life, do you?'

'No, but—Look, I don't really see that going to school's going to make any difference.I'm never going to catch up now. I don't think I'll ever get any O levels. Maybe I'm just too thick.'

'You thought you were too stupid to read once, remember?'

'Of course I remember. I loved those stories you made up for me, and the drawings.'

I've still got them folded up in my magic casket cardboard box. The paper is as flimsy as tissue now and every fold has had to be reinforced with sellotape.

'I can't draw for toffee,' says Davie. 'I'm not artistic. But you are. Look.' He picks up my pillow and fingers the embroidery, and waves at my patchwork quilt. 'Look at all this.'

'I didn't learn to sew at any school. I can still sell my things in the craft market.'

'How much do you make? Enough for your own flat? For food and clothes and little treats?'

I shrug because he's winning again.

'Go back to school. Do all the exams you can. Specialise in needlework. Go on to art college. Get a proper training. And *then* you'll be free. Free to live exactly the way you want.'

I sigh.

'I'm making sense, aren't I?'

'Do you really think I could go to art college? To sew?'

'I'm sure you could.'

'I hadn't thought of that.' I think about it now. I want to do it. But I still can't face the thought of school.

'It's Justin,' I explain.

'I know it is.'

'You know everything.'

'That's right. I know you'll go back to school today. I know it'll be awful when you first see him. I know it'll sort itself out. I know you'll go on to art school.'

'Don't stop. What else do you know?'

'I know I'm going to miss you a lot,' says Davie.

I get up on my knees and reach for him and hug him hard. Jay comes back and gasps. It is the most innocent of hugs. I could be Naomi hugging Gordon—and yet Jay looks at us, appalled.

'Amber, the bathroom's free. Go and get washed,' she says sharply.

I can't believe it. And yet when I walk past her in my nightie she hisses 'And wrap a shawl round you or something. You're too old to prance about like that.'

This is Jay speaking, my mother, the failed groupie. What did Peter the Potter call her once? The Middle-class Polo Mint.

I don't say anything. I don't need to. I look at her sour screwed-up face and I know something amazing. She's jealous of me.

Chapter 18

I WALK into the class-room. I feel as if I've jumped off a cliff. The walls whirl round me, the floor slopes. I clutch hold of a chair, breathless. Justin is sitting at his desk turning the pages of a book. He is not looking at me. I wait. No one looks at me. I sit at my own desk and get out a pen, a pencil, a ruler and set them out carefully, as if laying a table. My hand is shaking and the ruler clatters. Justin is still deep in his book.

'Here. Amber.'

It is only one of the girls. Claire. She comes over to me.

'We thought you'd left or something. Where've you been then?'

I shrug and gather my pen and pencil and ruler, dealing them out again in a new pattern.

'Nowhere,' I mutter.

'So what have you been up to?'

'I've been—ill.'

'What with?' It's Julie now. She comes and sits on my desk. 'Yeah, you look a bit thinner. You've lost weight, haven't you? Still a bit chubby-chops round the face but your figure's not bad now.'

Two of the boys behind us snigger. Justin takes no notice.

'What was it then?'

'That flu bug that's been going round.'

'You've been away ages!'

'Well, I had it badly.'

I don't say it firmly enough. Claire and Julie look at each other, eyebrows raised.

'What do you think she's been up to, Jules?'

'Something very suspect if you ask me. She's got much thinner, especially round the tum. Maybe she's been away having a little weeny Amberette.'

I mustn't panic. They are just messing about, being silly for the sake of it. They don't mean any of it. I try to ignore them. Justin ignores us all. He turns the pages of his book. He can't be reading it, not at that pace. I stop listening to the Claire and Julie Double Act and look at him properly.

He's had a haircut but it hasn't helped. He's wearing his Sleeve grey jersey and tight black trousers that show too much of his ankles. It looks as if he's grown even taller, and his toes are rubbing a hole in his old trainers. I stare at him and he senses it. He looks up from his book. Oh God. I can't smile. I can't say I'm sorry. I can't even look him in the face. I rearrange my pens and ruler as if their pattern has some mystic significance. They point at me accusingly. How can I ever get Justin to forgive me? I can't charm like Davie. He can make us all uncoil and sway to his tune. But I am not a charmer. I am the snake.

I have an idea. I search my desk, find my scissors and cut all round the hem of my green General Science overall. I can always re-hem it later, and it could do with shortening anyway. I take needle and thread and start sewing. Claire and Julie ask what I'm up to but I won't tell them. I sew surreptitiously through the lessons. It's easy enough on my lap and none of the teachers take much notice of me. Justin isn't noticing me either. He hasn't looked at me again. He seems much quieter than usual although he goes through the Sleeve routine several times in a subdued fashion.

He doesn't wait for me at lunch-time. I stay sitting in the class-room, sewing. I need some filling so I raid the Handiwork cupboard for kapok. The needlework teacher comes into the room as I'm on my way out, the kapok temporarily stuffing my sweater instead of my sewing. I panic but she's so surprisingly pleased to see me she doesn't notice my new forty inch bust.

'I didn't know what was wrong with you, and no one else seemed to know either. I knew you weren't the sort who'd simply stay away and someone said they thought you'd moved. I was so disappointed at the thought of losing my star pupil.'

Star pupil! I can't believe she's talking about me. She's never been like this in lessons. But now she's going on about A grades and special needlework prizes and I'm going twinkle twinkle.

I tell her the flu lie and she's so sympathetic I feel guilty. I want to get away, the kapok is starting to slip, but I have to ask her something first.

'Do you think there's a chance I could get into art school and do some sewing there?'

I'm scared she'll laugh at me but she doesn't seem to think it's such a daft idea.

'Of course you could, Amber.'

'But don't you need A levels? I don't think I'm ever going to manage more than two O levels.'

'Just wave that night-dress at the principal of any art college and I'm sure they'd take you like a shot,' she says. 'And there's the Royal College of Needlework and the Embroiderers' Guild. I'd better find out some details for you.'

I thank her and then dance off down the corridor. Davie was right. I'll sew something for him next. Maybe a new black and purple patchwork jacket. No, it would look awful nowadays. A plain blouson jacket in black cord. I'll have to go back to the craft market because the cord will cost a bit. Maybe I could appliqué a few funny bits on the lining where it won't show. Little pelicans.

But it's Justin's turn now. I get the stuffing finished before afternoon school and then I sew it into shape and it's ready well before the bell rings at four o'clock. Justin gets up hurriedly, throws his book in a tattered carrier and lopes towards the door. I could put it in his desk where he could find it tomorrow. No, I want to get it over with now. Then when I go home I can at least tell Davie that I tried. So I follow him, down the corridor, out into the yard. I reach out to catch hold of him, to press it into his hand, but we are jostled on all sides and I don't want anyone else to see. So I wait and watch and walk after Justin, right up the road and round the corner. This is getting ridiculous, I shall be following him all the way home at this rate.

'Justin.'

He hesitates in mid-stride but his trainers go on walking. Perhaps he didn't hear me.

'Justin!'

He's not going to stop. I don't suppose I blame him. So I run up to him and thrust my sewing inside his carrier-bag. I don't stop. I run away again, but when I get to the corner I look back over my shoulder. Justin is holding his present in his hand. It is a green snake with gold feather-stitching scales, beady black French-knot eyes and a forked tongue I plaited out of scarlet embroidery silk. I used red for the marking on the head too. A scarlet letter A. Adder. Adulterer. Amber. Justin can take his pick. The snake's body bends in complicated curves. They spell out a word. 'Sorry'.

Justin is staring at the snake. His head is bent and I can't see his expression. I have to know if it's going to be all right or not. I walk slowly back to him. I don't think he sees me coming. I feel as if I'm playing a game of grandmother's footsteps. My steps get slower and slower as I approach.

'Justin?'

He looks up, startled. He doesn't say anything. I'm the one who has to do the talking.

'I know it's pointless saying sorry. But I am. Terribly.'

He's looking at the snake, not at me. Some second-years barge past us and then turn round and stare.

'I don't know why I went with him,' I whisper. 'I don't even like him, Justin. I know it sounds stupid.'

'Yes.'

'I didn't want him—but I wanted him to want me.'

'Well he doesn't,' says Justin. 'He only did it because you were my friend. It was one of his little jokes.'

I wince. The words are like jagged glass. I don't know if it's true or not. Is he just saying it to hurt me?

'I don't care whether he did it for a joke or not,' I lie. 'All I care about is us.'

'Oh?'

'Yes. Can't we be friends again?'

'Don't be a fool.'

'Why is that so foolish? Look, if you'd done the same thing to me I'd be really angry and upset, of course I would, but I wouldn't hate you for ever.'

'I don't hate you, Amber. Don't be so childish,' says Justin. 'There's just no point continuing our relationship.'

He sounds so pompous that I want to kick him. 'Look, it's not my fault it happened.'

'Are you saying he raped you?'

'No. I'm saying it was partly your fault.'

'Oh I see. I was lying there ill in bed. You went off with my brother and in five minutes flat you were . . . . And it's *my* fault?'

'You made it absolutely plain you didn't want me. We've been friends for months and apart from that one kiss you've never even touched me.'

'What about our three golden rules?'

'Now who's being childish? Sex is stupid, romance is rubbish, love is lunacy. It sounds like a creed for six-year-olds. We just said all that because we were both scared.'

'I see. So it was an act of outstanding courage, was it, dropping your knickers for my brother?'

'No. It was stupid and hateful of both of us. And pointless too. Because it wasn't even much good.'

'Extremely stupid. And hateful,' says Justin, but there's a crack in his mask. He twiddles my 'sorry' snake round and round. 'But pointless? Do I take it the *Kama Sutra* Champ is starting to slip? Wasn't his performance quite up to the usual peak of perfection? Did the earth not move? Did it only give a half-hearted shiver and shake?'

'You make me sick. That's all you're interested in. Your bloody brother. You're obsessed with him. And I don't know why. He's not that special. He's handsome and clever, but so what?'

'So I'm ugly and thick.'

'Oh God! *Yes*. Why should I try to reassure you all the time? You don't do it to me. You've just made *me* feel ugly and unwanted all this time. And I'm sick of it. I'm sick of you. I don't know why I wasted my time sewing that stupid snake all day today. You can stick it up your jumper for all I care.'

I march off down the road. There's a whole crowd of second-years staring at us, giggling. I glare at them and stalk past.

'Young lady! *Young lady*!'

It's Sleeve's voice, high-pitched and imperious.

'*I'm* the only personage who lives up the lad's jumper. I can't possibly share my quarters with this overstuffed serpent.'

I turn round. I look at Justin and Sleeve and the little snake. The second-years are splitting their sides. I sigh. And smile.

'Do you want to come home with me?' Justin asks in his own voice.

'I can't tonight. But maybe tomorrow.'

Justin nods. He walks off, holding the snake. I hurry home, my smile growing into a great grin. I can't wait to tell Davie.

But he's not at home. Jay is. She didn't go to work today. She stayed away to be with Davie.

'Where is he?'

'He's gone.'

She's sitting on her mattress with her legs drawn up and her head resting on her knees. She's wearing her canary yellow dungarees. She's tied her hair into limp little plaits. I think she's trying to look cute.

'Gone out with Wendy and the girls?'
'Gone to some friends in Kentish Town.'
'But he's coming back here?'
'No he's not, actually.'
I can't hear her properly when she's all hunched up like that.
'Why isn't he? What's happened?'
'Nothing. He's going to go to Wales for a few days too. You know Davie. He never settles anywhere for very long.'
'I was sure he was staying a while this time.' I so badly wanted to tell him about Justin. How could he clear off without waiting to see if it was all right or not?
'Do shut up,' says Jay. 'I've got a splitting headache.' She rubs her head against her knees.
'You've been drinking,' I say coldly. She's still drinking. There's a bottle of Gordon's sherry beside her. She doesn't even *like* sherry.
'We went to the Swan for lunch,' Jay mutters.
'You and Davie?'
'Of course me and Davie.'
Was it just the two of them? The Swan is expensive. Davie doesn't have that sort of money and Jay certainly hasn't. So Gordon probably took the day off work too. I'm not going to ask in case I'm wrong. I don't want to think of Jay and Davie on their own together all day. Jay is obviously thinking of that now. She takes another swig of sherry. She doesn't even pour it into a glass, she swigs straight from the bottle. She's making the whole room reek of drink. I'd give anything in the world for my own room. I edge round her mattress and go to my own bed. I lie down on it, not caring about creasing my clothes. I shut my eyes and lie still. I can't *feel* still. My heart pounds as if I'm running a race. The disappointment is closing right over my head like a black blanket. I was so happy too. I'd made it almost all right with Justin. I wanted Davie to be proud of me. I want to get my secret casket and look at my marzipan tulip and the Christina Rossetti poem, but how can I with Jay here?

It's probably her fault he's gone. She must have bored him silly. She still fancies herself as some freaked-out *femme fatale* and yet what sort of success has she had with men? None of them have stayed for very long. I don't blame them. I'm not staying either. Just wait till I'm at art college. I'll get a grant, I'll get my own room, I'll still sell my stuff in one of the markets, I'll be *free*.

Thank goodness there's no baby after all. I put my hands on my tummy. The past month seems like a nightmare now. I can feel all the fear of it but the facts are mixed-up and misty. I'm not going to lie on this bed any more. I'm done with dreaming.

I get up, step over Jay and open the window. She screws up her eyes and shivers.

'What are you doing? It's freezing in here as it is.'

'We need some fresh air. Put a jumper on,' I say briskly. I rummage in the cupboard for my sewing things. I might as well make a start on Davie's jacket right away. 'Did he leave an address?'

'I know where he'll be in Wales. And I've got his Amsterdam address. He always keeps in touch. In his own way,' Jay says. She reaches for her old leather jacket and wraps it round her shoulders. It's split at the back and the style is horribly seventies, tight and spindly with a pointed collar. She's had that jacket as long as I can remember and I've always hated it.

'Why are you looking at me like that?' she asks and she takes another drink.

'Don't! You're drunk. It's only half-past four and here you are swigging sherry.'

'I'm not drunk. I wish I was but I'm not,' says Jay and puts the bottle down on the carpet so violently that it nearly spills. I take it from her and put it on top of the cupboard.

'It isn't even yours. It's Gordon's.'

'He won't mind.'

'I mind. I hate the way we keep taking their stuff. We ought to be more independent. You don't care about sponging off people but I do.'

'I don't care?'

'No.'

'What do you know about caring, Amber?' says Jay, and her voice is thick with self-pity. 'Maybe you should have had a baby after all. It might have helped you grow up a bit.'

'It didn't help you. You still act like a baby yourself. Look at you now.'

'Don't let's quarrel, please,' she says, kneading her forehead.

'You started it.'

'It was such a lovely day too,' she says, and she rocks herself backwards and forwards. 'Davie and I went for this long walk together and we talked about so many things. He's the only person I can ever really *talk* to. We're so close. I know I don't see him very often but it doesn't matter. When we're together we're like soul mates.'

I can't bear to listen to this maudlin rubbish. I gather up my sewing things and get up.

'Where are you going?'

'Downstairs. Out. This room smells like a brewery.'

Jay laughs out loud. I hate the way she throws back her head and gurgles like that, showing all the fillings in her teeth.

'That is my mother's voice exactly. You're turning into her, Amber. I ran away from one mother and now I'm lumbered with another.'

'Feel free to run away from me too,' I say. 'The sooner the better. I don't want you.'

She goes on laughing but it's a weird braying sound. She puts her head on her knees. She's not laughing now. She's crying.

'You're really drunk.'

She goes on crying. I want to walk out on her but I'm stuck staring at this sad clown of a mother crouching inside her creaking jacket.

'I didn't really mean that. It was just a joke.'

'I know you don't want me.'

'Don't cry like that. You'll make your headache worse.'

'No one wants me,' Jay sobs.

She's playing the same trick as Justin. It's pathetic at her age. But I go over to her and kneel beside her.

'Shall I make you a coffee?'

She shakes her head.

'We haven't got any aspirin.'

'No one wants me,' she repeats relentlessly.

I'm forced to go through the whole performance:

'Of course they do.'

'Who?'

'I do.'

'My mother said you'd have been much better off adopted. And I think she was right. I don't suppose you've had much of a chance with me. I didn't think it mattered about possessions or property, all that bourgeois stuff. All you need is love and all that jazz. But it hasn't been enough.'

'Yes it has.'

'I don't know what to do now. I don't seem to have got anywhere. I can't believe I've got so old. And there's my hair.' She holds out her ridiculous plaits. 'I don't know what to do with it any more. There were some kids today, they were actually laughing at me.'

'What rubbish,' I say. 'You're the one who's loopy now, not me. You're going paranoid. Your hair's all right.'

'What if I wore it up in a little bun, the way you do yours?'

'You could try.' It wouldn't suit her. It would look awful. And anyway it's *my* hair-style.

'I could always cut it off and have a decent perm,' Jay says in Grandma's voice. She wipes her cheeks with the back of her hand. 'Didn't she really mention me when you saw her?'

'She moaned a bit. She's getting very doddery. She kept going funny.'

'What sort of funny? She is all right? I mean she's not going senile or anything?'

'I don't think so.'

'I don't even know how old she is. I suppose she is getting on a bit. Oh God, what's going to happen if she gets so she can't look after herself?'

'She'll go into a home.'

'But who's going to organise it? Do you think I ought to go and see her? I know she hates me, she *certainly* doesn't want me, but if she's getting really frail—'

'She'll just think you're after her flat,' I say. 'Oh God, Jay, don't cry again. It was another joke.'

'I know. I'm just a bit down, take no notice. Look, you go round and see her again. Soon.'

'All right. Although I don't think she wants to see me either.'

'I wish my father was still alive,' says Jay, rocking again. 'Amber, do you think I really killed him?'

'What?'

'The shock of me getting pregnant, leaving home, all that. Don't you remember my mother said it was all my fault.'

'That was rubbish. It was right after the funeral, she didn't even know what she was saying.'

'We used to be really close, Dad and me. Well, I thought we were. It was a terrible shock when he turned against me. I couldn't believe he didn't want me any more.'

'Don't start all that no one wants me stuff again,' I say, rummaging in my sewing bag.

I find the badly-dyed black nightie. I could have another go at dyeing it and use it for the lining. I'll have to buy the black corduroy of course, but I've got black thread and big black buttons. I haven't got a pattern but they're boring anyway.

'I thought it was all right with Pete. Well it was until he started to get nasty. And it was O.K. with Tim, wasn't it, up in the mountains?'

Who is she trying to kid?

'All right, I know you never thought much of him but he

could be really sweet and gentle at times. Only he cleared off, didn't he? In the end. They all do. Even Davie.'

I don't want her to start talking about Davie. I sketch a rough design for a jacket on a scrap piece of paper, concentrating fiercely.

'I've always wanted Davie,' Jay whispers. 'There's always been such magic between us. It's not just the sex, it's—'

'Shut *up*, Jay. Don't go on about it.' I'm pressing so hard my pencil's right through the paper.

'Do you think he cares about me? He goes away, I know, he needs to be free, but he does always come back, doesn't he? He comes when I need him.'

He comes for *me*. He came this time because he thought I needed him. He wants me. How can she be such a fool? She saw for herself this morning. It's *me*.

'Amber? Do you think he loves me just a little?' Jay whispers.

'How should I know?'

She sags. She sighs. I wait, but at least she doesn't cry again. She sniffs instead, and absent-mindedly blows her nose on a scrap from my sewing bag.

'Do you mind? I'm going to use that.'

'Sorry.' She looks at my sketch. 'That looks good. What is it, a jacket?'

'Mm.'

'Are you going to make it out of that nightie?'

'No, of course not. It's going to be a proper jacket. I'm going to get some black corduroy as soon as I've got the money.'

She nods. 'I wish I could sew. Who's it for, this jacket?'

'Wait and see.' I think about it. We haven't got that long together after all. And I'd give anything to see the last of that old leather thing. 'Maybe it's for you.'

BREAKING TRAINING

Sandy Welch

Alison took the advertisement out of her bag and stuck it to her dressing table mirror. It was from the *Stage* and read: 'AUDITIONS: Female dancers and singers required. June 5th. Manchester.' You had to be over twenty-one, but that didn't matter, she looked much older. And she was pretty clever too, when she wanted to be; her idea about accompanying the school sports star, Tessa, to the race in Manchester was a good one, the ideal excuse. She shouldn't really have spent the money for her rail fare, but never mind, they could hitch up to Manchester easily enough . . .

Sandy Welch portrays in her stories the turbulent, frenetic and often bizarre world of teenage girls. She has captured their chatter and worries, foibles and obsessions with striking clarity and humour.

Waiting for the Sky to Fall

Jacqueline Wilson

Katherine's family seems different from others. Her father is dominant and demanding, her mother submissive and her sister increasingly unhappy and secretive. Katherine herself is worried sick about her 'O' level results. Things are further complicated and strained when she secretly starts meeting her first boyfriend. Soon, she is living in daily dread of the sky falling on top of her – and when it does the consequences are unexpected and dramatic.

'Superbly written' *Punch*

HEY, DOLLFACE

Deborah Hautzig

How do you separate loving as a friend and sexual love – or do they cross over sometimes? Val Hoffman knows that there is nothing wrong, or bad, in the way she feels about Chloe. They are friends, and their friendship has a trust and intimacy which is special for both of them. But sometimes outsiders, even family, can misjudge and label such friendships and labels are frightening because they distort the truth. In this perceptive, funny and wholly convincing novel about two teenage girls, young, unsure, and on the brink of sexual awakening, Deborah Hautzig charts that all-important time between adolescence and adulthood – that fragile moment when we first begin to learn about loving other people.

'This excellently constructed book is an honest documentary of the tribulations of becoming an adult. It is a sharp, credible and moving book.' *Learn*